# Advances and Technical Standards in Neurosurgery

## Volume 49

This series, which has earned a reputation over the years and is considered a classic in the neurosurgical  field, is now relaunched under the editorship of Professor Di Rocco, which relies on the collaboration of a renewed  editorial board.

Both volumes focused on recent advances in neurosurgery and on  technical standards, and monographs devoted to more specific subjects in the neurosurgical field will implement it. Written  by key opinion leaders, the series volumes will be useful for  young neurosurgeons in their postgraduate training but also for more experienced clinicians.

Concezio Di Rocco

Editor

# Advances and Technical Standards in Neurosurgery

## Volume 49

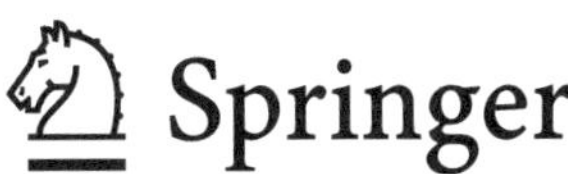 Springer

*Editor*
Concezio Di Rocco
International Neuroscience Institute
Hannover, Germany

ISSN 0095-4829　　　　　　　　ISSN 1869-9189　(electronic)
Advances and Technical Standards in Neurosurgery
ISBN 978-3-031-42400-7　　　　ISBN 978-3-031-42398-7　(eBook)
https://doi.org/10.1007/978-3-031-42398-7



This Springer imprint is published by the registered company Springer Nature Switzerland AG
The registered company address is: Gewerbestrasse 11, 6330 Cham, Switzerland

Paper in this product is recyclable.

# Contents

# Chapter 1
# Molecular Biomarkers Affecting Moyamoya Disease

**Yong-Kwang Tu and Yao-Ching Fang**

## Contents




Y.-K. Tu (✉)
Taipei Neuroscience Institute, Taipei Medical University, Taipei, Taiwan

Department of Neurosurgery, Shuang-Ho Hospital, Taipei Medical University, New Taipei City, Taiwan
e-mail: yktu@ntu.edu.tw

Y.-C. Fang
Taipei Neuroscience Institute, Taipei Medical University, Taipei, Taiwan



© The Author(s), under exclusive license to Springer Nature Switzerland AG 2024
C. Di Rocco (ed.), *Advances and Technical Standards in Neurosurgery*,
Advances and Technical Standards in Neurosurgery 49,
https://doi.org/10.1007/978-3-031-42398-7_1

## 1.1  Background

Moyamoya disease (MMD) is an idiopathic cerebrovascular disease featuring progressive steno-occlusive changes in the supraclinoidal internal carotid artery (ICA) and "moyamoya vessels," which are excessive, hazy, proximal collateral vessels developed from the perforating arteries [1]. These fragile, smoke-like arteriopathic vessels result in insufficient cerebral perfusion and various symptoms of ischemic and hemorrhagic stroke. Furthermore, these vessels can cause disability or death in children and adults [2–4].

If the progression of MMD is rapid, the speed at which the collateral vessels develop may be insufficient to compensate for the impaired cerebral perfusion, and the patient will exhibit ischemic symptoms early in life. Patients with slower MMD progression will experience the onset of symptoms after adolescence. Insufficient cerebral perfusion is more easily compensated in such patients. Rather than leading to ischemic symptoms, the moyamoya vessels develop from perforating arteries with thin arterial walls and progressively dilate to compensate for the insufficient cerebral perfusion until they have dilated beyond their limit and rupture, causing cerebral hemorrhage. Because of these factors, children and adolescents with MMD always exhibit ischemic stroke symptoms, whereas adults with MMD also exhibit hemorrhagic stroke symptoms.

Because of its notably high annual incidence in East Asia, particularly in Japan, China, Taiwan, and South Korea [5, 6]. MMD was proposed to be associated with genetic factors involving regional and ethnic characteristics [7]. The polymorphism R4810K in RNF213, a finger protein encoded by the Really Interesting New Gene 1 (RING), [8] was reported to be the gene most likely linked to MMD susceptibility and was associated with protein–protein interaction and ubiquitin–protein ligase activity [9, 10]. However, the RNF213 variant has not been identified in all patients with MMD. The "double hit hypothesis" was thus proposed, in which researchers indicated that the pathology of MMD cannot be explained by a single theory. Multiple gene abnormalities, immune and infectious triggers, and innate hemodynamic factors may play roles in the complex pathogenic pathway [11–13].

However, understanding of the pathology of MMD remains limited, and further research is required to identify the precise mechanism. This article discusses the research on abnormal circulating factors identified in patients with MMD and discusses the influences of these factors on pathogenic endothelial proliferation, smooth muscle cell (SMC) migration, and neovascularization in MMD.

## 1.2  Growth Factors

Increased levels or abnormal activity of growth factors in patients with MMD have been hypothesized to have a role in pathological angiogenesis and vasculogenesis, leading intimal hyperplasia and SMC migration in vessels. The related growth factors—vascular endothelial growth factor (VEGF), basic fibroblast growth factor (bFGF), hepatocyte growth factor (HGF), and platelet-derived growth factor (PDGF-BB)—are discussed in the following (Table 1.1).

**Table 1.1** Growth factors involved in MMD

| | Substance | Samples | Abn. findings in patients with MMD | Hypothetical pathogenetic pathway | Reference |
|---|---|---|---|---|---|
| Growth factor | VEGF | MMD Pt/ Plasma | VEGF ↑ | VEGF ↑ → vascular progenitor cell recruitment and coll. vessel fm. ↑ | [14] |
| | | MMD Pt/ Dura mater | VEGF ↑ | VEGF ↑ → vascular cell prolif., migr., and neovascularization ↑ | [15] |
| | | Pediatric MMD/Gene | VEGF−634CC ↓ → better post-op coll. Vessel fm. | VEGF−634G allele → poor coll. vessel fm. | [16] |
| | | MMD Pt/ Serum | sVEGF1-R and sVEGF2-R ↓ → better coll. vessel fm. | 1. VEGF2-R. → angiogenesis ↑ 2. VEGF1-R and VEGF2-R ↓. → path. angiogenesis ↓ | [18] |
| | bFGF | MMD Pt/ CSF | bFGF ↑ | bFGF ↑ → path. in MMD | [20] |
| | | MMD Pt/ CSF | bFGF ↑ (after neovascularization) | bFGF ↑ → mesoderm, neuroectoderm-derived cell, and SMC ↑ → ICA stenosis and occlusion | [21] |
| | HGF | MMD Pt/ CSF | HGF ↑ (in CSF/carotid intima/media) | HGF ↑ → ECs prolif. and SMC migr. ↑ | [24] |
| | PDGF-BB | MMD Pt/ plasma | PDGF-BB ↑ PDGF R ↓ (on SMCs) | PDGF-BB ↑ → SMC lineage ↑ → intimal hyperplasia | [14] |
| | | MMD Pt/ SMC strains | PDGF-AA and PDGF-BB → SMC migr. ↑ | PDGF ↑ → intimal thickening ↑ | [22] |
| | Endoglin | MMD Pt/ MCA samples | Staining in the endothelium ↑ | Endoglin ↑ → TGF-β1 signaling ↑ → intimal hyperplasia | [25] |
| | ANGs | MMD Pt/ MCA | 1. ANG-2 in MMD vessels ↑ 2. MMD serums induce ANG-2 ↑ | MMD serum → ANG-2 ↑ → endothelium integrity ↓ | [26] |
| | | HMMD Pt/ Serum | ANG-2 ↑ | ANG-2 ↑ → abn. angiogenesis → hemorrhage | [27] |

*Abn.* abnormal, *ANGs* angiopoietins, *bFGF* basic fibroblast growth factor, *coll.* collateral, *EC* endothelial cell, *fm.* formation, *HGF* hepatocyte growth factor, *HMMD* hemorrhage in adult-onset MMD, *ICA* internal carotid artery, *MCA* middle carotid artery, *migr.* migration, *MMD* moyamoya disease, *path.* pathological, *PDGF* platelet-derived growth factor, *post-op* post-operation, *prolif.* proliferation, *Pt* patients, *R* receptor, *SMC* smooth muscle cell, *VEGF* vascular endothelial growth factor, ↑: upregulated; ↓: downregulated; →: leading to

### 1.2.1 VEGF

VEGF has been reported to be significantly increased in the plasma and dura mater of patients with MMD. It is the only growth factor that directly facilitates vessel formation, and high VEGF expression can lead to the recruitment of vascular progenitor cells and thereby promote migration, proliferation, and neovascularization and result in pathological collateral vessel formation [14, 15].

Morphological differences in VEGF lead to pathological vasculogenetic responses. In one study, VEGF-634CC, which is less frequently expressed in the pediatric population with MMD than the corresponding adult population, was discovered to be associated with more favorable postoperative collateral vessel formation. By contrast, the VEGF-634G allele caused poor collateral vessel formation [16].

Expression of specific VEGF receptors (VEGFRs) can affect angiogenetic activity. VEGFR-2, the receptor responsible for endothelial development and vessel production, [17] was discovered to be decreased in patients with MMD and be associated with more favorable collateral vessel formation, indicating that an increased VEGFR-2 level may promote abnormal vessel formation and that blockage of VEGFR-2 may be a therapeutic target warranting further study [17, 18].

### 1.2.2 bFGF

Research has indicated that bFGF, a signal protein reported to activate the hypoxia-inducible factor (HIF)-$\alpha$ pathway and thus increase both endothelial cell motility and VEGF expression, promotes proliferation of the mesoderm, neuroectoderm-derived cells, and SMCs, eventually leading to ICA stenosis and occlusion [19].

Patients with MMD were discovered to have a higher bFGF level in the cerebrospinal fluid (CSF). Furthermore, an increased bFGF level was noted after neovascularization from indirect revascularization [20]. These results indicate that bFGF may participate in the pathological pathway of MMD and may serve as a predictor when evaluating the efficacy of surgery [21]. However, whether bFGF is a pathogenic factor of MMD or a product of defective MMD vessels under hypoxic conditions remains unclear [22].

### 1.2.3 HGF

Mediated by vascular endothelial cells, HGF is considered a strong angiogenic inducer that facilitates endothelial cell proliferation and SMC migration [23]. HGF is believed to be involved in the etiology of MMD. Considerably increased levels of HGF were detected in the CSF as well as the intima and media of the carotid fork in patients with MMD [24].

### *1.2.4   PDGF*

The several subtypes of PDGF have different homodimeric peptide chains. PDGF-BB was reported to stimulate both DNA synthesis and SMC migration in angiogenesis, whereas PDGF-AA was discovered to only stimulate DNA synthesis.

One study revealed that the PDGF-BB level was significantly higher in plasma obtained from patients with MMD that in plasma obtained from healthy individuals [14]. Another reported that both PDGF-AA and PDGF-BB extracted from SMC strains in patients with MMD stimulated cell migration activity; however, neither promoted DNA synthesis compared with that in the control group [22]. This indicates that excessive PDGF can stimulate differentiation between vascular progenitor cells and SMC linages. Therefore, when unscheduled migration of SMCs is increased, intimal hyperplasia and impaired arterial wall repair processes may be considered to be involved in the pathological pathway of MMD.

### *1.2.5   Endoglin*

Endoglin facilitates cellular responses to transforming growth factor (TGF)-$\beta$1. Furthermore, a higher level of endoglin was discovered to colocalize with HIF-1$\alpha$ and TGF-$\beta$3 in endothelia obtained from middle cerebral artery (MCA) samples of patients with MMD [25]. This could lead to pathological intimal hyperplasia.

### *1.2.6   Angiopoietins (ANGs)*

ANGs are protein ligands that modulate vascular network maturation and neovascularization. In addition to being significantly increased in MMD vessels, ANG-2 was discovered to be upregulated by MMD serum in vitro and to be accompanied by impaired endothelial integrity [26]. One study investigated hemorrhage in adult-onset MMD and reported increased serum ANG-2, which could contribute to the instability of vascular structures and cause hemorrhage [27].

Upregulated growth factors can lead to excessive activity, abnormal morphology, and aberrant responses to specific receptors and thus stimulate vascular progenitor cell recruitment, promote angiogenesis, and activate other growth factors through signaling pathways; this may explain their reported pathogenic connections to MMD.

## 1.3   Circulating Progenitor Cells

Circulating progenitor cells, including endothelial progenitor cells (EPCs) and smooth muscle progenitor cells (SPCs), were discovered to be overexpressed in MMD, with CD34$^+$ CD133$^+$, and VEGFR2$^+$ mostly present. Moreover, such cells were reported to be recruited and regulated by growth factors, particularly VEGF, and to promote vasculogenesis and vascular remodeling (Table 1.2) [11].

### 1.3.1   EPCs

The increased plasma EPCs in MMD can induce arteriogenesis and angiogenesis by activating resting endothelial cells and thereby cause vessel formation to be

**Table 1.2**  Circulating progenitor cells involved in MMD

|  | Substance | Samples | Abn. findings in patients with MMD | Hypothetical pathogenetic pathway | Reference |
|---|---|---|---|---|---|
| Circulating progenitor cells | EPCs | Pediatric MMD/ Peripheral blood | Tube fm. type ECFC ↓ Senescent-like ECFC ↑ | EPC ↓ → ineffective vasculogenesis | [31] |
|  |  | MMD Pt/ peripheral blood | ECFC ↑ | EPC ↑ → activate resting EC ↑ → arteriogenesis and angiogenesis ↑ | [28] |
|  |  | Pt with ICA/ MCA stenosis or occlusion/ peripheral blood | Circulating CD34+ cell ↑ | Circulating ECFC ↑ → path. neovascularization | [30] |
|  |  | MMD Pt/ peripheral blood | Abn. morphology and function in mito. of ECFCs | Abn. ECFC function → delayed repairing → vessel occlusion | [33] |
|  |  | Adult MMD/CFU and outgrowth cell | 1. CFU ↓ (advanced MMD) 2. EOC ↑ (early MMD) | Inefficient EPC → vascular occlusion and angiogenesis | [36] |
|  |  | Pediatric MMD/ ECFCs in vitro and vivo | ECFC *RALDH2* ↓ → capillary fm. ↓ | *RALDH2* ↓ → RA ↓ → defective tube fm. | [32] |
|  | SPCs | MMD Pt/ peripheral blood | *ACTA2* mutation → SMC prolif. ↑ | SMC ↑ → occlusive disease | [35] |
|  |  | MMD Pt/ peripheral blood | Irregularly arrangement and thickened tubules | Genes expressed differentially → irregular morphological SMCs | [34] |

*Abn.* abnormal, *CFUs* colony-forming units, *EC* endothelial cell, *ECFC* endothelial colony-forming cell, *EOC* endothelial outgrowth cell, *EPC* endothelial progenitor cell, *fm.* formation, *ICA* internal carotid artery, *MCA* middle carotid artery, *mito.* Mitochondria, *MMD* moyamoya disease, *path.* Pathological, *prolif.* Proliferation, *Pt* patients, *RA* retinoic acid, *SMC* smooth muscle cell, *SPC* smooth muscle progenitor cell, ↑: upregulated; ↓: downregulated; →: leading to ineffective [28]. However, the alteration ratios of different subtypes of EPC lead to similar responses.

Endothelial colony-forming cells (ECFCs), which are considered a subtype of EPCs, exhibit characteristics more specific to endothelial function than do other EPC subtypes [29] and may play a critical role in producing pathogenic MMD vessels. One study reported a higher circulating CD34+ cell level in patients with MMD with ICA–MCA stenosis or occlusion, indicating that highly expressed ECFCs can lead to pathological neovascularization in the ischemic brain [30]. An increased number of senescent-like and a decreased number of tube formation ECFC phenotypes were identified in the peripheral blood of pediatric patients with MMD. This may result in delayed reparation and aberrant differentiation in ischemic vessels [31]. In adult MMD, the EPC–colony-forming unit, an EPC subtype related to tube formation activities, and outgrowth cells, an EPC subtype responsible for regeneration and vasogenic activity in defect tissue, were discovered to be reduced in severe MMD and increased in early MMD.

Gene polymorphism can also affect tube formation. One study reported that knockdown of *RALDH2* mRNA in ECFCs obtained from pediatric patients with MMD downregulated the expression of retinoic acid, thereby decreasing the amount of typical capillary formation in vitro [32]. In addition, mitochondrial morphological and functional abnormalities in ECFCs were determined to be associated with delayed reparation of defect vessels, leading to occlusion in MMD [33].

## 1.3.2  SPCs

SPC proliferation can promote intimal thickening, which is a prominent histological characteristic of MMD. Studies have suggested that variant gene expression may result in atypical SPCs with irregular morphology and thus lead to abnormal arrangements and thickened tubules in MMD [34]. Another study reported that mutations in the *ACTA2* gene can lead to increased SMC proliferation, which can cause occlusive disease [35].

Both excessive progenitor cell proliferation and hyperplasia in progenitor cells' ineffective subgroups due to gene polymorphism or mitochondrial abnormalities can result in poor or atypical vessel formation and a thickened intima. These findings may explain the pathological mechanism underlying stenosis and occlusion in fragile MMD vessels.

## 1.4  Angiogenesis-Related Cytokines

Various circulating cytokines react with growth factors and stimulate neovascularization, steno-occlusive changes, and collateral vessel formation in moyamoya vessels (Table 1.3) [37].

**Table 1.3** Angiogenesis-related cytokines involved in MMD

| | Substance | Samples | Abn. findings in patients with MMD | Hypothetical pathogenetic pathway | Reference |
|---|---|---|---|---|---|
| Angiogenesis-related cytokines | TGF-β1 | MMD pt/SMCs | TGF-β1 ↑ (in SMCs and serum) | TGF-β1 ↑ → connective tissue gene ↑ → neovascularization ↑ | [38] |
| | | MMD pt./SMCs | TGF-β1 ↑ → elastin mRNA ↑ | TGF-β1 ↑ → elastin synthesis ↑ | [39] |
| | | MMD pt./ peripheral blood | Fr III Treg cell ↑ (lack suppressive functions) | Fr III Treg → TGF-β ↑ → VEGF ↑ | [40] |
| | CRABP-1 | Pediatric MMD/ CSF | CRABP-1 ↑ | CRABP-1 ↑ → RA ↓ → SMC migr. and prolif. ↑ | [42] |
| | MMPs | MMD Pt/Serum | MMP-9 autocrine activity ↑ | MMP-9 ↑ → gelatinase ↑ → angiogenesis ↑ | [43] |
| | | MMD Pt/ peripheral blood | Plasma MMP-9 ↑ | MMP-9 ↑ → intimal hyperplasia and coll. vessel fm. ↑ | [14] |
| | | MMD Pt/serum | Serum MMP ↑ | MMP-9 ↑ → path. angiogenesis and defect vessel → hemorrhage | [44] |
| | TIMP | MMD Pt/serum | Serum TIMP-1 and TIMP-2 ↓ | TIMP-1 and TIMP-2 ↓ → MMP-9 ↑ → SMC migr. ↑ and intimal thickening | [14] |
| | HIF-1α | MMD Pt/MCA sample | HIF-1α ↑ (in intima and endothelium) | HIF-1α ↑ → GF transcription and cytokine ↑ → intimal prolif. ↑ | [25] |
| | MCP-1 | MMD Pt/serum | MCP-1 ↑ | MCP-1 ↑ → stromal cells migr. ↑ → path. coll. vessel fm. | [14] |
| | SDF-1α | MMD Pt/serum and peripheral blood | 1. SDF-1α ↑ 2. CD34(+) CXCR4(+) cell ↑ | SDF-1α/CXCR4 axis ↑ → neovascularization ↑ | [45] |
| | CCL5 | MMD Pt/ECFCs and SPCs from peripheral blood | CCL5-intensified migr. of SPCs toward ECFCs | Impaired endothelial repair and CCL5 secretion → SPC recruitment↑ → neointimal hyperplasia | [46] |

*Abn.* abnormal, *CCL5* chemokine (C-C motif) ligand 5, *coll.* collateral, *CRABP-1* cellular RA-binding protein-1, *ECFC* endothelial colony-forming cell, *fm.* formation, *GF* growth factor, *migr* migration, *HIF-α* hypoxia-inducible factor-α, *MCP-1* monocyte chemoattractant protein-1, *MMD* moyamoya disease, *path.* pathological, *MMP-9* matrix metalloproteinase-9, *prolif.* proliferation, *Pt* patients, *RA* retinoic acid, *SDF-1α* stromal cell-derived factor-1α, *SMC* smooth muscle cell, *SPC* smooth muscle progenitor cell, *TGF-β1* transforming growth factor-β1, *TIMP* tissue inhibitor of metalloproteinase, *VEGF* vascular endothelial growth factor, ↑: upregulated; ↓: downregulated; →: leading to

### 1.4.1  TGF-β1

TGF-β1 was hypothesized to be an enhancer of atypical arteriogenesis in MMD. Higher levels of TGF-β1 were identified in SMCs obtained from the superficial temporal arteries and serum of patients with MMD [38]. One study reported TGF-β1-induced increased elastin mRNA expression in SMCs [39]. These findings indicate that the overexpression of TGF-β1 detected in SMCs or activated by inflammation may upregulate the expression of matrix genes, promoting elastin synthesis and pathological angiogenesis. Furthermore, an increase in defective circulating Treg cells lacking typical suppressive functions, as was identified in the peripheral blood of patients with MMD, could activate TGF-β1 expression [40].

### 1.4.2  Cellular Retinoid Acid (RA)-Binding Protein-1 (CRABP-1)

RA has a critical role in modulating normal angiogenesis in that it reduces the neointimal formation and proliferation of SMCs. However, RA is downregulated by CRABP-1, which induces RA-metabolizing enzyme production and accelerates RA degradation, thus enhancing the formation of atypical vessels in patients with MMD. A study reported higher CRABP-1 expression in the CSF of pediatric patients with MMD than in the CSF of pediatric patients without MMD [41, 42].

### 1.4.3  Matrix Metalloproteinase-9 (MMP-9) and Tissue Inhibitor of Metalloproteinase (TIMP)

MMP-9 is an angiopoietin that is closely associated with the bioavailability of VEGF. By targeting collagen IV and other extracellular matrices, MMP-9 modulates vasculogenic and angiogenic processes. MMP-9 enhances gelatinase activity and stimulates collagen IV degradation and remodeling, causing pathological angiogenesis in MMD [43]. Patients with MMD were reported to have elevated serum and plasma MMP-9 levels, suggesting that MMP-9 upregulation promotes intimal hyperplasia and excessive collateral vessel formation and that the defective vessel structures may cause further hemorrhaging in MMD [14, 44]. Furthermore, TIMP-1 and TIMP-2, which are natural inhibitors of MMPs, were both significantly decreased in serum retrieved from patients with MMD, suggesting that the imbalance between MMP and TIMP could be a pathogenic mechanism underlying MMD [14].

### *1.4.4 Others*

Patients with MMD were discovered to have higher expression of HIF-α in the intima and serum monocyte chemoattractant protein-1 (MCP-1). By activating the transcription of genes responsible for vascular regulation, such as those in the VEGF and TGF-β families, HIF-1 stimulates aberrant intima thickening [25]. Additionally, MCP-1 causes pathological collateral vessel formation by facilitating stromal cell migration [14]. Circulating stromal-cell-derived factor-1α, which interacts with CXCR4 receptors, was discovered to be increased and involved in neovascularization in patients with MMD [45]. Furthermore, chemokine (C-C motif) ligand 5 (CCL5) was discovered to intensify the migration of SPCs toward ECFCs, suggesting that CCL5 secretion may result in greater SPC recruitment and thus promote neointimal hyperplasia in patients with MMD [46].

Cytokines were hypothesized to cause intimal hyperplasia and the formation of excessive, defective, and fragile vessels through extracellular matrix dysregulation or interference with regular angiogenesis. However, whether cytokines are causative or the consequence of the pathophysiology of MMD remains unclear [12].

## 1.5 Inflammatory and Immune Mediators

Proinflammatory and anti-inflammatory cytokines are mediated by immune cells, such as M2 macrophages and Treg cells, and participate in inflammatory responses, stimulating intimal hyperplasia and neovascularization and leading to stenosis, vessel occlusion, and further collateral formation, all of which are characteristics of MMD. This suggests that the pathology of MMD may be related to the immune-mediated inflammatory pathway (Table 1.4) [47].

### *1.5.1 Autoimmune Activity and Autoantibodies*

M2 macrophages are involved in angiogenesis in the inflammatory response. As an activation marker of M2 macrophages, sCD163 was reported to be higher in the serum of patients with MMD than in that of healthy controls. Moreover, a higher level of CXCL5, a cytokine associated with the severity of autoimmune reactions, was reported in these patients [48]. This suggests that M2 macrophages may promote autoimmune activity and be involved in the pathogenic pathway of MMD. An increased level of IL-1β, which is secreted by macrophages, was also identified in patients with MMD. Elevated IL-1β was reported to stimulate the proliferation of macrophages, endothelial cells, and SMCs and thereby increase vascular permeability and endothelial dysfunction [14].

**Table 1.4** Inflammatory mediators involved in MMD

| | Substance | Samples | Abn. findings in patients with MMD | Hypothetical pathogenetic pathway | Reference |
|---|---|---|---|---|---|
| Inflammatory mediators | IgG immune complex | MMD Pt/ Intracranial vessels | IgG & S100A4 protein↑ | IgG immune complex deposition ↑ → S10A4+ SMC migr. into intima → vessel stenosis and occlusion | [49] |
| | M2 macrophage | MMD Pt/ Serum | CD163+ M2-Mφ and CXCL5 ↑ | M2 Mφ ↑ → autoimmune activity ↑ | [48] |
| | IL-1β | MMD Pt/ Peripheral blood | IL-1β ↑ | IL-1β ↑ → Mφ, ECs, and SMC ↑ → vascular permeability ↑ and endothelial dysfunction↑ | [14] |

*EC* endothelial cell, *Ig* immunoglobin, *migr.* migration, *MMD* moyamoya disease, *Mφ* macrophage, *Pt* patient, *SMC* smooth muscle cell, ↑: upregulated; ↓: downregulated; →: leading to

Inflammation-induced deposition of antibodies can also destroy vessel structures. Excessive levels of immunoglobulin G (IgG) and S100A4 proteins were identified in the intracranial vascular walls of patients with MMD, suggesting that IgG deposition may lead to defective internal elastic lamina and S100A4 + SMC migration, which may cause vessel stenosis and compensatory vessel formation [49]. One study identified autoantibodies against APP, GPS1, STRA13, CTNNB1, ROR1, and EDIL3 in the serum of patients with MMD. This was considered to indicate impaired DNA damage responses, aberrant angiogenesis, and neuronal impairment. However, the actual pathogenic mechanism underlying the influence of autoantibodies requires further study [50].

Although inflammation and immune activities were determined to cause defects in intima and vessel stenosis, which coincides with the characteristics of MMD, MMD has been defined as a noninflammatory disease because no inflammatory cells or macrophage infiltration are detected in the subintimal layer in patients with the disease. However, even if inflammatory activities do not directly contribute to the pathogenesis of MMD, they may still influence *RNF213* and stimulate curative angiogenesis [47].

## 1.6  Other Factors (Table 1.5)

### *1.6.1  Caveolin-1 (Cav-1)*

Cav-1, a scaffolding protein located on the cell membrane, modulates numerous signaling pathways. In patients with MMD, particularly those with variants of the RNF213 gene, Cav-1 is significantly decreased. Cav-1 has been hypothesized to attenuate typical angiogenesis in endothelial cells and to activate apoptosis in SMCs, resulting in negative arterial remodeling and impaired angiogenesis in MMD [51, 52].

### *1.6.2  Nitric Oxide (NO) Metabolites*

NO is an angiogenetic factor modulated by Cav-1. Colocalized in caveolae, endothelial NO synthase (eNOS) and VEGFR-2 are repressed by Cav-1, decreasing NO production and tube formation in mice [53]. A decrease in Cav-1 leads to a decline in the suppression function of eNOS, which may lead to abundant NO production and thus promote excessive angiogenesis. CSF obtained from patients with MMD contained increased levels of NO metabolites (nitrate and nitrite), and NO metabolite levels were reported to be lower after bypass surgery. These findings indicate that in states of chronic ischemic circulation, upregulated NO metabolites may stimulate moyamoya vessel development by dilating collateral vessels and promoting collateral circulation [54]. However, no significant differences were identified in plasma NO metabolites levels or eNOS polymorphisms of patients with MMD

**Table 1.5**  Other biomarkers involved in MMD

| | Substance | Samples | Abn. findings in patients with MMD | Hypothetical pathogenetic pathway | Reference |
|---|---|---|---|---|---|
| Others | Caveolin-1 | MMD Pt/ serum | Serum Cav-1 ↓ | Cav-1 ↑<br>→ typical angiogenesis ↓ and SMC apoptosis ↑<br>→ impaired angiogenesis | [52] |
| | | MMD Pt/? | Caveolin-1 ↓ (in RNF213 variant carriers) | Cav-1 is a crucial mediator in MMD | [51] |
| | NO metabolites | MMD Pt/ CSF | 1. CSF NO metabolites ↑<br>2. NO metabolite ↓ (after bypass surg.) | Defect coll. vessel Fm. → NO metabolite ↑ | [54] |
| | Haptoglobin | MMD Pt/ CSF | Haptoglobin ↑ | Inflammation and ischemia<br>→ haptoglobin ↑<br>→ angiogenesis and coll. Vessel fm. ↑ | [56] |

*Coll* collateral, *CSF* cerebrospinal fluid, *fm* formation, *MMD* moyamoya disease, *Mφ* macrophage, *Pt* patient, *SMC* smooth muscle cell, *surg.* surgery, ↑: upregulated; ↓: downregulated; →: leading to versus a healthy control group, suggesting that the interaction between NO and MMD pathogenesis warrants further investigation [12, 55].

### *1.6.3 Haptoglobin*

Under conditions of inflammation and ischemia, haptoglobin activates angiogenesis and tissue repair. One study reported that haptoglobin was overexpressed in the CSF of patients with MMD, indicating that haptoglobin may be involved in the pathogenesis of MMD [56].

## 1.7 Interaction of Circulating Factors

The pathological mechanism underlying MMD may be significantly associated with excessive levels and activities of growth factors promoting the recruitment of vascular progenitor cells, which would lead to excessive and defective collateral vessel formation (Fig. 1.1). Because they are the result of inflammation and an

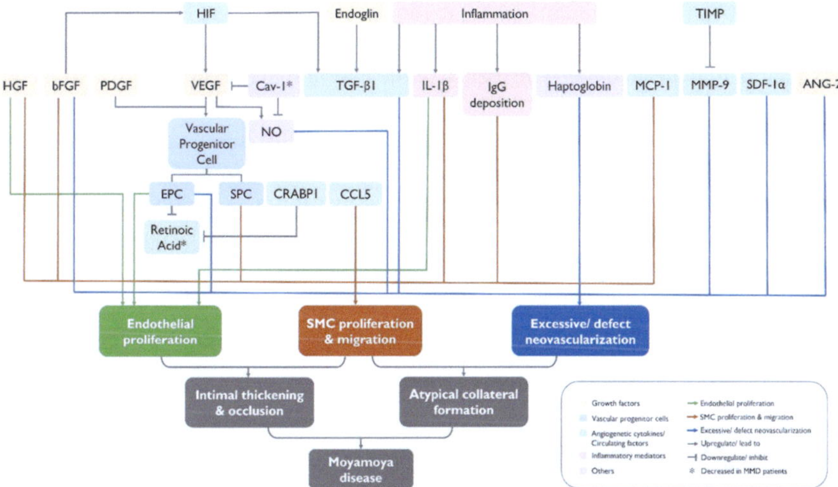


**Fig. 1.1** Interaction between various circulating factors collectively working to stimulate endothelial proliferation and smooth muscle cell (SMC) proliferation and migration, leading to excessive but defective neovascularization, intimal thickening and occlusion, and compensatory atypical collateral formation, both of which occur in moyamoya disease. *ANG-2* angiopoietin-2, *bFGF* basic fibroblast growth factor, *Cav-1* caveolin-1, *CCL5* chemokine (C-C motif) ligand 5, *CRABP-1* cellular retinoic acid-binding protein, *EPC* endothelial progenitor cell, *HGF* hepatocyte growth factor, *HIF* hypoxia-inducible factor, *IgG* immunoglobin G, *IL-1β* interleukin-1β, *MCP-1* monocyte chemoattractant protein-1, *MMP-9* matrix metalloproteinase 9, *PDGF* platelet-derived growth factor, *SDF-1αTM* stromal cell-derived factor-1α, *SPC* smooth muscle progenitor cell, *TGF-β1* transforming growth factor, *TIMP* tissue inhibitor of metalloproteinase, *VEGF* vascular endothelial growth factor

ischemic environment, cytokines and immune mediators have been suggested to be involved in abnormal angiogenesis and arteriogenesis.

Moreover, of the growth factors, VEGF is considered to have the most determining role in vascular formation because it interacts with other angiogenetic cytokines and progenitor cells [14, 15]. VEGF modulates EPC and SMC activities and stimulates endothelial cell proliferation and SMC migration, leading to intimal hyperplasia and neovascularization [17]. Both morphological differences and aberrant receptor expression, which could result from a genetic susceptibility or be a response to inflammatory stimuli, have been suggested to be strongly associated with pathological angiogenesis in MMD [4, 16–18]. Moreover, VEGF was discovered to be upregulated by TGF-β1 and HIF-1α, the expression of which is increased in MMD [37]. The finding that VEGFR2 and eNOS are suppressed by Cav-1, the level of which is lower in patients with MMD, [54] also emphasizes the essentiality of VEGF modulation through various pathways in partially preventing excessive neovascularization in MMD.

Other growth factors—such as bFGF, HGF, and PDGF—have been determined to be higher in patients with MMD and to promote endothelial hyperplasia, SMC migration, and collateral formation. Moreover, bFGF has been reported to activate the HIF-α signaling pathway and indirectly upregulate VEGF; [18, 19] PDGF-BB was reported to induce vascular progenitor cell differentiation into an SMC lineage, thereby strengthening intimal hyperplasia [14]. In addition, the single nucleotide polymorphism (SNP) rs382861 [A/C] in the promoter region of PDGFRB was identified in DNA obtained from European patients with MMD, suggesting that genetic risk factors may be an underlying cause of the aberrant expression of growth factors and MMD development [57].

Excessive accumulation of growth factors and cytokines can also result from altered endothelial barrier properties due to endothelial injury [4, 58]. Cerebral inflammation and ischemia can trigger the activation and expression of various circulating factors (such as angiogenetic cytokines), immune complex deposition, and other associated biomarkers, which may lead to consequential intimal hyperplasia and compensatory collateral formation. Elevated TGF-β and MMP-9 were determined to regulate the extracellular matrix of vessel walls and to, respectively, cause an imbalance in elastin and collagen IV levels. These actions may result in defects being created in vessel structures during pathological neovascularization [14, 21, 33, 34, 36, 40]. Another factor that may decrease endothelial integrity is ANG-2, which may contribute to hemorrhaging in MMD [26, 27].

Furthermore, in addition to causing endothelial dysfunction by enhancing vascular permeability, IL-1β can activate SMC proliferation, which leads to intimal occlusion and compensatory collateral formation. Other cytokines and immune complex deposits—including CCL5, MCP-1, and IgG—can also facilitate SMC recruitment and migration [14, 38, 46]. Patients with MMD were discovered to have attenuated levels of retinoic acid, which is a protective factor for typical vascular formation because it prevents excessive proliferation of SMCs. This was determined to be connected to the knockdown of *RALDH2* mRNA in ECFCs in patients with MMD and the higher level of CRABP-1 detected in such patients' CSF and may thus be a pathological mechanism of MMD [30, 32, 41, 42, 52]. However, in the promoter region of CRABP1 (15q25.1), no significant association was identified between the rs2280367 or rs3813573 SNP and MMD [57].

## 1.8 Conclusions

This article has outlined the factors that have been hypothesized to be significantly associated with MMD. However, whether the pathogenesis of MMD can be attributed to these factors or the factors are merely the consequence of compensatory collateral formation, inflammation, and ischemic status in the brain remains unclear.

Gene mutation is a strongly suspected pathological factor. The RING finger protein *RNF213* was identified in familial cases, exhibited a strong ethnicity effect, and is therefore frequently discussed as a gene making an individual susceptible to MMD. Several subtypes of MMD, such as the ischemic and hemorrhagic subtypes, were determined to be attributable to the *RNF213 p.4810 K* variant [3]. However, differences in subtypes and onset age groups could not be explained by findings on angiogenetic factors. Therefore, determining whether an association exists between genetic variation and aberrant angiogenetic factors is required.

The interaction and intermolecule regulation mediated by angiogenetic growth factors, vascular progenitor cells, inflammation or immune-related cytokines, and other relative circulating biomarkers were determined to be strongly associated with endothelial proliferation, SMC migration, and excessive neovascularization with defect structures, leading to intimal thickening or occlusion and compensatory formation of albeit fragile vessels, both of which are notable characteristics of MMD. However, research has not yet thoroughly explained the pathogenic mechanism of MMD. Therefore, further studies, such as those employing animal models or conducting gene research on RNF213-associated factors, are required to elucidate this complex pathway.

## References


1. Suzuki J, Takaku A. Cerebrovascular "moyamoya" disease. Disease showing abnormal net-like vessels in base of brain. Arch Neurol. 1969;20(3):288–99.
2. Scott RM, Smith ER. Moyamoya disease and moyamoya syndrome. N Engl J Med. 2009;360(12):1226–37.
3. Shang S, et al. Progress in moyamoya disease. Neurosurg Rev. 2020;43(2):371–82.
4. Dorschel KB, Wanebo JE. Genetic and proteomic contributions to the pathophysiology of moyamoya angiopathy and related vascular diseases. Appl Clin Genet. 2021;14:145–71.
5. Goto Y, Yonekawa Y. Worldwide distribution of moyamoya disease. Neurol Med Chir (Tokyo). 1992;32(12):883–6.
6. Kuroda S, Houkin K. Moyamoya disease: current concepts and future perspectives. Lancet Neurol. 2008;7(11):1056–66.

7. Kamada F, et al. A genome-wide association study identifies RNF213 as the first moyamoya disease gene. J Hum Genet. 2011;56(1):34–40.

8. Freemont PS, The RING, finger. A novel protein sequence motif related to the zinc finger. Ann N Y Acad Sci. 1993;684:174–92.

9. Elangovan M, et al. The ubiquitin-interacting motif of 26S proteasome subunit S5a induces A549 lung cancer cell death. Biochem Biophys Res Commun. 2007;364(2):226–30.

10. Liu W, et al. Identification of RNF213 as a susceptibility gene for moyamoya disease and its possible role in vascular development. PLoS One. 2011;6(7):e22542.

11. Houkin K, et al. Review of past research and current concepts on the etiology of moyamoya disease. Neurol Med Chir (Tokyo). 2012;52(5):267–77.

12. Bang OY, Fujimura M, Kim SK. The pathophysiology of moyamoya disease: an update. J Stroke. 2016;18(1):12–20.

13. Fujimura M, et al. Genetics and biomarkers of moyamoya disease: significance of RNF213 as a susceptibility gene. J Stroke. 2014;16(2):65–72.

14. Kang HS, et al. Plasma matrix metalloproteinases, cytokines and angiogenic factors in moyamoya disease. J Neurol Neurosurg Psychiatry. 2010;81(6):673–8.

15. Sakamoto S, et al. Expression of vascular endothelial growth factor in dura mater of patients with moyamoya disease. Neurosurg Rev. 2008;31(1):77–81. discussion 81.

16. Park YS, et al. The role of VEGF and KDR polymorphisms in moyamoya disease and collateral revascularization. PLoS One. 2012;7(10):e47158.

17. Olsson AK, et al. VEGF receptor signalling—in control of vascular function. Nat Rev Mol Cell Biol. 2006;7(5):359–71.

18. He J, et al. Expression of circulating vascular endothelial growth factor-antagonizing cytokines and vascular stabilizing factors prior to and following bypass surgery in patients with moyamoya disease. Exp Ther Med. 2014;8(1):302–8.

19. Jaipersad AS, et al. The role of monocytes in angiogenesis and atherosclerosis. J Am Coll Cardiol. 2014;63(1):1–11.

20. Takahashi A, et al. The cerebrospinal fluid in patients with moyamoya disease (spontaneous occlusion of the circle of Willis) contains high level of basic fibroblast growth factor. Neurosci Lett. 1993;160(2):214–6.

21. Yoshimoto T, et al. Angiogenic factors in moyamoya disease. Stroke. 1996;27(12):2160–5.

22. Yamamoto M, et al. Differences in cellular responses to mitogens in arterial smooth muscle cells derived from patients with moyamoya disease. Stroke. 1998;29(6):1188–93.

23. Morishita R, et al. Impairment of collateral formation in lipoprotein(a) transgenic mice: therapeutic angiogenesis induced by human hepatocyte growth factor gene. Circulation. 2002;105(12):1491–6.

24. Nanba R, et al. Increased expression of hepatocyte growth factor in cerebrospinal fluid and intracranial artery in moyamoya disease. Stroke. 2004;35(12):2837–42.

25. Takagi Y, et al. Expression of hypoxia-inducing factor-1 alpha and endoglin in intimal hyperplasia of the middle cerebral artery of patients with Moyamoya disease. Neurosurgery. 2007;60(2):338–45. discussion 345

26. Blecharz KG, et al. Autocrine release of angiopoietin-2 mediates cerebrovascular disintegration in Moyamoya disease. J Cereb Blood Flow Metab. 2017;37(4):1527–39.

27. Yu J, et al. Significance of serum angiopoietin-2 in patients with hemorrhage in adult-onset Moyamoya disease. Biomed Res Int. 2020;2020:8209313.

28. Rafat N, et al. Increased levels of circulating endothelial progenitor cells in patients with Moyamoya disease. Stroke. 2009;40(2):432–8.

29. Paschalaki KE, Randi AM. Recent advances in endothelial colony forming cells toward their use in clinical translation. Front Med (Lausanne). 2018;5:295.

30. Yoshihara T, et al. Increase in circulating CD34-positive cells in patients with angiographic evidence of moyamoya-like vessels. J Cereb Blood Flow Metab. 2008;28(6):1086–9.

31. Kim JH, et al. Decreased level and defective function of circulating endothelial progenitor cells in children with moyamoya disease. J Neurosci Res. 2010;88(3):510–8.

32. Lee JY, et al. Deregulation of retinaldehyde dehydrogenase 2 leads to defective angiogenic function of endothelial colony-forming cells in Pediatric moyamoya disease. Arterioscler Thromb Vasc Biol. 2015;35(7):1670–7.
33. Choi JW, et al. Mitochondrial abnormalities related to the dysfunction of circulating endothelial colony-forming cells in moyamoya disease. J Neurosurg. 2018;129(5):1151–9.
34. Kang HS, et al. Smooth-muscle progenitor cells isolated from patients with moyamoya disease: novel experimental cell model. J Neurosurg. 2014;120(2):415–25.
35. Guo DC, et al. Mutations in smooth muscle alpha-actin (ACTA2) cause coronary artery disease, stroke, and Moyamoya disease, along with thoracic aortic disease. Am J Hum Genet. 2009;84(5):617–27.
36. Jung KH, et al. Circulating endothelial progenitor cells as a pathogenetic marker of moyamoya disease. J Cereb Blood Flow Metab. 2008;28(11):1795–803.
37. Tokunaga K, Date I. Moyamoya disease. Brain Nerve. 2008;60(1):37–42.
38. Hojo M, et al. Role of transforming growth factor-beta1 in the pathogenesis of moyamoya disease. J Neurosurg. 1998;89(4):623–9.
39. Yamamoto M, et al. Increase in elastin gene expression and protein synthesis in arterial smooth muscle cells derived from patients with Moyamoya disease. Stroke. 1997;28(9):1733–8.
40. Weng L, et al. Association of increased Treg and Th17 with pathogenesis of moyamoya disease. Sci Rep. 2017;7(1):3071.
41. Boylan JF, Gudas LJ. The level of CRABP-I expression influences the amounts and types of all-trans-retinoic acid metabolites in F9 teratocarcinoma stem cells. J Biol Chem. 1992;267(30):21486–91.
42. Kim SK, et al. Elevation of CRABP-I in the cerebrospinal fluid of patients with Moyamoya disease. Stroke. 2003;34(12):2835–41.
43. Blecharz-Lang KG, et al. Gelatinolytic activity of autocrine matrix metalloproteinase-9 leads to endothelial de-arrangement in Moyamoya disease. J Cereb Blood Flow Metab. 2018;38(11):1940–53.
44. Fujimura M, et al. Increased expression of serum Matrix Metalloproteinase-9 in patients with moyamoya disease. Surg Neurol. 2009;72(5):476–80. discussion 480
45. Ni G, et al. Increased levels of circulating SDF-1alpha and CD34+ CXCR4+ cells in patients with moyamoya disease. Eur J Neurol. 2011;18(11):1304–9.
46. Phi JH, et al. Chemokine ligand 5 (CCL5) derived from endothelial colony-forming cells (ECFCs) mediates recruitment of smooth muscle progenitor cells (SPCs) toward critical vascular locations in Moyamoya disease. PLoS One. 2017;12(1):e0169714.
47. Mikami T, et al. Influence of inflammatory disease on the pathophysiology of moyamoya disease and quasi-moyamoya disease. Neurol Med Chir (Tokyo). 2019;59(10):361–70.
48. Fujimura M, et al. Increased serum production of soluble CD163 and CXCL5 in patients with moyamoya disease: involvement of intrinsic immune reaction in its pathogenesis. Brain Res. 2018;1679:39–44.
49. Lin R, et al. Clinical and immunopathological features of Moyamoya disease. PLoS One. 2012;7(4):e36386.
50. Sigdel TK, et al. Immune response profiling identifies autoantibodies specific to Moyamoya patients. Orphanet J Rare Dis. 2013;8:45.
51. Bang OY, et al. Caveolin-1, Ring finger protein 213, and endothelial function in Moyamoya disease. Int J Stroke. 2016;11(9):999–1008.
52. Chung JW, et al. Cav-1 (Caveolin-1) and arterial remodeling in adult Moyamoya disease. Stroke. 2018;49(11):2597–604.
53. Sonveaux P, et al. Caveolin-1 expression is critical for vascular endothelial growth factor-induced ischemic hindlimb collateralization and nitric oxide-mediated angiogenesis. Circ Res. 2004;95(2):154–61.
54. Noda A, et al. Elevation of nitric oxide metabolites in the cerebrospinal fluid of patients with moyamoya disease. Acta Neurochir. 2000;142(11):1275–9. discussion 1279-80

55. Park YS, et al. Age-specific eNOS polymorphisms in moyamoya disease. Childs Nerv Syst. 2011;27(11):1919–26.
56. Kashiwazaki D, Uchino H, Kuroda S. Downregulation of apolipoprotein-E and apolipoprotein-J in moyamoya disease-a proteome analysis of cerebrospinal fluid. J Stroke Cerebrovasc Dis. 2017;26(12):2981–7.
57. Roder C, et al. Polymorphisms in TGFB1 and PDGFRB are associated with Moyamoya disease in European patients. Acta Neurochir. 2010;152(12):2153–60.
58. Bedini G, et al. Vasculogenic and angiogenic pathways in moyamoya disease. Curr Med Chem. 2016;23(4):315–45.

# Chapter 2
# Current Applications of VR/AR (Virtual Reality/Augmented Reality) in Pediatric Neurosurgery

Nirali Patel, Katherine Hofmann, and Robert F. Keating

## Contents



## 2.1   Introduction

Neurosurgical procedures are some of the most complex procedures in medicine and since the advent of the field, planning, performing, and learning them has challenged the neurosurgeon. Virtual reality (VR) and augmented reality (AR) are making these challenges more manageable. VR refers to a virtual digital environment that can be experienced usually through use of stereoscopic glasses and controllers. AR, on the other hand, fuses the natural environment with virtual images, such as superimposing a preoperative MRI image on to the surgical field [1]. They initially


N. Patel · K. Hofmann · R. F. Keating (✉)
Department of Neurosurgery, Children's National Medical Center, George Washington University School of Medicine, Washington, DC, USA
e-mail: rkeating@cnmc.org





C. Di Rocco (ed.), *Advances and Technical Standards in Neurosurgery*,
Advances and Technical Standards in Neurosurgery 49,
https://doi.org/10.1007/978-3-031-42398-7_2

were used primarily as neuronavigational tools but soon their potential in other areas of surgery, such as planning, education, and assessment, was noted and explored. Through this chapter, we outline the history and evolution of these two technologies over the past few decades, describe the current state of the technology and its uses, and postulate future directions for research and implementation.

The initial utilization of VR can be found in the early 1830s when it was used for panoramic pictures, but the first simulator, a flight simulator, was introduced almost a century later. After the advent of head-mounted displays in the 1960s, these technologies were mainly targeted for entertainment purposes and it was not until the late 1990s that the first use of this technology for medical purposes, treatment of arachnophobia, was documented [2, 3]. Around the same time, use of VR for neurosurgical procedures, especially in terms of neuronavigation, was initially documented. Grimson et al., working out of Brigham and Women's Hospital in Boston, demonstrated how VR could be used to build "detailed, patient-specific models of anatomy and augment those models with other information, such as functional properties." They argued that this information could be registered with actual patient position and would allow the surgeon to plan optimal trajectories as well as obtain real time feedback regarding position of instruments [4]. However, it was not until the new millennium that this technology was first utilized in a neurosurgical procedure.

In the first direct patient use (in 2009), David Clarke used a NeuroTouch neurosurgical simulator to excise a left frontal meningioma [5]. This unleashed a storm of innovation and research that worked to incorporate VR and AR into neurosurgical procedures and training. Since 2009, there have been dozens of publications describing the use of VR and AR for neurosurgical procedures. These technologies are now being leveraged to improve all aspects of neurosurgery including planning, training, patient education, and neuronavigation.

## 2.2 Current State/Research

### 2.2.1 VR/AR Systems in Use

Multiple VR and AR systems are currently available for neurosurgery, including devices that utilize multifunctional head-mounted displays (HMD: Microsoft HoloLens, VSI PE, Google Glass), haptic feedback (NeuroVR, Immersive Touch, Procedicus Vascular Interventional System Trainer (VIST)), surgical planning software (Surgical Theater, Dextroscope, VPI Reveal, Synaptive Medical, BrainLab, Vesalius, Perspectus VR), and VOSTARS (video and optical see-through augmented reality surgical systems) HMD-based surgical navigation platforms [1]. These systems are currently being used in operative planning, neurosurgical training, intraoperative neuronavigation, patient education, and assessment of surgeon performance. New systems are being developed almost daily and are being employed to make the technology even more efficient and accessible. Virtual interactive presence and augmented reality (VIPAR), for instance, is a recent development that allows "a remote surgeon to deliver real-time virtual assistance to a local surgeon, over a standard internet connection" [6]. Table 2.1 lists these different systems. Given this, the above list should be considered a starting point and not an all-inclusive list for those looking for more information.

### 2.2.2  Neurosurgical Planning and VR/AR

Proper surgical planning requires that the neurosurgeon has a precise understanding of patient-specific anatomy. VR and AR, as visualization technologies, have easily found their way into neurosurgery, acting as a way for physicians to view and model unique patient anatomy in 3D, leading to improved efficiency and outcomes. Although VR neurosurgical planning has been improving intracranial operative strategies for over two decades [7, 8], more recent advances have improved the accuracy and efficiency of VR planning technology, leading to shorter procedure times and improved surgeon anatomical understanding, resulting in better patient outcomes.

Utilization of VR in preoperative planning and rehearsal has been shown to reduce procedure lengths. In 2021, a controlled retrospective study used Surgical Theater to evaluate outcomes and procedure lengths of minimally invasive middle cerebral artery (MCA) aneurysm clipping [9]. Surgical Theater is a VR and AR system that constructs 3D anatomical models based on DICOM imaging. Using the Surgical Theater planning platform (shown in Fig. 2.1), 360VR models were constructed from patient-specific CTA scans. In conjunction with Oculus VR headsets, surgeons were able to view and manipulate the VR models for presurgical planning and rehearsal. For MCA clipping surgeries that used VR preoperatively, procedure time was significantly shorter than in the control group, by about 80 minutes (a 24% reduction in procedure time) [9]. Reduction in procedure time is associated with

**Table 2.1**  Current VR/AR systems being used in surgical education, planning, and research

| **Head-Mounted Displays** | | |
|---|---|---|
| Microsoft HoloLens | VSI Patient Education | Google Glass |
| **Haptic Feedback** | | |
| NeuroVR | Immersive Touch | Procedicus Vascular Interventional System Trainer (VIST) |
| **Surgical Planning Software** | | |
| Surgical Theater | Dextroscope | VPI Reveal |
| Synaptive Medical | Vesalius | Perspectus VR |
| BrainLab | | |
| **Video and Optical See-Through Augmented Reality Surgical Systems** | | |

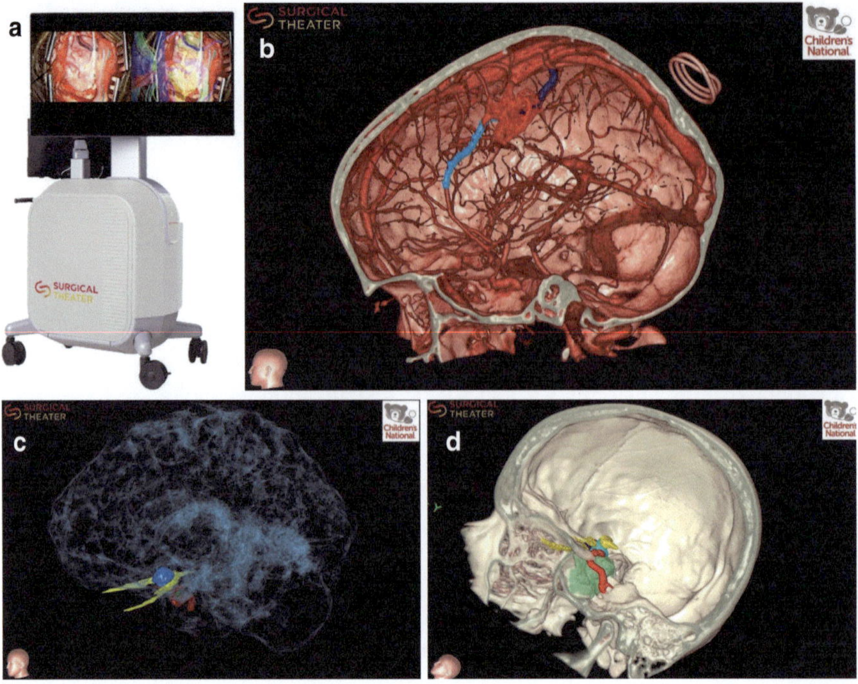

**Fig. 2.1** (**a**) The surgical theater VR system, (**b**) 3D model of a patient with a right frontoparietal arteriovenous malformation (AVM) with the feeding artery shown in light blue and the primary draining vein shown in dark blue. (**c**) Model of a patient with optic tract meningioma with the optic nerves and chiasm in yellow, tumor in blue, and the carotids shown in red. (**d**) 3D model fused with CT scan of a patient with pituitary lesion with the lesion shown in green, the optic nerves and tracts shown in yellow, the carotids shown in red, and the pituitary gland shown in blue

less time under anesthesia and less risk of heart attack, blood pressure changes, venous thromboembolism, or stroke [9–12]. Less OR time for each patient can lead to increased efficiency for surgeons and reduction of hospital expenses for patients [10, 11]. Therefore, use of VR for presurgical planning may result in improved patient outcomes, better allocation of resources, and more OR space.

VR technology can also help improve the surgeon's understanding of patient-specific anatomy. One prospective study analyzed subjective and objective data regarding the effectiveness of the BananaVision VR modeling program, a platform that can rapidly generate virtual 3D models using patient CT or MRI images in less than 2 min [13]. Questionnaires given to surgeons operating on cerebrovascular disease (CVD) showed that the VR sessions were evaluated as "effective" for increasing understanding of patient-specific anatomy in 83.3% of cases [13]. Objective measures (comparisons of surgeon presurgical illustrations to intraoperative video) demonstrated that use of VR planning significantly improved their illustrations, indicating their increased understanding of the patient's anatomy [13].

Patient outcomes in general have been shown to improve with use of VR surgical planning. The Dextroscope is a VR stereoscopic visualization and planning

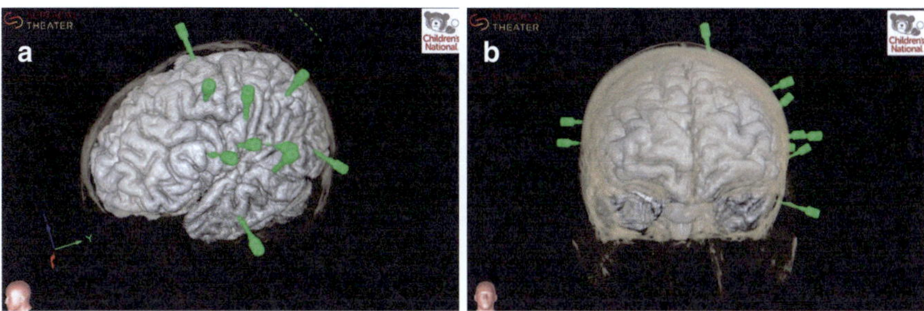

**Fig. 2.2** Plans for an SEEG electrode placed in a patient at our institution using the Surgical Theater VR system in sagittal (**a**) and coronal (**b**) cuts

workstation that uses natural 3D hand movements instead of the mouse or keyboard to work with 3D images generated by MRI or CT images [14]. The first multicenter study to evaluate the clinical outcomes associated with regular use of VR planning, the Dextroscope, was used by 9 surgeons—7 of which had clipped fewer than 20 aneurysms—to plan the clipping of 115 aneurysms (85 unruptured, 28 ruptured) in 105 patients [14]. The study found that at the 6-month follow-up, Dextroscope-planned surgeries resulted in a 97.4% favorable outcome rate with zero mortality in the unruptured aneurysm group and 92.9% in the ruptured aneurysm group [14]. Because this was a retrospective study with no control group, the results were compared to benchmarks already published in literature. The rates of favorable outcomes in those with unruptured aneurysms in this study were similar to those published in the literature, while favorable outcomes in those with ruptured aneurysms were slightly higher in this study compared to the published benchmarks. This demonstrates the key advantage of advanced 3D planning in cases where subarachnoid blood and edematous brain obscures anatomy and prevents further exploration, especially for the less experienced surgeon [14].

Although widely used in tumor or vascular cases, neurosurgical planning with VR has also proven useful in the epilepsy-related procedures [15]. Surgical Theater, for example, has been used by neurosurgeons in preoperative planning, such as in planning the placement of stereotactic electroencephalography (SEEG) depth electrodes for patients undergoing SEEG monitoring [15]. Figure 2.2 demonstrates certain trajectories devised using Surgical Theater for placement of these SEEG depth electrodes. Future research is needed, however, to evaluate and validate the effectiveness of VR preoperative planning technology in epilepsy procedures.

### 2.2.3  VR/AR in Intraoperative Neuronavigation

Localization of anatomic landmarks and pathology of interest have always been a challenge for neurosurgeons, and they must rely on pre-operative images. Prior to VR and AR, these images were on a remote computer or TV screen and the surgeon often had to disrupt their flow to consult them [16]. The images displayed are also in 2D

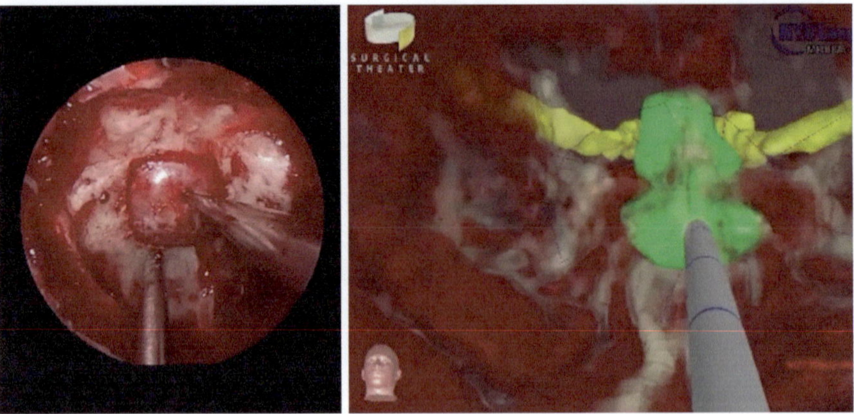


**Fig. 2.3** SyncAR, a new innovation from Surgical Theater, allows direct overlay of critical anatomy and pathology onto the microscope oculars

and must be interpreted by the surgeon [17]. However, with VR and AR, it is becoming easier for the surgeon to focus on the surgical field while still being able to obtain the relevant information even while using the surgical microscope [18] (Fig. 2.3).

In the area of neurooncology, the use of VR/AR for neuronavigation has been shown to improve the extent of resection and, thus, overall survival. Sun et al. demonstrated that combining VR and AR based on intraoperative MRI and functional imaging can help enhance extent of resection while preserving neural function in patients with gliomas adjacent to eloquent structures [19]. They studied 134 patients with glioma and noted 69.6% of the patients who underwent surgery using VR/AR protocols had a complete resection as opposed to only 36.4% of control subjects. At 2 weeks and 3 months, patients who underwent surgery with VR/AR protocols also had higher neural function (motor, visual field, and language) compared to control patients [19]. The intraoperative brain imaging system (IBIS) was created in 2012 and validates intraoperative ultrasound through AR. Updated patient models can be obtained quickly, and this system has been used in vascular neurosurgery, neurooncology, electrode implantation for DBS/epilepsy, and, most importantly, to assess brain shift during surgery [20].

VR and AR neuronavigation has also been steadily gaining ground in spinal surgery where the worldwide market for navigation systems was valued at $600 million in 2019 [21]. The appeal of VR/AR in spinal procedures is mainly due to the ability for more precise instrumentation and decreasing exposure to ionizing radiation for the operating room staff [21]. Head-mounted displays (HMD) are often the VR/AR of choice for these procedures and Microsoft HoloLens is the most frequently used system for spinal procedures [22–25], whereas Google Glass is reportedly the most often used HMD overall [26]. Many studies show that AR increases accuracy of pedicle screw placement during spinal surgeries though there is some variability amongst currently published studies regarding outcome measures and further studies are needed [21, 27]. Most of these studies document difficulties with registration and calibration difficulties which also need to be addressed prior to wider adaptation [21] .

New results demonstrate that this technology is clearly and unequivocally superior to older methods. Haemmerli et al. recently had success showing that AR is superior to the more standard pointer-based navigation and even in those operators who may not be familiar with AR techniques. They utilized a 3D-printed skull that was fused with a reference MRI and CT scan showing a frontal sinus defect and 26 subjects (all of whom had little to no AR experience) were asked to target the center of the lesion. The "median distance to target was statistically lower for AR than for the stereotactic navigation module" in these subjects [28]. Other studies assessing variance from target have achieved similar results showing that VR/AR could be used for several procedures including small needle biopsies of deep brain sites [29].

### 2.2.4  VR/AR in Educating Surgical Trainees

After the requirement of an 80-hour work week in 2003, surgical residents now spend significantly less time in the operating room (OR) than before, reducing operative experience to approximately one third of the pre-2003 amount [30]. Some evidence has suggested increased complication rates in neurosurgical procedures as a result of this change [31, 32]. To improve patient safety, there has been a push for technologies that allow neurosurgical residents to gain more surgical practice outside of the OR, and developments in neurosurgical simulators can facilitate operative experience through artificial 3D learning environments. Just as VR and AR assist in neurosurgical planning and rehearsal, simulated surgeries can enhance the anatomical understanding, spatial reasoning, and surgical skill development of the neurosurgical resident, while posing no risk to patients [33–36].

Various forms of neurosurgical simulations are already widely used in training, including plastic, animal, and cadaveric models. These models, however, are not ideal because plastic and cadaveric models do not respond in the same way as live tissue, and animal model anatomy differs from human anatomy [37]. VR simulations offer a better alternative because they are based on the movement illusion from visuospatial input and vestibular system stimulation to create graphic renderings, tissue deformation, and haptic feedback, allowing the simulation to be as realistic as possible [38–40]. VR simulations are also advantageous in that they do not suffer from repeated use, and therefore do not require continuous replacement of the plastic, cadaver, or animal models, resulting in lower costs [41, 42]. The programmable aspect of VR models also means that they can be used to mimic a wide range of anatomic and physical variance, providing residents with experience in uncommon procedures [33, 41].

VR simulations allow residents to practice complex technical skills without the associated risks to patients. The ImmersiveTouch system, for example, is commonly used for ventriculostomy and percutaneous spinal needle placement simulations [42–45]. Evidence suggests that after completing VR ventriculostomy or spinal needle placement simulations using ImmersiveTouch, residents demonstrated significant improvement in burr hole placement ($p < .03$), final location of the catheter ($p = .05$), and procedure completion time ($p < .004$), or in performance accuracy of needle placement ($p = .04$), respectively [43, 45]. Other systems, such as the NeuroVR (previously NeuroTouch) haptic simulation platform, have been associated with an increase in resident performance scores in the operating room for endoscopic endonasal surgeries ($p = 0.0045$) [46]. These studies indicate that the application of VR and AR simulations in neurosurgical resident education can improve the operative skills of residents and allows them to practice outside of the OR.

### 2.2.5  Limitations and Barriers of VR and AR in Neurosurgery

As with any new technology, VR and AR have not been without their challenges. The predominant barriers are due to the enormous difficulties associated with designing and implementing clinically relevant models. Most of the VR models developed have issues with feasibility, especially in real-life scenarios, and have prevented widespread adaptation of this technology into standard practice [1]. Additionally, most of the VR/AR hardware is custom-made for each laboratory investigating the product or institution using it in their clinical practice. This makes it difficult to generalize findings of one lab or experience of one institution to others and prevents collaboration in both further research and resolving challenges mentioned above [47].

Specific to their use in neuronavigation, VR and AR are prone to registration errors and system delays. In neurosurgical procedures where even a one-millimeter error can be critical, this is a major impediment to adaptation. Issues with calibration of the instruments used and optical distortions of the image also often plague those using these technologies. Lastly, as with all neuronavigation, tissue movement, especially as surgery progresses, can result in significant errors in image alignment and localization [48, 49]. With the invention of increasingly powerful microcomputers behind the VR and AR software, these issues should eventually be resolved, but again will face challenges as long as each laboratory and institution have their own customized programs [40]. Advances are already being made to incorporate methods to compensate for spatial drift intraoperatively while using AR technology [50].

Lastly, the challenges associated with acquiring and implementing VR and AR programs within individual institutions cannot be ignored. The significant learning curve as surgeons and operating room staff initially begin to use the multiple variations of software and devices can add substantial time and resources to already stressed systems [1]. The cost of acquiring these programs is also not inconsequential and though studies show that over time we see a reduction in overall costs due to decreased complications, the upfront cost cannot be ignored. As further iterations of these systems are designed, it is imperative to make these devices more user friendly and easily accessible.

## 2.3  Future Directions

As virtual and augmented reality technology continues to evolve and become more accessible, its uses will only expand. Though it is already being efficiently used in neurosurgical planning, neuronavigation, and improvement of outcomes, there are several other aspects that can be enhanced with the use of VR/AR. Optimizing resources to assist impoverished areas, mapping cognitive functions during awake craniotomies, and patient education are all fields which we believe hold significant promise.

### 2.3.1  *Optimizing Neurosurgical Resources Using VR/AR*

Almost 5 million people each year in low- and middle-income countries do not have access to safe and affordable neurosurgical interventions [51]. The lack of care has only been exacerbated by the COVID-19 pandemic, as UN efforts to increase neurosurgical capacity were disrupted by travel restrictions, increasing the demand for virtual solutions [51, 52]. VR and AR systems make it possible to train and proctor neurosurgeons across the world to improve patient outcomes globally.

VR simulation platforms can assist in remote neurosurgical training of neurosurgeons worldwide. As also seen in resident education, VR neurosurgical simulators reduce the learning curve of complex procedures. The use of VR compared to physical simulators is especially critical in low-resource settings, where replacing plastic, cadaver, and animal models becomes expensive. In this way, VR simulation systems may be a better way to conserve supplies while improving patient outcomes [51].

By allowing information to be superimposed onto a neurosurgeon's visual field, AR technology can be used in remote tele-proctoring. With tele-proctoring, an experienced neurosurgeon can virtually assist with procedures from anywhere in the world [51–53]. Although tele-proctoring has been used for neurosurgeries, its use is limited since proctors can only verbally instruct remote surgeons [54]. When integrated with AR, however, tele-proctoring enhances unidirectional video communication, as the AR uses optical see-through displays, allowing the proctor to see and virtually interact in the remote surgeon's visual field [55, 56]. This AR tele-proctoring technology has been used to assist in many remote neurosurgeries without complications, including intracranial balloon angioplasty, carotid stenting, intracranial stenting, and endoscopic third ventriculostomy [54, 57].

Adopting VR and AR technologies in low-resource settings can be challenging due to the cost of the equipment, however recent innovations are trying to overcome this barrier by making AR and VR compatible with existing software and equipment, such mobile devices [51]. The virtual interactive presence and augmented reality (VIPAR) system, for example, is an iPad-based platform which allows proctoring surgeons to project their hands into the visual field of the remote surgeons wherever wireless internet connection is available [51, 57]. Other AR and VR devices can be used with smartphones as well, such as the low-cost ($15) Google Cardboard headset, which like other VR systems can be used for neurosurgical training and patient education in low- and middle- income countries [51].

### 2.3.2 Mapping Cognitive Functions During Awake Craniotomies

When faced with lesions in eloquent areas, awake craniotomies are often used to map and preserve neurological functions, especially language and motor. These surgeries allow increased resection margins while simultaneously decreasing the risk of injury [58, 59]. However, certain tracts, such as optic radiations, are difficult to map with conventional tactics during awake surgeries due to their diffuse connectivity [60, 61]. Work is now being done to map these highly diffuse and individual networks using VR/AR technology. One promising approach was pioneered by Mazerand et al. who used VR-based intraoperative visual field assessment during direct subcortical stimulation intraoperatively. The patient presented in their paper was blind in his right eye and had a left parietotemporal glioblastoma. Using their VR protocol, their team was able to accurately identify the optic radiations and the patient had no postoperative deficits [62]. Their team is continuing to test their protocol in larger number of patients, while others have attempted to map more complex cognitive functions.

Social cognition, especially interpretation of nonverbal cues during social interactions, has often been an overlooked and misunderstood casualty of neurosurgery [63, 64]. There are certain networks that are implicated in the processing of these social cues, but anatomical localization during surgery is difficult [65, 66]. VR headsets are now being used to simulate social interactions during awake craniotomies and test feasibility of mapping these cognitive networks intraoperatively [66–68]. These preliminary studies demonstrate that patients can be safely and effectively be immersed in a VR environment during awake craniotomies. Though further studies are needed with proof of concept for these protocols and actual mapping of these networks, they show a promising start in this aspect of VR.

### 2.3.3 Patient Education Using VR/AR

Valid informed consents (IC) for surgery require that the patient fully understands the intervention, including all the possible risks, benefits, and alternatives. IC today, however, is often either overly simplified or is too technically complex for patients to fully comprehend the proposed procedure [69]. Studies evaluating the neurosurgical informed consent process have demonstrated that, on average, patients remember only 18–44% of procedural information and only 15–33% of risks [70–73]. Furthermore, neurosurgery generates the highest rate of claims and legal issues among the surgical specialties, with lack of adequate and thorough consent being the one of the most frequent causes of malpractice suits [74–76]. To improve patient comprehension and memory of the neurosurgical procedures and risks, new technologies using VR and 3D models can be beneficial.

In a 2021 randomized controlled clinical trial, Perin *et al.* evaluated virtual reality immersions systems Surgical Theater and Vesalius, which can both construct 3D models of patients' unique DICOM images [76]. Surgical Theater uses the Oculus Rift headset to allow patients to navigate through their brain and locate the surgically relevant structures, while Vesalius creates a 3D phantom-hologram that can be visualized and dissected by using 3D glasses and a 3D screen [76]. Perin *et al.* found for patients undergoing brain tumor surgery, use of the Surgical Theater and Vesalius VR systems led to greater global patient comprehension and comprehension of risks compared to standard MR or CT 2D DICOM images [76]. To aid in decision making, some institutions use VR software to create "flythrough" videos of the planned surgery. With the Surgical Theater platform, a specialist can generate a 3D videos that demonstrate their unique anatomy and can be sent home with patients and families to allow them to come to a decision regarding surgery in their own time [15].

Use of VR in the neurosurgical consent process can also lead to decreased anxiety levels and increased patient satisfaction. The Virtual Surgery Intelligence Patient Education (VSI PE) tool uses the mixed reality Microsoft HoloLens glasses to view 3D projections of MRIs and CT scans [58]. When both the physician and patient wear HoloLenses, the doctor can show a 3D virtual model of the patient's head and demonstrate how the brain lesion or region will be accessed, with the patient always viewing the same orientation as the physician [77]. House *et al.* found that not only did the VSI PE system increase comprehension of the surgery for both patients and relatives compared to physical models, but the use of VR also significantly reduced anxiety for patients undergoing implantation of electrodes for deep brain stimulation or stereo-EEG [77]. Reduction of anxiety maybe be due to an improvement in the patient–physician relationship. One study demonstrated that when Surgical Theater VR models were used in the IC process for patients undergoing elective craniotomy for aneurysm or tumor resection, patient satisfaction, and measures of physician–patient alliance both increased [78].

Recent research in the IC process has found that using multiple modalities—various combinations of video, booklet, discussion, physical models, interactive groups, teach-backs, etc.—led to greater comprehension and satisfaction for neurosurgical patients [79, 80]; however, there is a paucity in the literature of use of VR-IC with additional modalities. Further research is also needed to explore how demographic factors such as socioeconomic status or education level impacts patient satisfaction and comprehension with VR.

## 2.4  Conclusions

From the simple flight simulators of the early 1900s to the complex systems that allow experienced surgeons to remotely proctor difficult surgeries, VR and AR have traversed a long path. Since the first clinical use in the excision of a left frontal meningioma by David Clarke in 2009, VR/AR have been used in every aspect of neurosurgery, including navigation, operative planning, surgical training, patient education, and skill assessment. Dozens of studies over the past few years have demonstrated clear benefits of these technologies. When used to plan surgeries pre-operatively, VR/AR help shorten surgical time, increase favorable outcomes, and decrease morbidity [9–12, 14]. Several studies have also demonstrated that use of VR/AR for neuronavigation intraoperatively during tumor surgeries increases extent of resection and is associated with better functional status for patients [19]. In the area of spine surgery, head-mounted devices are being utilized to increase accuracy of instrumentation [21, 27]. VR simulations are increasingly being used to train the next generation of neurosurgeons given its ability to mimic a wide variety of pathologies as well as creating a more realistic experience through graphic renderings, tissue deformation, and haptic feedback. Currently, accessibility, cost, and system delays are all major limitations of these technologies, but future iterations strive to resolve these issues. Though it has already revolutionized most aspects of neurosurgery, VR/AR continues to evolve and will be used in progressively creative ways to solve the issues facing neurosurgeons today. Optimizing resources and reaching impoverished areas, mapping cognitive networks, and educating patients are only some of these novel indications. Future generations will, undoubtedly, leverage these resources to provide increasingly better care for our patients.

## References


1. Mishra R, Narayanan K, Umana G, Montemurro N, Chaurasia B, Deora H. Virtual reality in neurosurgery: beyond neurosurgical planning. Int J Environ Res Public Health. 2022;19:1719. https://doi.org/10.3390/ijerph19031719.
2. Madhavan K, Kolcun JP, Chieng LO, Wang M. Augmented-reality integrated robotics in neurosurgery: are we there yet? Neurosurg Focus. 2017;42(5):E3. https://doi.org/10.3171/2017.2.FOCUS177.
3. Garcia-Palacios A, Hoffman H, Carlin A, Furness T, Botella C. Virtual reality in the treatment of spider phobia: a controlled study. Behav Res Ther. 2002;40:983–93.
4. Grimson E, Leventon M, Lorigo L, Kapur T, Kikinis R. Image guided surgery. Sci Am. 1999;280:62–9.
5. Clarke D, D'Arcy RC, Delorme S, Laroche D, Godin G, Hajra S, Brooks R, DiRaddo R. Virtual reality simulator: demonstrated use in neurosurgical oncology. Surg Innov. 2013;20(2):190–7. https://doi.org/10.1177/1553350612451354.
6. Shenai M, Dillavou M, Shum C, Ross D. Virtual interactive presence and augmented reality (VIPAR) for remote surgical assistance. Neurosurgery. 2011;68(1):200–7. https://doi.org/10.1227/NEU.0b013e3182077efd.
7. Kockro RA, Serra L, Tseng-Tsai Y, Chan C, Yih-Yian S, Gim-Guan C, Lee E, et al. Planning and simulation of neurosurgery in a virtual reality environment. Neurosurgery. 2000;46(1):118–35.

8. Kockro RA, Stadie A, Schwandt E, Reisch R, Charalampaki C, Ng I, et al. A collaborative virtual reality environment for neurosurgical planning and training. Neurosurgery. 2007;61(5):379–91. https://doi.org/10.1227/01.neu.0000303997.12645.26.

9. Steineke TC, Barbery D. Microsurgical clipping of middle cerebral artery aneurysms: preoperative planning using virtual reality to reduce procedure time. Neurosurg Focus. 2021;51(2):E12.

10. Liu J, Gormley N, Dasenbrock H, Aglio L, Smith T, Gormley W, Robertson F. Cost-benefit analysis of transitional care in neurosurgery. Neurosurgery. 2019;85(5):672–9. https://doi.org/10.1093/neuros/nyy424.

11. McLaughlin N, Upadhyaya P, Buxey F, Martin N. Value-based neurosurgery: measuring and reducing the cost of microvascular decompression surgery. J Neurosurg. 2014;121(3):700–8. https://doi.org/10.3171/2014.5.JNS131996.

12. Kim J, Khavanin N, Rambchan A, McCarthy R, Mlodinow A, De Oliveria G, et al. Surgical duration and risk of venous thromboembolism. JAMA Surg. 2015;150(2):110–7. https://doi.org/10.1001/jamasurg.2014.1841.

13. Sugiyama T, Clapp T, Nelson J, Eitel C, Motegi H, Nakayama N, et al. Immersive 3-dimensional virtual reality modeling for case-specific presurgical discussions in cerebrovascular neurosurgery. Oper Neurosurg. 2021;20(3):289–99. https://doi.org/10.1093/ons/opaa335.

14. Kockro R, Killeen T, Ayyad A, Glaser M, Stadie A, Reisch R, et al. Aneurysm surgery with preoperative three-dimensional planning in a virtual reality environment: technique and outcome analysis. World Neurosurg. 2016;96:489–99. https://doi.org/10.1016/j.wneu.2016.08.124.

15. Phan T, Prakash K, Elliott R, Pasupuleti A, Gaillard W, Keating R, Oluigbo C. Virtual reality based 3-dimensional localization of stereotactic EEG (SEEG) depth electrodes and related brain anatomy in pediatric epilepsy surgery. Childs Nerv Syst. 2022;38(3):537–46. https://doi.org/10.1007/s00381-021-05403-5.

16. Lee C, Wong G. Virtual reality and augmented reality in the management of intracranial tumors: a review. J Clin Neurosci. 2019;62:14–20.

17. Meola A, Cutolo F, Carbone M, Cagnazzo F, Ferrari M, Ferrari V. Augmented reality in neurosurgery: a systematic review. Neurosurg Rev. 2017;40(4):537–48. https://doi.org/10.1007/s10143-016-0732-9.

18. Contreras Lopez W, Navarro P, Crispin S. Intraoperative clinical application of augmented reality in neurosurgery: a systematic review. Clin Neurol Neurosurg. 2019;177:6–11. https://doi.org/10.1016/j.clineuro.2018.11.018.

19. Sun GC, Wang F, Chen XL, Yu XG, Ma XD, Zhou DB, et al. Impact of virtual and augmented reality based on intraoperative magnetic resonance imaging and functional neuronavigation in glioma surgery involving eloquent areas. World Neurosurg. 2016;96:375–82.

20. Drouin S, Kochanowska A, Kersten-Oertel M, Gerard IJ, Zelmann R, De Nigris D, et al. IBIS: an OR ready open-source platform for image-guided neurosurgery. Int J Comput Assist Radiol Surg. 2017;12:363–78.

21. Sakai D, Joyce K, Sugimoto M, Horikita N, Hiyama A, Sato M, et al. Augmented, virtual and mixed reality in spinal surgery: a real-world experience. J Ortho Surg. 2020;28(3):1–12.

22. Urakov TM, Wang MY, Levi AD. Workflow caveats in augmented reality-assisted pedicle instrumentation: cadaver lab. World Neurosurg. 2019;126:e1449–55.

23. Liebmann F, Roner S, von Atzigen M, Scaramuzza D, Sutter R, Snedeker J, et al. Pedicle screw navigation using surface digitization on the Microsoft HoloLens. Int J Comput Assist Radiol Surg. 2019;14(7):1157–65.

24. Gibby J, Swenson S, Cvetko S, Rao R, Javan R. Head-mounted display augmented reality to guide pedicle screw placement utilizing computed tomography. Int J Comput Assist Radiol Surg. 2019;14(3):525–35.

25. Muller F, Roner S, Liebmann F, Spirig J, Furnstahl P, Farshad M. Augmented reality navigation for spinal pedicle screw instrumentation using intraoperative 3D imaging. Spine J. 2020;20(4):621–8.

26. Rahman R, Wood M, Qian L, Price C, Johnson A, Osgood G. Head-mounted display use in surgery: a systematic review. Surg Innov. 2020;27(1):88–100.

27. Felix B, Kalatar S, Moatz B, Hofstetter C, Karsy M, Parr R, Gibby W. Augmented reality spine surgery navigation: increasing pedicle screw insertion accuracy for both open and minimally

invasive spine surgeries. Spine. 2022; https://doi.org/10.1097/BRS.0000000000004338. Online ahead of print

28. Haemmerli J, Davidovic A, Meling T, Chavaz L, Schaller K, Bijlenga P. Evaluation of the precision of operative augmented reality compared to standard neuronavigation using 3D-printed skull. Neurosurg Focus. 2021;50(1):E17.

29. Gibby W, Cvetko S, Gibby A, Gibby C, Sorensen K, Andrew E, et al. The application of augmented reality-based navigation for accurate target acquisition of deep brain sites: advances in neurosurgical guidance. J Neuosurg. 2021:1–7. https://doi.org/10.3171/2021.9.JNS21510.

30. Ahmed N, Devitt K, Keshet I, Spicer J, Imrie K, Feldman L, et al. A systematic review of the effects of resident duty hour restrictions in surgery. Ann Surg. 2014;259(6):1041–53.

31. Dumont T, Rughani A, Penar P, Horgan M, Tranmer B, Jewell R. Increased rate of complications on a neurological surgery service after implantation of the accreditation council for graduate medical education work-hour restriction. J Neurosurg. 2012;116(3):483–6. https://doi.org/10.3171/2011.9.JNS116.

32. Hoh B, Neal D, Kleinhenz D, Hoh D, Mocco J, Barker F. Higher complications and no improvement in mortality in the ACGME resident duty-hour restriction era: an analysis of more than 107,000 neurosurgical trauma patients in the nationwide inpatient sample database. Neurosurgery. 2012;70(6):1369–81.; discussion 1381-2. https://doi.org/10.1227/NEU/0b013e3182486a75.

33. Pelargos P, Nagasawa D, Lagman C, Tenn S, Demos J, Lee S, et al. Utilizing virtual and augmented reality for educational and clinical enhancements in neurosurgery. J Clin Neurosci. 2017;25:1–4. https://doi.org/10.1016/j.jocn.2016.09.002.

34. Malone H, Syed O, Downes M, D'Ambrosio A, Quest D, Kaiser M. Simulation in neurosurgery: a review of computer-based simulation environments and their surgical applications. Neurosurgery. 2010;67(4):1105–16. https://doi.org/10.1227/NEU.0b013e3181ee46d0.

35. Chen T, Zhang Y, Ding C, Ting K, Yoon S, Sahak H, et al. Virtual reality as a learning tool in spinal anatomy and surgical techniques. N Am Spine Soc J. 2021;6:10063. https://doi.org/10.1016/j.xnsj.2021.100063.

36. Zaed I, Chibbaro S, Ganau M, Tinterri B, Bossi B, Peschillo S, et al. Simulation and virtual reality in intracranial aneurysms neurosurgical training: a systematic review. J Neurosurg Sci. 2022; https://doi.org/10.23736/S0390-5616.22.05526-6.

37. Alaraj A, Lemole M, Finkle J, Yudkowsky R, Wallace A, Luciano C, et al. Virtual reality training in neurosurgery: review of current status and future applications. Surg Neurol Int. 2011;2:52. https://doi.org/10.4103/2152-7806.80117.

38. Oliveira LM, Figueiredo EG. Simulation training methods in neurological surgery. Asian J Neurosurg. 2019;14(2):364–70.

39. Cohen A, Lohani S, Manjila S, Natsupakpong S, Brown N, Cavusoglu M. Virtual reality simulation: basic concepts and use in endoscopic neurosurgery training. Childs Nerv Syst. 2013;29(8):1235–44. https://doi.org/10.1007/s00381-013-2139-z.

40. Robison RA, Liu CY, Apuzzo ML. Man, mind, and machine: the past and future of virtual reality simulation in neurologic surgery. World Neurosurg. 2011;76(5):419–30.

41. Konakondla S, Fong R, Schirmer CM. Simulation training in neurosurgery: advances in education and practice. Adv Med Educ Pract. 2017;8:465–73.

42. Lemole GM, Banerjee PP, Luciano C, Neckrysh S, Charbel F. Virtual reality in neurosurgical education: part-task ventriculostomy simulation with dynamic visual and haptic feedback. Neurosurgery. 2007;61(1):142–8. discussion 148-9

43. Schirmer C, Elder JB, Roitberg B, Lobel D. Virtual reality-based simulation training for ventriculostomy: an evidence-based approach. Neurosurgery. 2013;73(Suppl 1):66–73.

44. Alaraj A, Charbel F, Birk D, Tobin M, Luciano C, Banerjee P, et al. Role of cranial and spinal virtual and augmented reality simulation using immersive touch modules in neurosurgical training. Neurosurgery. 2013;72(Suppl 1(01)):115–23.

45. Luciano C, Banerjee P, Sorenson J, Foley K, Ansari S, Rizzi S, et al. Percutaneous spinal fixation simulation with virtual reality and haptics. Neurosurgery. 2013;72(Suppl 1): 89–96.

46. Thawani J, Ramayya A, Abdullah K, Hudgins E, Vaughan K, Piazza M, et al. Resident simulation training in endoscopic endonasal surgery utilizing haptic feedback technology. J Clin Neurosci. 2016;34:112–6.
47. Cannizzaro D, Zaed I, Safa A, Jelmoni A, Composto A, Bisoglio A, et al. Augmented reality in neurosurgery, state of art and future projections: a systematic review. Front Surg. 2022;9:864792.
48. Zhu E, Hadadgar A, Masiello I, Zary N. Augmented reality in healthcare education: an integrative review. PeerJ. 2014;2:e469.
49. Guha D, Alotaibi N, Nguyen N, Gupta S, McFaul C, Yang V. Augmented reality in neurosurgery: a review of current concepts and emerging applications. Can J Neurol Sci. 2017;44:235–45.
50. Zhou Z, Yang Z, Jiang S, Zhuo J, Zhu T, Ma S. Augmented reality surgical navigation system based on the spatial drift compensation method for glioma resection surgery. Med Phys. 2022; https://doi.org/10.1002/mp.15650.
51. Higginbotham G. Virtual connections: improving global neurosurgery through immersive technologies. Front Surg. 2021;8:629963.
52. Majmundar N, Ducruet A, Wilkinson DA, Catapano J, Patel J, Baranoski J, et al. Telemedicine for endovascular neurosurgery consultation during the COVID-19 Era: patient satisfaction survey. World Neurosurg. 2021;158:e577–82.
53. McCullough M, Kulber L, Sammons P, Santos P, Kulber D. Google glass for remote surgical tele-proctoring in low- and middle-income countries: a feasibility study from Mozambique. Plast Reconstr Surg Glob Open. 2018;6(12):e1999.
54. Hassan A, Desai S, Georgiadis A, Tekle W. Augmented reality enhanced tele-proctoring platform to intraoperatively support a neuro-endovascular surgery fellow. Interv Neuroradiol. 2022;28(3):277–82. https://doi.org/10.1177/15910199211035304.
55. Rai AT, Deib G, Smith D, Boo S. Teleproctoring for neurovascular procedures: demonstration of concept using optical see-through head-mounted display, interactive mixed reality, and virtual space sharing – a critical need highlighted by the COVID-19 pandemic. AJNR AM J Neuroradiol. 2021;42(6):1109–15.
56. Greenfield M, Luck J, Billingsley M, Heyes R, Smith O, Mosahebi A, et al. Demonstration of the effectiveness of augmented reality telesurgery in complex hand reconstruction in Gaza. Plast Reconstr Surg Glob Open. 2018;6(3):e1708.
57. Davis M, Can D, Pindrik J, Rocque B, Johnston J. Virtual interactive presence in global surgical education: international collaboration through augmented reality. World Neurosurg. 2016;86:103–11.
58. Duffau H. Resecting diffuse low-grade gliomas to the boundaries of brain functions: a new concept in surgical neuro-oncology. J Neurosurg Sci. 2015;59(4):361–71. Epub 2015 Apr 24
59. Delion M, Terminassian A, Lehousse T, Aubin G, Malka J, Guyen S, et al. Specificities of awake craniotomy and brain mapping in children for resection of supratentorial tumors in the language area. World Neurosurg. 2015;84(6):1645–52. https://doi.org/10.1016/j.wneu.2015.06.073.
60. Gras-Combe G, Moritz-Gasser S, Herbet G, Duffau H. Intraoperative subcortical electrical mapping of optic radiations in awake surgery for glioma involving visual pathways. J Neurosurg. 2012;117(3):466–73. https://doi.org/10.3171/2012.6.JNS111981.
61. Wolfson R, Soni N, Shah A, Hosein K, Sastry A, Bregy A, Komotar R. The role of awake craniotomy in reducing intraoperative visual field deficits during tumor surgery. Asian J Neurosurg. 2015;10(3):139–44. https://doi.org/10.4103/1793-5482.161189.
62. Mazerand E, Le Renard M, Hue S, Lemee JM, Klinger E, Menei P. Intraoperative subcortical electrical mapping of the optic tract in awake surgery using a virtual reality headset. World Neurosurg. 2017;97:424–30.
63. Herbet G, Lafargue G, Moritz-Gasser S, Menjot DCN, Costi E, Bonnetblanc F, Duffau H. A disconnection account of subjective empathy impairments in diffuse low-grade glioma patients. Neuropsychologia. 2015;70:165–76. https://doi.org/10.1016/j.neuropsychologia.2015.02.015.
64. Milesi V, Cekic S, Peron J, Fruhholz S, Cristinzio C, Seeck M, Grandjean D. Multimodal emotion perception after anterior temporal lobectomy (ATL). Front Hum Neurosci. 2014;8:275. https://doi.org/10.3389/fnhum.2014.00275.

65. Bernard F, Lemee J, Ter MA, Menei P. Right hemisphere cognitive functions: from clinical and anatomical bases to brain mapping during awake craniotomy Part I: clinical and functional anatomy. World Neuosurg. 2018;118:360–7. https://doi.org/10.1016/j.wneu.2018.07.099.

66. Bernard F, Lemee JM, Aubin G, Ter Minassian A, Menei P. Using a virtual reality social network during awake craniotomy to map social cognition: prospective trial. J Med Internet Res. 2018;20(6):e10332.

67. Delion M, Klinger E, Bernard F, Aubin G, Ter AM, Menei P. Immersing patients in a virtual reality environment for brain mapping during awake surgery: safety study. World Neuosurg. 2020;134:e937–43. https://doi.org/10.1016/j.wneu.2019.11.047.

68. Katsevman G, Greenleaf W, Garcia-Garcia R, Perea M, Ladera V, Sherman J, Rodriguez G. Virtual reality during brain mapping for awake patient brain tumor surgery: proposed tasks and domains to test. World Neurosurg. 2021;152:e462–6. https://doi.org/10.1016/j.wneu.2021.005.118.

69. Bernat JL, Peterson LM. Patient-centered informed consent in surgical practice. Arch Surg. 2006;141(1):86–92.

70. Shlobin NA, Sheldon M, Lam S. Informed consent in neurosurgery: a systematic review. Neurosurg Focus. 2020;49(5):E6.

71. Krupp W, Spanehl O, Laubach W, Siefert V. Informed consent in neurosurgery: patients' recall of preoperative discussion. Acta Neurochir. 2000;142(3):233–8.; discussion 283-9. https://doi.org/10.1007/s007010050030.

72. Knifed E, Lipsman N, Mason W, Bernstein M. Patients' perception of the informed consent process for neurooncology clinical trials. Neuro Oncol. 2008;10(3):348–54. https://doi.org/10.1215/15228517-2008-007.

73. Herz DA, Looman JE, Lewis SK. Informed consent: is it a myth? Neurosurgery. 1992;30(3):453–8.

74. Epstein NE. A review of medicolegal malpractice suits involving cervical spine: what can we learn or change? J Spinal Disord Tech. 2011;24(1):15–9.

75. Jena A, Seabury S, Lakdawalla D, Chandra A. Malpractice risk according to physician specialty. N Engl J Med. 2011;365(7):629–36.

76. Perin A, Galbiati T, Ayadi R, Gambatesa E, Orena EF, Riker N, et al. Informed consent through 3D virtual reality: a randomized clinical trial. Acta Neurochir. 2021;163(2):301–8. https://doi.org/10.1007/s00701-020-04303-y.

77. House P, Pelzi S, Furrer S, Lanz M, Simova O, Voges B, et al. Use of the mixed reality tool "VSI Patient Education" for more comprehensible and imaginable patient educations before epilepsy surgery and stereotactic implantation of DBS or stereo-EEG electrodes. Epilepsy Res. 2020;159:106247. https://doi.org/10.1016/j.eplepsyres.2019.106247.

78. Wright J, Raghavan A, Wright C, Shammassian B, Duan Y, Sajatovic M, Selman W. Back to the future: surgical rehearsal platform technology as a means to improve surgeon-patient alliance, patient satisfaction, and resident experience. J Neurosurg. 2020:1–8. https://doi.org/10.3171/2020.6.JNS201865.

79. Shlobin N, Clark J, Hoffman S, Hopkins B, Kesavabhotla K, Dahdaleh N. Patient education in neurosurgery: part 2 of a systematic review. World Neurosurg. 2021;147:190–201 .e1. https://doi.org/10.1016/j.wneu.2020.11.169.

80. Coelho G, Trigo L, Faig F, Vieira E, Gomes da Silva H, Acacio G, et al. The potential applications of augmented reality in fetoscopic surgery for antenatal treatment of myelomeningocele. World Neurosurg. 2022;159:27–32. https://doi.org/10.1016/j.wneu.2021.11.133.

# Chapter 3
# Diagnosis and Management of Tethered Cord Syndrome

**Takeshi Hara, Yukoh Ohara, and Akihide Kondo**

## Contents



## 3.1  Introduction

Tethered cord syndrome is a condition in which the spinal cord is tethered by pathological structures such as a tight filum terminale, intradural lipomas with or without a connecting extradural component, intradural fibrous adhesions, diastematomyelia, and adherence of the neural placode following the closure of a myelomeningocele [1]. Since the spinal cord is not buffered by the filum terminale when it is tethered, body movement exerts traction on the spinal cord. The spinal cord blood flow is impaired, resulting in various disabling changes and neurological symptoms. The most widely recognized causes of tethered cord syndrome include neoplastic lesions and elongation of the spine during development. Tethered cord syndrome also occurs in spinal cord injury [2]. Cases of adult-onset tethered cord syndrome also exist; however, several patients have yet to receive accurate diagnoses, as it is not


T. Hara (✉) · Y. Ohara · A. Kondo
Department of Neurosurgery, Spine and Spinal Cord Center, Juntendo University School of Medicine, Tokyo, Japan
e-mail: tkhara@juntendo.ac.jp





C. Di Rocco (ed.), *Advances and Technical Standards in Neurosurgery*,
Advances and Technical Standards in Neurosurgery 49,
https://doi.org/10.1007/978-3-031-42398-7_3

well understood. Although tethered cord syndrome usually progresses slowly, its symptoms may be unnoticed and become irreversible over time. It is, therefore, important to take note of the time symptoms appear and their progression. It is also crucial to understand that the symptoms of patients with childhood-onset cases are different from those of cases that predominantly occur during adulthood. Early diagnosis and treatment of tethered cord syndrome require that health care providers know its symptoms and pathophysiology. In both children and adults, the symptoms of tethered cord syndrome are often exacerbated by trauma [3]. Symptom onset and progression are also believed to be provoked by degenerative conditions, such as degenerative disc disease and lumbar spinal stenosis. Although untethering is performed to arrest the progression of the tethered cord syndrome, it has been pointed out that multiple surgeries can worsen postoperative outcomes [4–6]. In recent years, there have been several reports on treatment methods other than untethering for recurrent cases. In the following chapter, we will describe the conceptual and clinical aspects of tethered cord syndrome, adult-onset tethered cord syndrome, and the latest surgical outcomes.

## 3.2  Embryology and Anatomy

To understand the pathophysiology of tethered cord syndrome, it is necessary to understand the mechanisms of spinal cord development. The neural tube develops during days 13–28 of gestation when the ectoderm first envelops the spinal cord. The central part of the ectoderm thickens to form the neural plate, and the median section that is in contact with the notochord is suppressed to form the neural groove. The neural fold bends toward the median side and gradually approaches and fuses with the median side to form the neural tube. Once the neural tube is closed, the ectoderm separates into the cutaneous and neural ectoderms, which differentiate to form the primary neural tube [7, 8].

The caudal cell mass, a population of cells with various differentiation potentials, develops caudally from the second sacral medulla to form the secondary neural tube, which is the origin of the caudal spinal cord and the filum terminale. The secondary neural tube joins the caudal side of the primary neural tube to form the filum terminale from the sacral cord [9].

Because the spine grows faster than the spinal cord, the position of the inferior end of the conus medullaris rises with fetal age, and the conus medullaris reaches the L2/3 intervertebral level at birth. When a disorder occurs at the time of primary neural tube closure, it prevents the separation of the neuroectoderm from the cutaneous ectoderm. The formation of abnormal structures between the spinal cord and the skin prevents the physiological ascending of the spinal cord with growth, resulting in spinal cord tethering [9].

The filum terminale is an elastic structure that stabilizes the conus medullaris and prevents traction forces from being applied to the spinal cord by allowing the filum terminale to freely extend when the spine is flexed or extended [10]. In normal anatomy, the filum terminale is formed on the most caudal side of the conus medullaris and attaches to the caudal end of the dural sac. The filum terminale is composed of two segments that are intradural and extradural and extends from the conus medullaris to the periosteum of the coccyx [11]. As the body and spine move, the filum terminale elongates, preventing the spinal cord from stretching. However, in conditions where the buffering ability of the filum terminale is impaired, either because the filum terminale is not structurally formed or because it has turned into a lipoma, the spinal cord is subjected to stretching forces in daily life. In addition, as children grow taller, they are constantly being subjected to stretching forces in daily life. This leads to a gradual impairment of spinal cord blood flows and damage to spinal cord neurons, resulting in symptoms.

## 3.3  Pathophysiology

There have been previous experimental studies on how tethering affects the spinal cord. When the spinal cord is subjected to a tractional force in the cephalocaudal direction, the conus medullaris is affected the most. In an experimental study, the conus medullaris was found to be the most vulnerable region of the spinal cord to traction [12].

In a study by Selçuki et al., histological examination of the filum terminale obtained from patients with dysuria showed that the abnormal filum was characterized by dense collagen fibers, dilated and increased capillaries, and hyaline formation [13]. Other studies have histologically searched for the filum terminale, as tethered cord syndrome may be caused by a lack of buffering of the filum terminale [14–17].

Although histological evidence has demonstrated changes in the filum terminale, the mechanism of these changes is not yet known and awaits further study.

Another study that used lateral radiography on the lumbar spine of adults found that the length of the spinal canal was extended by 7.4% in hyperflexion and shortened by 3.1% in hyperextension [18]. In addition, Tani et al. found that when the spinal cord and filum terminale of cats were loaded and traction was applied, the filum terminale of the spinal cord was significantly stretched while the caudal spinal cord was not. Another imaging study using cats demonstrated that the increased elasticity of the filum terminale can impair the buffering effect of the spinal cord, resulting in tethered cord syndrome independent of the position of the conus [19].

Yamada et al. used a dual-wavelength reflection spectrophotometer to measure the redox ratio of cytochrome aa3, which is an indicator of the metabolic state and overall activity level of cells in the central nervous system. They reported that a stronger traction force was associated with a greater reduction of cytochrome aa3. Conversely, a stronger traction was associated with lower recovery levels, even after release. In a clinical study, the redox ratio of cytochrome aa3 was measured intraoperatively using dual-wavelength reflection spectrophotometry. They found that changes in the redox ratio correlated with the severity of clinical symptoms before surgery, as well as the recovery of symptoms after surgery [20–22].

Regarding the relationship between spinal cord tethering and spinal cord blood flow, Kang et al. evaluated blood flow in the tethered spinal cord using somatosensory evoked potentials (SEP) in an experiment on cats. They found that 2 weeks of spinal cord traction resulted in a 32% decrease in spinal cord blood flow, and 10 weeks of traction resulted in a 67% decrease in blood flow [23]. These results suggest that spinal cord traction causes spinal cord blood flow disturbance, which in turn causes various pathological changes around the spinal cord cone, resulting in the development of symptoms. Surgical release of the tethering may free the patient from this pathological state, thereby improving blood flow disturbance and arresting the progression of symptoms [24, 25].

## 3.4  Symptoms

The clinical manifestations in patients with tethered cord syndrome reflect neurological deficits in the lumbosacral spinal cord and include motor deficits, lower-extremity deformities such as in the perianal and buttock region, lower-leg sensory deficits, pain in the lower extremities, back pain, and dysuria. These symptoms tend to progressively worsen after onset. A rare symptom is fecal incontinence [26]. In addition to neurological symptoms originating from the conus medullaris and the surrounding lumbosacral spinal cord, the following symptoms of tethered cord syndrome occur: (1) the extent of the associated sensory disturbances does not follow the dermatome and is often discontinuous (i.e., is a patchy pattern); (2) dysuria becomes irreversible before motor and sensory dysfunction become irreversible; (3) scoliosis and lumbar hypokyphosis occur [21, 27].

Of the above characteristics, sensory disturbances are similar to lumbar back pain and lower extremity pain. This can facilitate a proper diagnosis [28].

Lumbosacral cutaneous signs are essential findings to aid in the diagnosis of tethered cord syndrome (Fig. 3.1).

Typical cutaneous signs in the lumbosacral region include a duplicated or bifurcated gluteal fold, gluteal asymmetry, coccygeal pit, lumbar hair, Mongolian spot on the back, sacral dimple, and hemangioma, among others. In the presence of these findings, we should proceed with a close examination of tethered cord syndrome by spinal ultrasound, MRI, or urodynamic study [29, 30].

The tight filum terminale test (TFT) assesses pain provocation from tethered cord syndrome. In 2004, Komagata et al. proposed the TFT as a diagnostic technique for a tight filum terminale, which is difficult to diagnose using imaging alone. The test is positive when forward bending of the trunk and neck induces pain, such as back and lower extremity pain, and when the pain is relieved by forward bending of the neck [31] (Fig. 3.2). It is important to evaluate the distribution of sensory deficits because they often have a skip lesion appearance that does not follow the dermatome or is discontinuous [30].

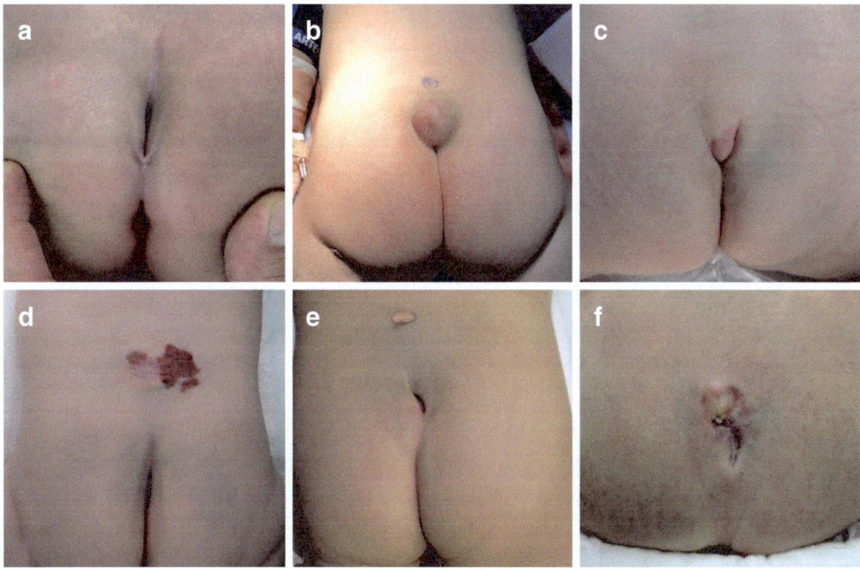

**Fig. 3.1** Cutaneous stigmata of occult spina bifida. (**a**) Dimple. (**b**) Subcutaneous mass. (**c**) Deviated gluteal cleft. (**d**) Hemangioma. (**e**) Skin tag and dimple. (**f**) Scar

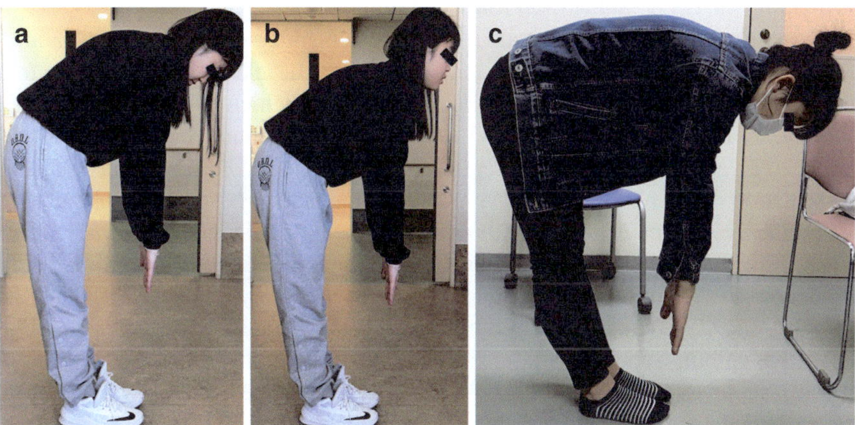

**Fig. 3.2** Tight filum terminale(TFT) test. The test is positive when forward bending of the trunk and neck induces pain (**a**), such as back and lower extremity pain, and when the pain is relieved by forward bending of the neck (**b**). Postoperatively, the patient was able to perform lumbar forward bending without back pain (**c**)

The clinical manifestations tof tethered cord syndrome differ between pediatric and adult cases [9, 22, 32, 33]. In adult cases, symptoms frequently include lower back and leg pain, which is treated relatively effectively with untethering surgery [33–35]. Low back and leg pain are characterized by tingling or aching pain that appears to radiate from the deep muscles of the back, lower legs, and unilateral lower extremities. According to Yamada et al., certain movements cause the lumbar alignment to shift from lordosis to straight. When there is a loss of filum terminale elasticity due to pathological factors, spinal canal lengthening causes the spinal cord to stretch, resulting in pain. Examples of such movements include sitting with legs crossed, bending over the sink to wash dishes or brush teeth, carrying a heavy object, lying on the back, and bending over to sit in a chair [22]. Pain may also occur in the feet and heels; however, these symptoms are thought to occur in areas consistent with the sclerotomes. We reviewed the symptoms of 30 adult-onset tethered cord syndrome cases that were operated on at Juntendo University hospital between 1994 and 2018. Our results showed that pain was the most frequent symptom (reported by 56.6% of the patients;17/30), followed by motor weakness (53.3%; 16/30), dysuria (46.6%; 14/30), and sensory disturbances (40%; 12/40).

The mechanisms underlying later development during adulthood are thought to be as follows: increased activity during adulthood leads to increased spinal mobility and stretching of the spinal cord; the formation of osteophytes and thickening in the flavum prevents the spinal cord from moving toward the head [36]; and sudden stretching of the spinal cord, such as from a direct blow to the back or trauma from an automobile accident, can result in the resolution of symptoms [3, 33].

Patients with asymptomatic tethered cords should be educated to recognize that symptoms can occur and worsen following trauma [3].

Symptoms in childhood include a neurogenic bladder, motor weakness, numbness, spasticity, differences in the length of the right and left lower limbs, foot deformity, and pain. In addition, painless ulceration, which is a useful diagnostic finding, is often observed in the foot [10]. Pain is less common, but may be mistakenly perceived as irritation due to reporting inaccuracies and difficulty in obtaining information from children [37]. A neurogenic bladder has symptoms such as incontinence, urgency, increased/abnormal frequency, and recurrent urinary infections. In addition to those with obvious symptoms, there are also mild and subclinical cases. Therefore, urodynamic studies are necessary for accurate evaluation [38, 39]. In pediatric patients, urodynamic studies have been used to evaluate preoperative voiding function, and the sensitivity of the urodynamic study for diagnosing sphincter dyssynergia has been reported to be 100% [40]. Even in asymptomatic patients, urodynamic studies sometimes show decreased voiding function [41].

Foot deformity, leg length difference, gluteal asymmetry, vertebral abnormalities, lamina defects, bifid vertebra, hemivertebra, split cord malformation, sacral malformation, sacral agenesis, segmentation errors, and scoliosis were present in 90% of the cases, while scoliosis alone was present in 25% [37].

In pediatric cases, symptoms are easily recognized, as they often consist of worsening neurological conditions. In adults, however, pain is a subjective symptom, and treatment may be continued without an appropriate diagnosis. Therefore, it is necessary to be aware of the characteristic symptoms of tethered cord syndrome.

## 3.5 Imaging

Magnetic resonance imaging (MRI) is useful for identifying tethering lesions that lead to tethered cord syndrome such as spina bifida occulta, thickened filum terminale, and other pathological conditions. In addition, understanding the location of the conus medullaris is important during MRI evaluation [42].

Tethered cord syndrome may be associated with minimal changes in imaging despite symptom progression [43]. Therefore, it is often difficult to determine whether symptoms are caused by the tethered cord, even if they appear. More recently developed imaging methods have been used to solve this problem.

For example, Sankhe et al. reported the usefulness of constructive interference in steady-state (CISS) sequences as a screening test for tethered cord syndrome. In their study, the sensitivity was 99.17%, which is higher than those of T2-weighted images (WI) (71.48%) and the assessment of tight filum terminale. It is also useful for the detection of a fibrous spur in cases of split cord malformation, and detection of the dorsal dermal sinus [44].

If there is no ventral conus motion on prone position MRI, a tethered cord is considered to be present [45, 46]. Stamates et al. reported the usefulness of prone position MRI as a method for assessing the presence or absence of a tethered cord, determined by a lack of ventral conus motion. They suggested a canal width motion of 10% as a threshold to separate the tethered and non-tethered groups [45].

Several cases of syringomyelia are associated with tethering [47–49]. The mechanism of cavity formation has been theorized; however, the relationship between tethered cord syndrome and syringomyelia remains unclear. Syringomyelia is a destructive lesion, and once it causes symptoms, it is intractable, and surgical interventions will not be effective. Since untethering can cause nerve damage, one method to consider is to not forcibly untether the spinal cord but to shunt the cavity. However, there is no relationship between the disappearance or improvement of the cavity and the improvement of symptoms. Moreover, there are reports that the cavity does not shrink when the tethered spinal cord is released. The presence or absence of a cavity should not determine the indication for surgery. Instead, clinicians should focus on the presence or absence of symptoms due to tethering [43, 48]. Symptoms suggestive of re-tethering include lower extremity muscle weakness, lower extremity spasticity, gait disturbance, progression of scoliosis, other orthopedic deformities, back pain, and worsening of or changes in urological function [5].

Over the years, spinal deformities often occur in patients with tethered cord syndrome, including kyphotic change, scoliosis, increased sacral angle, and changes in spinopelvic alignment, which can be evaluated using plain X-ray [27, 50, 51]. According to a report investigating sagittal spinopelvic alignment in patients with tethered cord syndrome due to fatty filum and split cord malformation, lumbar lordosis was statistically significantly increased, compared with normal values [27]. This is thought to be due to increased lumbar lordosis aimed at relieving spinal cord stretching.

There are cases of tethered cord syndrome in which the presence of a tethered cord is suggested, but no abnormalities such as a low-lying conus or spina bifida can be detected on imaging. This has been proposed as "Occult" tethered cord syndrome (OTCS) [52–57]. Although no abnormalities can be detected on imaging, histopathological studies have shown adipocyte invasion, fibrosis, and loss of meningothelial cell architecture in the filum terminale [52, 58]. Thus, as in a typical case of tethered cord syndrome, the pathogenesis may be associated with a decrease or loss of the buffering effect of the filum terminale.

As no abnormality can be detected by normal imaging, evaluation of the medical history and physical examination are necessary for diagnosis. The TFT test reported by Komagata et al. is also useful for the diagnosis of occult tethered cord syndrome [31, 59]. It is also useful for detecting bladder dysfunction with urodynamic testing [54, 60].

For cases of suspected occult tethered cord syndrome, prone position MRI revealed an anterior shift of the caudal nerve and posterior displacement of the filum terminale, and supine MRI revealed anteriorly shifted caudal nerves and posteriorly displaced endings, termed the "sunrise appearance" [45, 56, 61, 62] (Fig. 3.3).

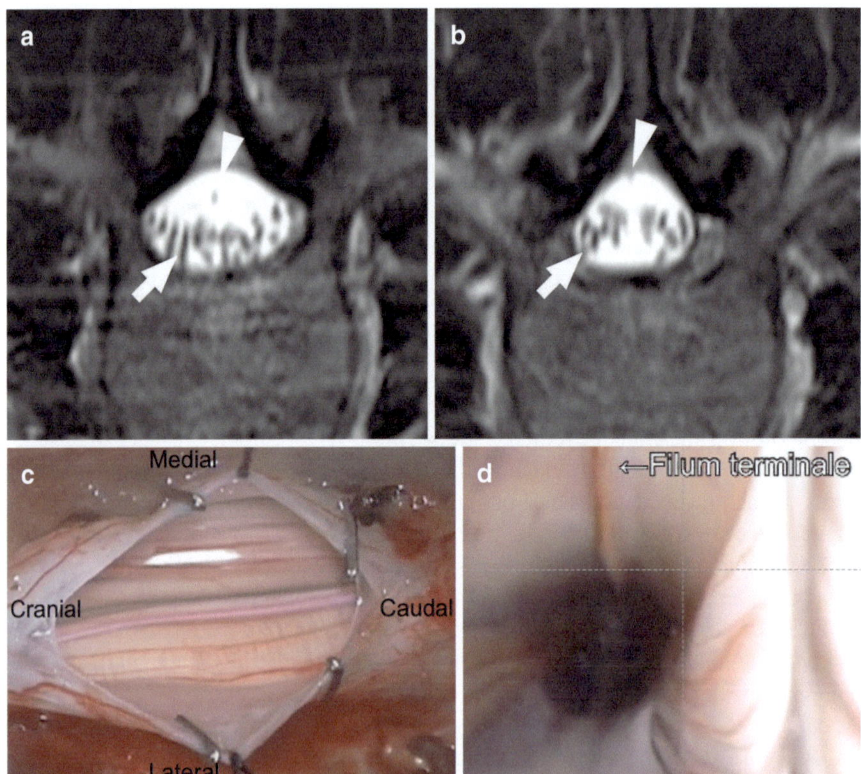


**Fig. 3.3** Axial T2-weighted MR images of L4/5 (**a**) and L5/S (**b**) of a patient with occult tethered cord syndrome. The cauda equina (arrow) is shifted anteriorly, whereas the filum terminale (arrowhead) is shifted dorsally. (**c**) Intraoperative images of the patients. The filum terminale had a macroscopically normal appearance. (**d**) Intraoperative endoscopic images of the same patient. The filum terminale ran along the dorsal aspect of the dural sac

## 3.6 Surgery

### 3.6.1 Untethering Surgery

#### 3.6.1.1 Neuromonitoring

Prepare BCR (bulbo-cavernous reflex) and nerve stimulator.

BCR is a method that enables simultaneous stimulation of input from the pubic nerve and monitoring of the output state and is useful for manipulating the nerves around the spinal cord during untethering [63].

#### 3.6.1.2 Details of surgery

Spinal Lipoma

To prevent the occurrence of CSF leak after surgery as much as possible, dissection is performed to prevent creating a dead space under the skin [64]. The lamina is exposed at a level where the normal structure is maintained without bifurcation. Laminectomy of this lamina is performed, and the dura mater is incised to expose the spinal cord with a normal structure. The spinal cord and lipoma are subsequently dissected from the surrounding tissue in a cephalocaudal direction. The lipoma is dissected at the border of the spinal cord, the so-called white line, and is, as much as possible, removed to reduce the lipoma volume [65].

To prevent postoperative CSF leak, dissection is performed without exposing the dural defect as much as possible. To prevent the severing of functioning nerves during dissection, nerve stimulation is performed as necessary, and dissection is performed after confirmation. In addition, dissection is performed while continuing to monitor the BCR because of the strain on the spinal cord during the surgical procedure (at intervals of 30 s to 1 min).

The dura mater is closed if primary closure is possible. If dural plasty is necessary, we use the autologous fascia. In this case, we also try to avoid creating a dead space under the skin as much as possible.

Filar Type Lipoma or Occult Tethered Cord Syndrome

The filum is dissected where it runs dorsal to the dural sac most on MRI, and it is exposed through a laminectomy and dural incision. The filum is cut after confirming that there is no response to nerve stimulation. When the filum is dissected, it is retracted cephalad or caudally. This means that the spinal cord is engaged and tension is applied.

### 3.6.1.3 Surgical Outcome

According to a recent meta-analysis of adult-onset tethered cord syndrome patients, postoperative pain improved in 81%, motor deficits in 61%, sensory deficits in 45%, bladder dysfunction in 45%, and bowel dysfunction in 32%; pain was the most likely symptom to improve in adult-onset cases. On the other hand, bladder function did not change in 41% but worsened in 2% of the patients. Additionally, bowel symptoms were unchanged in 36% and worsened in 3%. As such, bladder function and bowel dysfunction are deemed difficult to improve [66].

Of the 30 adult patients who underwent untethering surgery at our institute, 23 (76%) showed improvement in symptoms. Pain improved in 13 cases (76%), dysuria improved in five of 14 cases (35.7%), sensory disturbance improved in three of 12 cases (25.0%), and muscle weakness improved in 1 of 16 cases (6.2%). Our surgical results also showed a high rate of pain improvement.

Kang et al. reported on the surgical outcome of untethering surgery for tethered cord syndrome, with a 58.3% improvement in school-aged children, adolescents, and young adults. They also reported that the surgical outcomes for pain and motor weakness were satisfactory, but those for bowel and bladder dysfunction were not [1]. Surgery for tethered cord syndrome is beneficial for children and adults. The key to good outcomes is early diagnosis and complete spinal cord untethering [67].

After the onset of the disease, some symptoms can be expected to improve with untethering, while others cannot. Therefore, the option of prophylactic untethering before symptoms appear can be considered, but it should be kept in mind that the results of untethering may vary depending on the characteristics of the disease, as various conditions present with tethered cord syndrome.

Currently, it is unclear whether prophylactic surgery for asymptomatic patients can prevent future worsening of neurological symptoms. Recent studies have shown that asymptomatic patients become symptomatic in 3–4% per year [68, 69].

On the other hand, some reports have shown the efficacy of prophylactic surgery in pediatric cases. Seki et al. performed prophylactic surgery in asymptomatic children with spinal lipomas and myelomeningoceles. After a mean observation duration of 94 months, delayed neurological deficits occurred in two patients. They concluded that there is a preventive effect for a certain period, but strict follow-up is necessary because the natural course is still unknown [70]. For spinal cord lipoma, a study evaluating the urological outcome of prophylactic untethering in asymptomatic patients reported a mean of 14.2 years. The results showed that even with prophylactic surgery, 19% required CIC and 11% had urinary incontinence. In addition, the outcome differed with the type of lipoma, with the transitional type tending to have a worse prognosis [71].

The surgery performed for OTCS is filum sectioning, and the total improvement rate of clinical symptoms is 70–100% [72]. While there have been several reports of the benefits of surgery, there is also a randomized control study that shows no difference in urological outcomes between the medication and control groups [57]. The indications for surgical treatment of OTCS are still controversial.

There have been scattered reports of pain control with spinal cord stimulation therapy, which is expected to be a treatment for patients who have difficulty with untethering [73, 74].

Assessing the effectiveness of untethering surgery is challenging due to the various pathological conditions that can coexist with tethered cord syndrome. More complex diseases coexisting with a tethered cord are associated with more difficult untethering. This is especially true for spina bifida occulta, which is the most common form of tethered cords. Based on the results of these reports, it is important to inform patients of the symptoms expected to improve after untethering and those that are not.

### 3.6.2  Spine Shortening Osteotomy

In recent years, there have been several reports that vertebral column subtraction osteotomy (VCSO) can shorten the length of the spinal canal in patients with tethered cord syndrome, reducing traction on the spinal cord and improving symptoms [75, 76]. It may be an effective treatment for cases in which untether cannot be completed due to morphological or technical reasons, or when untethering is expected to be difficult. Usually, an osteotomy is performed at the lower thoracic or upper lumbar level. This is because the curve of the thoracolumbar transition is often straight, making shortening easier, preserving the range of motion compared to lower lumbar fusion, and reducing mechanical stress, compared with lower lumbar fusion [75, 77].

According to a recent meta-analysis, the postoperative improvement rates were 61–94% for motor function, 60–96% for pain and numbness, 27–75% for sensory function, and 18–100% for urinary and defecatory function. In addition, the complication rate was 0–7%, which was comparable to that for untethering [75].

According to a report that measured the tension on the neural elements of VCSO using a human cadaver, a 20–25-mm shortening was able to reduce the tension on the spinal cord, root, and filum terminale [78]. If blood flow is impaired, causing adhesions or scarring, shortening is unlikely to show improvement.

The advantage of VCSO is that it does not directly manipulate the nerve tissue, and there is a lower risk of cerebrospinal fluid leakage. This method indirectly reduces tension on the nerve tissue, and the effect is permanent once bone fusion is achieved. However, it is a highly invasive procedure with the possibility of excessive root traction, dural injury, and postoperative spinal deformity.

With the recent development of the minimally invasive surgical technique, surgery using the lateral retropleural approach for spinal shortening has also been performed. This approach allows direct entry into the vertebrae to be removed. This is thought to effectively reduce blood loss, shorten hospital stay, soft tissue damage, and postoperative pain [79].

## 3.7 Conclusion

Tethered cord syndrome has been recognized as a major cause of spina bifida, usually due to retethering after surgery for subclinical or manifested cases. If this is not acknowledged in daily practice, the diagnosis may be missed, and inappropriate treatment may be continued for chronic low back pain or sciatica. Because the diagnosis of tethered cord syndrome is difficult based on imaging alone, it is essential to evaluate changes in clinical symptoms. Such changes are often minor and progress slowly, requiring a long-term evaluation to achieve an accurate diagnosis. Defining a standardized approach to diagnosing and managing tethered cord syndrome would lead to early diagnosis and appropriately timed therapeutic interventions [80].

**Acknowledgments** We would like to thank Editage (www.editage.com) for English language editing.

## References


1. Kang J-K, Yoon K-J, Ha S-S, Lee I-W, Jeun S-S, Kang S-G. Surgical management and outcome of tethered cord syndrome in school-aged children, adolescents, and young adults. J Korean Neurosurg Soc. 2009;46:468–71.
2. Stenimahitis V, Fletcher-Sandersjöö A, Tatter C, Elmi-Terander A, Edström E. Long-term outcome following surgical treatment of posttraumatic tethered cord syndrome: a retrospective population-based cohort study. Spinal Cord. 2022;60:516–21.
3. Liang QC, Yang B, Song YH, Gao PP, Xia ZY, Bao N. Real spinal cord injury without radiologic abnormality in pediatric patient with tight filum terminale following minor trauma: a case report. BMC Pediatr. 2019;19:513.
4. Maher CO, Goumnerova L, Madsen JR, Proctor M, Scott RM. Outcome following multiple repeated spinal cord untethering operations. J Neurosurg. 2007;106:434–8.
5. Caldarelli M, Boscarelli A, Massimi L. Recurrent tethered cord: radiological investigation and management. Childs Nerv Syst. 2013;29:1601–9.
6. Sun J, Zhang Y, Wang H, Wang Y, Yang Y, Kong Q, Xu X, Shi J. Clinical outcomes of primary and revision untethering surgery in patients with tethered cord syndrome and spinal bifida. World Neurosurg. 2018;116:e66–70.
7. Eagles ME, Gupta N. Embryology of spinal dysraphism and its relationship to surgical treatment. Can J Neurol Sci. 2020;47:736–46.
8. American J of Med Genetics Pt C—2005—Sadler—Embryology of neural tube development.pdf.
9. Hertzler DA 2nd, DePowell JJ, Stevenson CB, Mangano FT. Tethered cord syndrome: a review of the literature from embryology to adult presentation. Neurosurg Focus. 2010;29:E1.
10. Sanchez T, John RM. Early identification of tethered cord syndrome: a clinical challenge. J Pediatr Health Care. 2014;28:e23–33.
11. Pinto FCG, Fontes RBDV, Leonhardt MDC, Amodio DT, Porro FF, Machado J. Anatomic study of the filum terminale and its correlations with the tethered cord syndrome. Neurosurgery. 2002;51:725–9. discussion 729–30
12. Fujita Y, Yamamoto H. An experimental study on spinal cord traction effect. Spine (Phila Pa 1976). 1989;14:698–705.

13. Selçuki M, Vatansever S, Inan S, Erdemli E, Bağdatoğlu C, Polat A. Is a filum terminale with a normal appearance really normal? Childs Nerv Syst. 2003;19:3–10.
14. Hendson G, Dunham C, Steinbok P. Histopathology of the filum terminale in children with and without tethered cord syndrome with attention to the elastic tissue within the filum. Childs Nerv Syst. 2016;32:1683–92.
15. Morioka T, Murakami N, Suzuki SO, Mukae N, Shimogawa T, Kurogi A, Shono T, Mizoguchi M. Surgical histopathology of a filar anomaly as an additional tethering element associated with closed spinal dysraphism of primary neurulation failure. Surg Neurol Int. 2021;12:373.
16. Liu F-Y, Li J-F, Guan X, Luo X-F, Wang Z-L, Dang Q-H. SEM study on filum terminale with tethered cord syndrome. Childs Nerv Syst. 2011;27:2141–4.
17. Thompson EM, Strong MJ, Warren G, Woltjer RL, Selden NR. Clinical significance of imaging and histological characteristics of filum terminale in tethered cord syndrome: clinical article. J Neurosurg Pediatr. 2014;13:255–9.
18. Tani S, Yamada S, Fuse T, Nakamura N. Changes in lumbosacral canal length during flexion and extension—dynamic effect on the elongated spinal cord in the tethered spinal cord. No To Shinkei. 1991;43:1121–5.
19. Tani S, Yamada S, Knighton RS. Extensibility of the lumbar and sacral cord. Pathophysiology of the tethered spinal cord in cats. J Neurosurg. 1987;66:116–23.
20. Yamada S (ed) 3 pathophysiology of tethered cord syndrome. Tethered Cord Syndrome in Children and Adults 2010.
21. Yamada S, Won DJ, Yamada SM. Pathophysiology of tethered cord syndrome: correlation with symptomatology. Neurosurg Focus. 2004;16:E6.
22. Yamada S, Lonser RR. Adult tethered cord syndrome. J Spinal Disord. 2000;13:319–23.
23. Kang JK, Kim MC, Kim DS, Song JU. Effects of tethering on regional spinal cord blood flow and sensory-evoked potentials in growing cats. Childs Nerv Syst. 1987;3:35–9.
24. Filippidis AS, Kalani MY, Theodore N, Rekate HL. Spinal cord traction, vascular compromise, hypoxia, and metabolic derangements in the pathophysiology of tethered cord syndrome. Neurosurg Focus. 2010;29:E9.
25. Schneider SJ, Rosenthal AD, Greenberg BM, Danto J. A preliminary report on the use of laser-Doppler flowmetry during tethered spinal cord release. Neurosurgery. 1993;32:214–7. discussion 217–8
26. Behaine J, Abdel Latif AM, Greenfield JP. Fecal incontinence as a predominant symptom in a case of multiply recurrent tethered cord: diagnosis and operative strategies. J Neurosurg Pediatr. 2015;16:748–51.
27. Karaaslan B, Gulsuna B, Toktaş O, Borcek AO. Sagittal spinopelvic alignment in tethered cord syndrome and split cord malformation. Br J Neurosurg. 2022:1–6.
28. Robbins JW, Lundy PA, Gard AP, Puccioni MJ. Perineal pain secondary to tethered cord syndrome: retrospective review of single institution experience. Childs Nerv Syst. 2015;31:2141–4.
29. Shields LBE, Mutchnick IS, Peppas DS, Rosenberg E. Importance of physical examination and imaging in the detection of tethered cord syndrome. Glob Pediatr Health. 2019;6:2333794X19851419.
30. Lew SM, Kothbauer KF. Tethered cord syndrome: an updated review. Pediatr Neurosurg. 2007;43:236–48.
31. Komagata M, Endo K, Nishiyama M, Ikegami H, Imakiire A. Management of tight filum terminale. Minim Invasive Neurosurg. 2004;47:49–53.
32. Yamada S (2010) 4 neurological assessment of tethered spinal cord. Tethered cord syndrome in children and adults, 2nd. Thieme, New York.
33. Pang D, Wilberger JE Jr. Tethered cord syndrome in adults. J Neurosurg. 1982;57:32–47.
34. Klekamp J. Tethered cord syndrome in adults. J Neurosurg Spine. 2011;15:258–70.
35. Sofuoglu OE, Abdallah A, Emel E, Ofluoglu AE, Gunes M, Guler B. Management of tethered cord syndrome in adults: experience of 23 cases. Turk Neurosurg. 2017;27:226–36.
36. Yamada S (2010) 15 tethered cord syndrome in adult and late-teenage patients without neural spinal dysraphism. Tethered cord syndrome in children and adults, 2nd. Thieme, New York.

37. Bui CJ, Tubbs RS, Oakes WJ. Tethered cord syndrome in children: a review. Neurosurg Focus. 2007;23:1–9.
38. Morizawa Y, Satoh H, Arai M, Iwasa S, Sato A, Fujimoto K. Urodynamics findings pre- and post-untethering surgery in children with filum lipoma: a single-institution experience. Int J Urol. 2022; https://doi.org/10.1111/iju.14931.
39. Park K. Urological evaluation of tethered cord syndrome. J Korean Neurosurg Soc. 2020;63:358–65.
40. Hsieh MH, Perry V, Gupta N, Pearson C, Nguyen HT. The effects of detethering on the urodynamics profile in children with a tethered cord. J Neurosurg(5 Suppl). 2006;105:391–5.
41. Broderick KM, Munoz O, Herndon CDA, Joseph DB, Kitchens DM. Utility of urodynamics in the management of asymptomatic tethered cord in children. World J Urol. 2015;33:1139–42.
42. Raghavan N, Barkovich AJ, Edwards M, Norman D. MR imaging in the tethered spinal cord syndrome. AJR Am J Roentgenol. 1989;152:843–52.
43. Halevi PD, Udayakumaran S, Ben-Sira L, Constantini S. The value of postoperative MR in tethered cord: a review of 140 cases. Childs Nerv Syst. 2011;27:2159–62.
44. Sankhe S, Dang G, Mathur S, Muzumdar D. Utility of CISS imaging in the management of tethered cord syndrome. Childs Nerv Syst. 2021;37:217–23.
45. Stamates MM, Frim DM, Yang CW, Katzman GL, Ali S. Magnetic resonance imaging in the prone position and the diagnosis of tethered spinal cord. J Neurosurg Pediatr. 2018;21:4–10.
46. Singh S, Behari S, Singh V, Bhaisora KS, Haldar R, Krishna Kumar G, Mishra P, Phadke RV. Dynamic magnetic resonance imaging parameters for objective assessment of the magnitude of tethered cord syndrome in patients with spinal dysraphism. Acta Neurochir. 2019;161:147–59.
47. Hsu AR, Hou LC, Veeravagu A, Barnes PD, Huhn SL. Resolution of syringomyelia after release of tethered cord. Surg Neurol. 2009;72:657–61.
48. Bruzek AK, Starr J, Garton HJL, Muraszko KM, Maher CO, Strahle JM. Syringomyelia in children with closed spinal dysraphism: long-term outcomes after surgical intervention. J Neurosurg Pediatr. 2019;25:1–7.
49. Caird J, Flynn P, McConnell RS. Significant clinical and radiological resolution of a spinal cord syrinx following the release of a tethered cord in a patient with an anatomically normal conus medullaris. Case report. J Neurosurg Pediatr. 2008;1:396–8.
50. Oktay K, Ozsoy KM, Gezercan Y, Cetinalp NE, Erman T. Progressive kyphosis associated with tethered cord syndrome treated by posterior vertebral column resection in a pediatric patient. Pediatr Neurosurg. 2017;52:323–6.
51. Tubbs RS, Naftel RP, Rice WC, Liechty P, Conklin M, Oakes WJ(2006) The patient with symptoms following resection of a lipomyelomeningocele: do increases in the lumbosacral angle indicate a tethered spinal cord? J.Neurosurg.(1 Suppl Pediatrics) 105:62–64.
52. Tu A, Steinbok P. Occult tethered cord syndrome: a review. Childs Nerv Syst. 2013;29:1635–40.
53. Warder DE, Oakes WJ. Tethered cord syndrome and the conus in a normal position. Neurosurgery. 1993;33:374–8.
54. Tsiptsios D, Sysoev K, Anastasiadis A, Tsamakis K, Rizos E, Kandilakis E. Occult tethered cord syndrome: a reversible cause of paraparesis not to be missed. Childs Nerv Syst. 2020;36:2089–92.
55. Yang J, Won J-K, Kim KH, Lee JY, Kim S-K, Shin H-I, Park K, Wang K-C. Occult tethered cord syndrome: a rare, treatable condition. Childs Nerv Syst. 2021;38:387. https://doi.org/10.1007/s00381-021-05353-y.
56. Veronesi V, Calderone M, Sacco C, Donati R. Prone position magnetic resonance imaging and transhiatal approach to filum Terminale Externum sectioning in adolescents with occult tethered cord syndrome: report of four cases. Pediatr Neurosurg. 2020;55:432–8.
57. Steinbok P, MacNeily AE, Hengel AR, Afshar K, Landgraf JM, Hader W, Pugh J. Filum section for urinary incontinence in children with occult tethered cord syndrome: a randomized, controlled pilot study. J Urol. 2016;195:1183–8.

58. Tehli O, Hodaj I, Kural C, Solmaz I, Onguru O, Izci Y. A comparative study of histopathological analysis of filum terminale in patients with tethered cord syndrome and in normal human fetuses. Pediatr Neurosurg. 2011;47:412–6.
59. Sato T, Eguchi Y, Enomoto K, Murata Y. Treating difficult-to-diagnose tight filum terminale: our experience with four patients. BMJ Case Rep. 2021;14:e239184. https://doi.org/10.1136/bcr-2020-239184.
60. Kearns JT, Esposito D, Dooley B, Frim D, Gundeti MS. Urodynamic studies in spinal cord tethering. Childs Nerv Syst. 2013;29:1589–600.
61. Nakanishi K, Tanaka N, Kamei N, Nakamae T, Izumi B-I, Ohta R, Fujioka Y, Ochi M. Use of prone position magnetic resonance imaging for detecting the terminal filum in patients with occult tethered cord syndrome. J Neurosurg Spine. 2013;18:76–84.
62. Kamei N, Nakamae T, Nakanishi K, Morisako T, Harada T, Maruyama T, Adachi N. Comparison of the electrophysiological characteristics of tight filum terminale and tethered cord syndrome. Acta Neurochir. 2022;164:2235–42.
63. Morota N. Intraoperative neurophysiological monitoring of the bulbocavernosus reflex during surgery for conus spinal lipoma: what are the warning criteria? J Neurosurg Pediatr. 2019;23:1–9.
64. Lim JX, Low SY, Ng LP, Seow WT. Prevention and treatment of CSF leaks in congenital complex spinal lipomas. Acta Neurochir. 2022; https://doi.org/10.1007/s00701-021-05095-5.
65. Pang D, Zovickian J, Oviedo A. Long-term outcome of total and near-total resection of spinal cord lipomas and radical reconstruction of the neural placode, part II: outcome analysis and preoperative profiling. Neurosurgery. 2010;66:253–72. discussion 272–3
66. O'Connor KP, Smitherman AD, Milton CK, Palejwala AH, Lu VM, Johnston SE, Homburg H, Zhao D, Martin MD. Surgical treatment of tethered cord syndrome in adults: a systematic review and meta-analysis. World Neurosurg. 2020;137:e221–41.
67. Hüttmann S, Krauss J, Collmann H, Sörensen N, Roosen K. Surgical management of tethered spinal cord in adults: report of 54 cases. J Neurosurg. 2001;95:173–8.
68. Kulkarni AV, Pierre-Kahn A, Zerah M. Conservative management of asymptomatic spinal lipomas of the conus. Neurosurgery. 2004;54:868–73. discussion 873–5
69. Wykes V, Desai D, Thompson DNP. Asymptomatic lumbosacral lipomas—a natural history study. Childs Nerv Syst. 2012;28:1731–9.
70. Seki T, Hida K, Yano S, Houkin K. Surgical outcomes of pediatric patients with asymptomatic tethered cord syndrome. Asian Spine J. 2018;12:551–5.
71. Hayashi C, Kumano Y, Hirokawa D, Sato H, Yamazaki Y. Long-term urological outcomes of spinal lipoma after prophylactic untethering in infancy: real-world outcomes by lipoma anatomy. Spinal Cord. 2020;58:490–5.
72. Rezaee H, Keykhosravi E. Effect of untethering on occult tethered cord syndrome: a systematic review. Br J Neurosurg. 2021:1–9.
73. Musick S, Ferguson J, Muizelaar JP. Successful treatment of chronic back and leg pain with lower than usual placement of high-frequency spinal cord stimulation in a patient with uncorrected tethered cord: case report. Neurosurg Open. 2021; https://doi.org/10.1093/neuopn/okab012.
74. Novik Y, Vassiliev D, Tomycz ND. Spinal cord stimulation in adult tethered cord syndrome: case report and review of the literature. World Neurosurg. 2019;122:278–81.
75. Lin W, Xu H, Duan G, Xie J, Chen Y, Jiao B, Lan H. Spine-shortening osteotomy for patients with tethered cord syndrome: a systematic review and meta-analysis. Neurol Res. 2018;40:340–63.
76. Aldave G, Hansen D, Hwang SW, Moreno A, Briceño V, Jea A. Spinal column shortening for tethered cord syndrome associated with myelomeningocele, lumbosacral lipoma, and lipomyelomeningocele in children and young adults. J Neurosurg Pediatr. 2017;19:703.
77. Hsieh PC, Stapleton CJ, Moldavskiy P, Koski TR, Ondra SL, Gokaslan ZL, Kuntz C. Posterior vertebral column subtraction osteotomy for the treatment of tethered cord syndrome: review

of the literature and clinical outcomes of all cases reported to date. Neurosurg Focus. 2010;29:E6.

78. Grande AW, Maher PC, Morgan CJ, Choutka O, Ling BC, Raderstorf TC, Berger EJ, Kuntz C 4th. Vertebral column subtraction osteotomy for recurrent tethered cord syndrome in adults: a cadaveric study. J Neurosurg Spine. 2006;4:478–84.

79. Steinberg JA, Wali AR, Martin J, Santiago-Dieppa DR, Gonda D, Taylor W. Spinal shortening for recurrent tethered cord syndrome via a lateral retropleural approach: a novel operative technique. Cureus. 2017;9:e1632. https://doi.org/10.7759/cureus.1632.

80. Bradko V, Castillo H, Janardhan S, Dahl B, Gandy K, Castillo J. Towards guideline-based management of tethered cord syndrome in spina bifida: a Global Health paradigm shift in the era of prenatal surgery. Neurospine. 2019;16:715–27.

# Chapter 4
# Management of Low and High Grades Spondylolisthesis

Jesus Lafuente, Juan Diego Patino, and Lucas Capo

## Contents




J. Lafuente (✉)
Associate Profedsor Neurosurgery, Director Spine center Hospital del Mar, Barcelona, Spain

J. D. Patino
Consultant Neurosurgeon Hospital de Sant Pau, Barcelona, Spain

L. Capo
Fellow Neurosurgeon Hospital de Sant Pau, Barcelona, Spain



© The Author(s), under exclusive license to Springer Nature Switzerland AG 2024
C. Di Rocco (ed.), *Advances and Technical Standards in Neurosurgery*,
Advances and Technical Standards in Neurosurgery 49,
https://doi.org/10.1007/978-3-031-42398-7_4

## 4.1 Introduction

Spondylolisthesis is defined as the displacement or misalignment of the vertebral bodies one on top of the other. It comes from the Greek spondlylos, which means vertebra, and olisthesis, which means sliding on a slope. The nomenclature used to refer to spondylolisthesis consists of the following elements: vertebral segment (vertebrae involved), degree of sliding of one vertebral body over the other, the position of the upper vertebral body with respect to the lower one (anterolisthesis/retrolisthesis), and finally the etiology [1].

It has been shown that many spondylolistheses are precipitated by lysis of the pars articularis since it is usually the weakest portion of the posterior vertebral arch. Although there is a greater predominance of spondylolytic spondylolisthesis in men, it has been seen that there is a greater risk of progression in women, especially during growth and adolescence [2].

Most of the lytic spondylolisthesis that occur in the young population occur due to lysis in the pars interarticularis at the level of L5/S1 predominantly. In adulthood, the most frequent cause is degenerative spondylolisthesis, which is six times more common in women than in men [3, 4]. The most predominantly associated level is usually L4/L5 [5].

## 4.2 Classification

The first classification was made by Neugebauer in 1882, he described spondylolisthesis as congenital or acquired according to the presence or absence of L5-S1 facet dysplasia. The first comprehensive classification system was described by Newman and Stone [6] in 1963 and included five groups:

1. Congenital (type I).
2. Spondylolytic (type II).
3. Traumatic (type III).
4. Degenerative (type IV).
5. Pathological (type V).

Later it was expanded by Wiltse and Winter [7] in 1976, as shown in Table 4.1. The Wiltse-Newman classification, based on etiology and anatomy, continues to be the most accepted in clinical practice and research. In 1982, Marchetti and Bartolozzi [8] developed a new classification of spondylolisthesis, later modified in 1994, which is based on two fundamental groups: developmental and acquired spondylolisthesis. Developmental spondylolisthesis includes all dysplastic forms and is divided into high or low dysplastic types, with lysis or elongation subtypes.

**Table 4.1**  Callsification of spondylolisthesis

| Wiltse-Newman classification of spondylolisthesis | |
| --- | --- |
| Dysplastic/congenital (type 1) | Congenital abnormalities of the upper sacrum or the arch of L5 permit the olisthesis to occur |
| | Type IA: Dysplastic posterior elements and facets usually associated with spina bifida |
| | Type IB: Dysplastic articular process with sagittal-oriented facet joints |
| | Type IC: Other congenital abnormalities, such as failure of formation or segmentations producing spondylolisthesis |
| Isthmic (type II) | Lesion within the pars interarticularis |
| | Type MIA: Lytic fatigue fracture |
| | Type IIB: Elongation (microfracture healed with elongation) |
| | Type IIC: Acute fracture secondary to trauma |
| Degenerative (type III) | Long-standing intersegmental instability, such as within the apophyseal joints, permitting shippage |
| Traumatic (type IV) | Due to fractures in areas of the bony hook other than the pars |
| Pathologic (type V) | Results from generalized or localized bone disease (i.e., osteogenesis imperfecta, Paget's disease) |

The Wiltse-Newman and Marchetti-Bartolozzi classification systems have been shown to have high intra- and interobserver reliability [8–11]. However, neither the Wiltse-Newman nor the Marchetti-Bartolozzi system take into account sacropelvic balance, which has been shown to be an important predictor of progression [11–20]. Labelle et al. proposed a classification that takes into account the risk of progression and surgical management of spondylolisthesis, as shown in Table 4.2.

## 4.3  Biomechanics

Biomechanical studies have shown that, under normal conditions, the lumbar vertebral bodies and discs support 80–90% of the axial load, while the remaining 10–20% of the load is supported by the posterior elements. The anterior forces through the spine are the combined result of the action of gravity on a tilted sacrum and the contraction of the lumbar musculature. These forces are mainly counteracted by intact posterior elements via a tension band principle and by the ligamentous function of the annulus fibrosus [21]. When bilateral fractures have occurred at the level of the pars, the shearing forces cause a tendency toward anterior displacement of the vertebral body, as well as the anterior superior fragment of the pars, especially during flexion [22–24]. Displacement after a unilateral defect is less common, allowing healing to occur in some patients.

**Table 4.2** Labelle classification

| Grade | Dysplasia | Sacro-pelvic balance |
|---|---|---|
| Low-grade (<50% slip) | *Low dysplastic*:<br>• Minimal lumbosacral kyphosis<br>• Almost rectangular L5<br>• Minimal sacral doming<br>• Relatively normal sacrum<br>• Minimal posterior element dysplasia<br>• Relatively normal transverse process | *Low PI/low SS*<br>• Sacral slope $\leq 40°$<br><br>*High PI/high SS*<br>• Sacral slope $> 40°$ |
| | *High dysplastic*:<br>• Lumbosacral kyphosis<br>• Trapezoidal L5<br>• Sacral doming<br>• Sacral dysplasia and kyphosis<br>• Posterior element dysplasia<br>• Small transverse process | *Low PI/low SS*<br>• Sacral slope $\leq 40°$<br><br>*High PI/high SS*<br>• Sacral slope $> 40°$ |
| High-grade (≥50% slip) | *Low dysplastic*:<br>• Minimal lumbosacral kyphosis<br>• Almost rectangular L5<br>• Minimal sacral doming<br>• Relatively normal sacrum<br>• Minimal posterior element dysplasia<br>• Relatively normal transverse process | *High SS/low PT (balanced pelvis)*<br>• Balanced sacrum<br>• Sacral slope $\geq 50°$<br>• Pelvic tilt $\leq 35°$<br><br>*Low SS/high PT (unbalanced pelvis)*<br>• Vertical sacrum<br>• Sacral slope $< 50°$<br>• Pelvic tilt $\geq 25°$ |
| | *High dysplastic*:<br>• Lumbosacral kyphosis<br>• Trapezoidal L5<br>• Sacral doming<br>• Sacral dysplasia and kyphosis<br>• Posterior element dysplasia<br>• Small transverse process | *High SS/low PT (balanced pelvis)*<br>• Balanced sacrum<br>• Sacral slope $\geq 50°$<br>• Pelvic tilt $\leq 35°$<br><br>*Low SS/high PT (unbalanced pelvis)*<br>• Vertical sacrum<br>• Sacral slope $< 50°$<br>• Pelvic tilt $\geq 25°$ |

## 4.4  Diagnosis

The correct study when there is a suspicion of spondylolisthesis includes anteroposterior (AP) and lateral radiographs of the lumbar spine. Oblique views can also help detect spondylolysis, with a sensitivity of 84%, demonstrating the characteristic finding of "Scotty the dog's broken collar or neck" [25–27].

To assess the stability of the segment, it is helpful to request flexion-extension radiographs, in order to thus assess the progression of listhesis in movement.

As complementary studies, computed tomography (CT) and magnetic resonance imaging (MRI) can be performed to also assess the degree of stenosis of the associated canal or foraminal.

### *4.4.1  Grading of Lumbar Spondylolisthesis*

The forward slip of the vertebra above is measured by one of two methods [28]. The first is the method of Myerding. The anteroposterior (AP) diameter of the superior surface of the lower vertebra is divided into quarters, and a grade of I–IV is assigned to slips of one, two, three, or four quarters of the superior vertebra, respectively (Fig. 4.1a). The other method, first described by Taillard, expresses the degree of slip as a percentage of the AP diameter of the top of the lower vertebra (Fig. 4.1b).

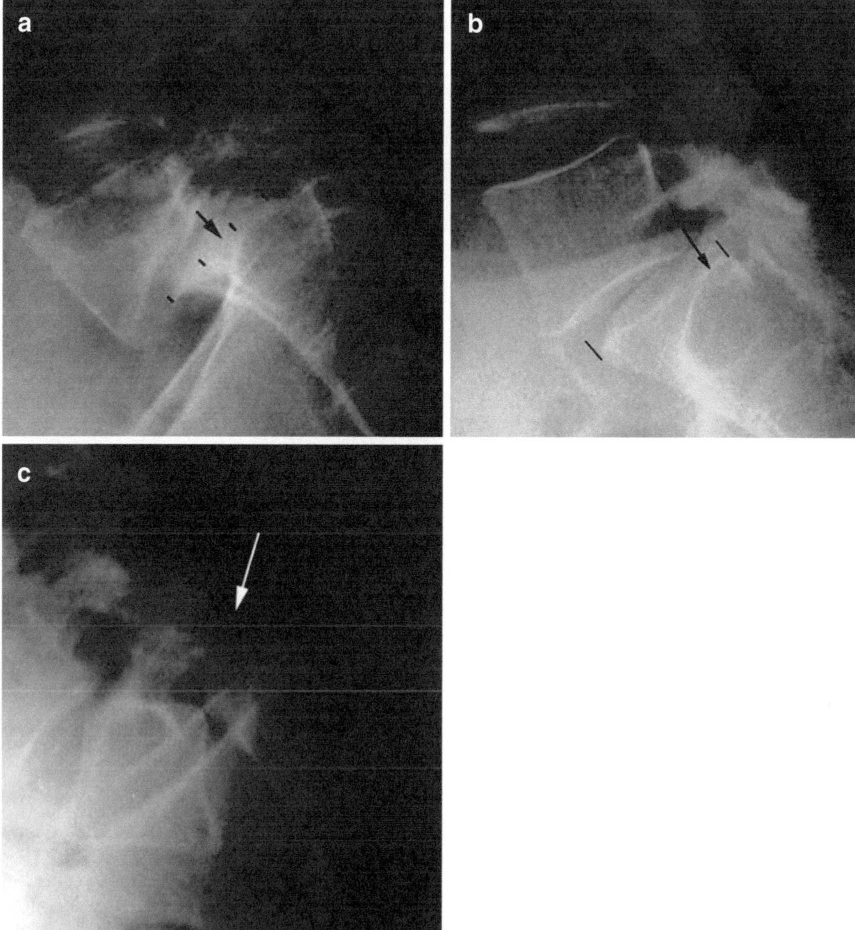

**Fig. 4.1**  Methods of grading lumbar spondylolisthesis. (**a**) The method of Myerding: lateral radiograph of the lumbosacral junction in type 1 spondylolisthesis shows a Grade III slip. (**b**) The method of Taillard: lateral radiograph of the lumbosacral junction shows a type 2 spondylolisthesis with an approximately 15° slip. (**c**) Spondyloptosis of L5 on S1. Note the wide defect in the pars interarticularis (arrow)

Complete slip of L5 on S1 is termed spondyloptosis (Fig. 4.1c). The second method is favored by most authors as it is more accurately reproducible. Measurement of the slip and its apparent progression, however, should be viewed with caution. Studies have shown that there can be inter- and intra-observer error of up to 15%. This variation can increase if there is an element of rotation. Therefore, only a progression of greater than 20% slip can be reliably assessed [29, 30].

## 4.5   Classification and Images

### 4.5.1   Type 1, Dysplastic (Congenital) Spondylolisthesis

Type 1a. The articular processes of L5 and S1 are dysplastic, having a horizontal rather than coronal orientation. There is rounding of the superior vertebral endplate of S1, and there may be spina bifida occulta affecting S1 or L5 or both (Figs. 4.2 and 4.3).

Type 1b. The orientation of the facet joints is sagittal and the facets are malformed, allowing spondylolisthesis to occur typically in adult life (Fig. 4.4).

Type 1c includes other congenital malformations of the lumbar spine which permit spondylolisthesis (Fig. 4.5).

### 4.5.2   Type 2, Isthmic (Lytic) Spondylolisthesis

The pars interarticularis is the part of the neural arch that joins the superior and inferior articular processes. Isthmic spondylolisthesis occurs in the presence of bilateral pars defects, which can result from a variety of causes (Figs. 4.6 and 4.7). Wiltse, in his original description, divided this category into three subtypes Table 4.2.

### 4.5.3   Type 3, Degenerative Spondylolisthesis

This is the commonest cause of lumbar spondylolisthesis above the age of 50 years. The neural arch is intact and the slip occurs because of degenerative changes in the facet joints with associated disc degeneration (Figs. 4.8 and 4.9).

**Fig. 4.2** Type 1a
dysplastic
spondylolisthesis. (**a**)
Anteroposterior radiograph
demonstrates the
'Napoleon's hat' sign. (**b**)
Lateral radiograph
demonstrates
approximately 70% slip,
with posterior wedging of
L5 and rounding of the
superior endplate of S1.
Note the pars defect of L5
(arrows)

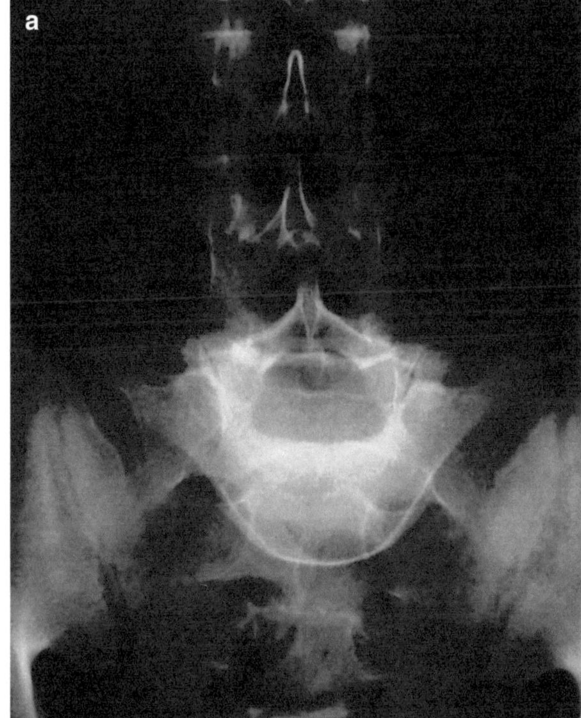

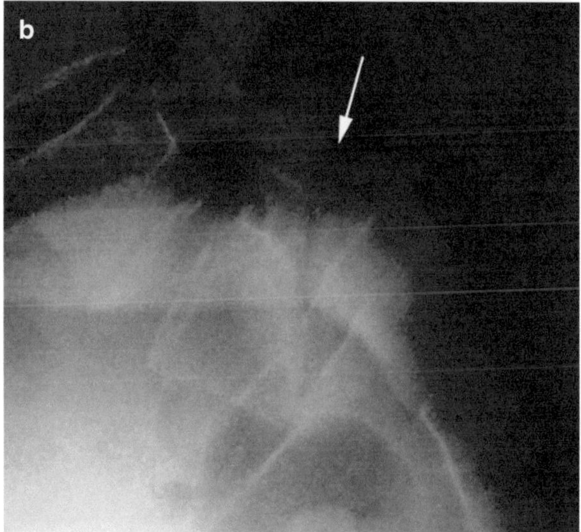

**Fig. 4.3** Type 1a dysplastic spondylolisthesis. (**a**) Midline sagittal T2W FSE MRI demonstrates a degenerate pseudobulging lumbosacral disc with severe compression of the cauda equina between the neural arch of L4 and the superoposterior aspect of the sacrum. (**b**) Parasagittal T1W SE MRI at the level of the intervertebral foramen shows severe compression of the exiting L5 nerve root

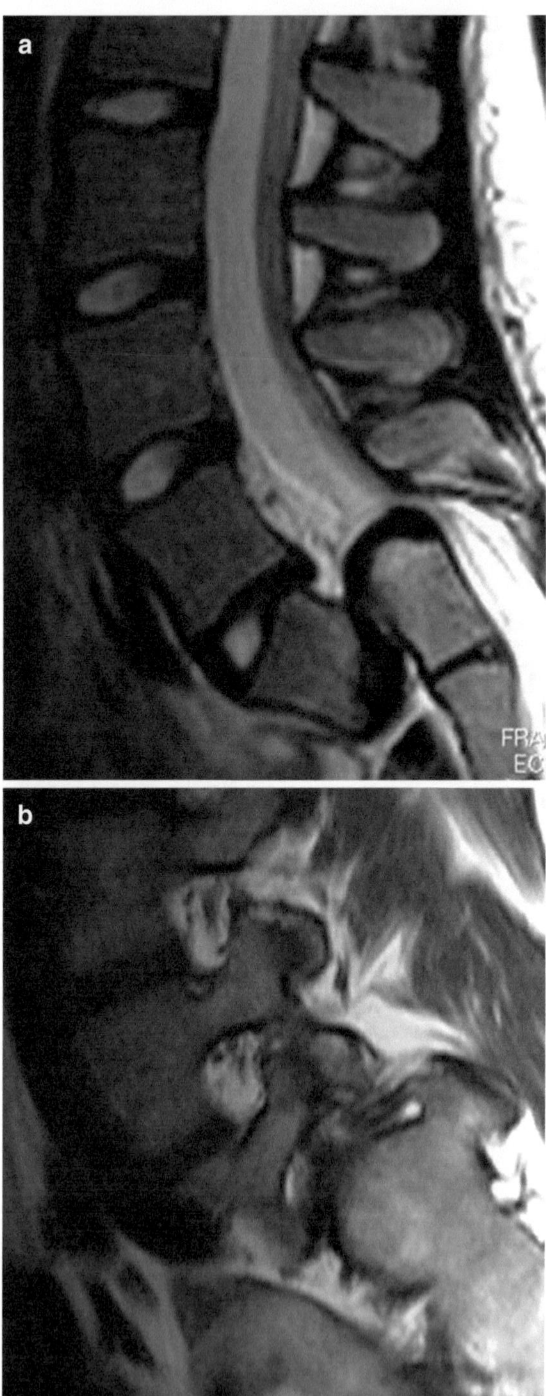

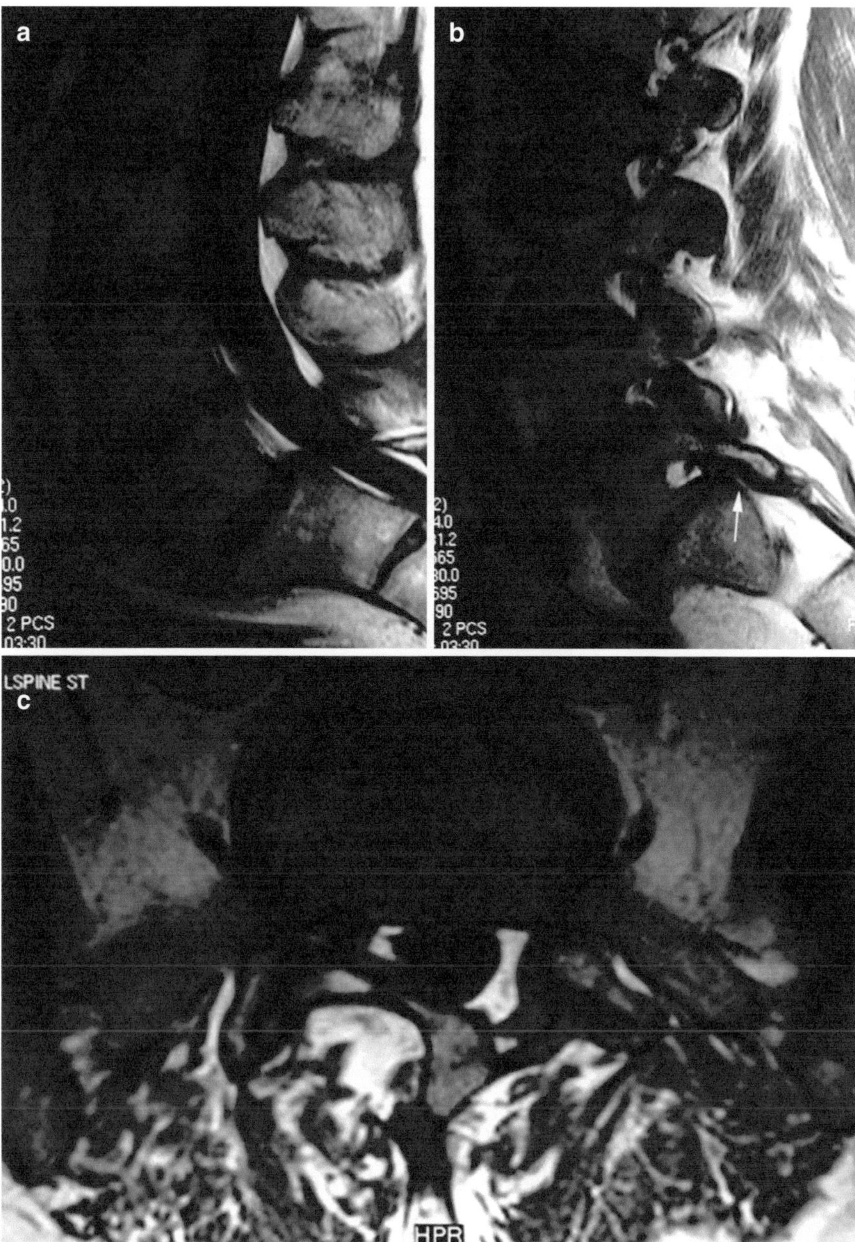


**Fig. 4.4** Type 1b dysplastic spondylolisthesis in an adult. (**a**) Sagittal T1W SE MRI demonstrates a grade 1 spondylolisthesis. The L4/5 and L5/S1 discs are degenerate. (**b**) Parasagittal T1W SE MRI demonstrates marked hypoplasia of the S1 superior articular facet and elongation of the L5 pars interarticularis. (**c**) Axial T1W SE MRI demonstrates a dysplastic L5 neural arch. Note also the asymmetry of facet joint orientation (facet tropism)

                                                    

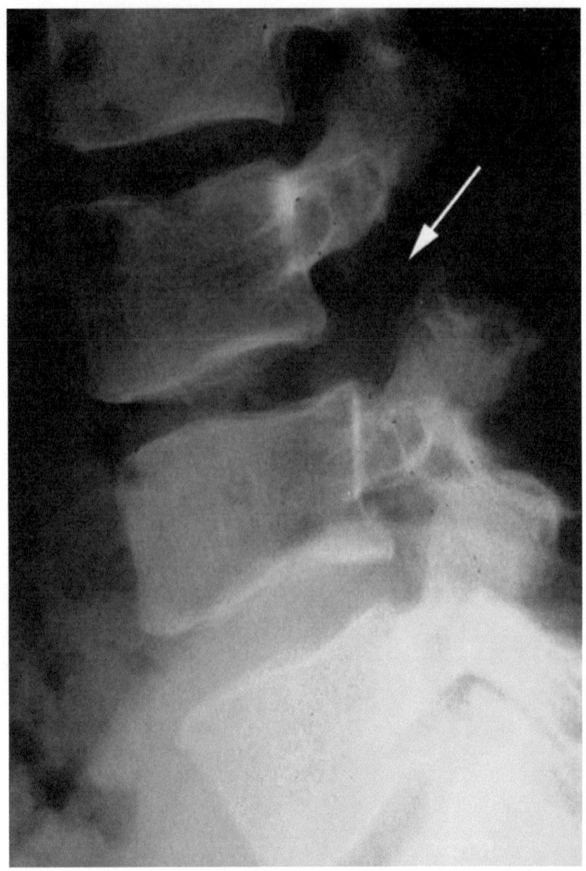

**Fig. 4.5** Type 1c dysplastic spondylolisthesis. Lateral radiograph demonstrates congenital absence of the inferior articular processes of L3 with associated grade 1 L3/4 spondylolisthesis

### 4.5.4   *Type 4, Traumatic Spondylolisthesis*

Traumatic spondylolisthesis is rare and results from fractures or dislocations involving any part of the neural arch except the pars interarticularis, for example, the pedicle or the facet joints (Fig. 4.10).

### 4.5.5   *Type 5, Pathological Spondylolisthesis*

Type V can occur when a generalized bone disease weakens the spine. Examples include Paget's disease (Fig. 4.11), osteoporosis, osteogenesis imperfecta, achondroplasia, arthrogryposis, and osteopetrosis.

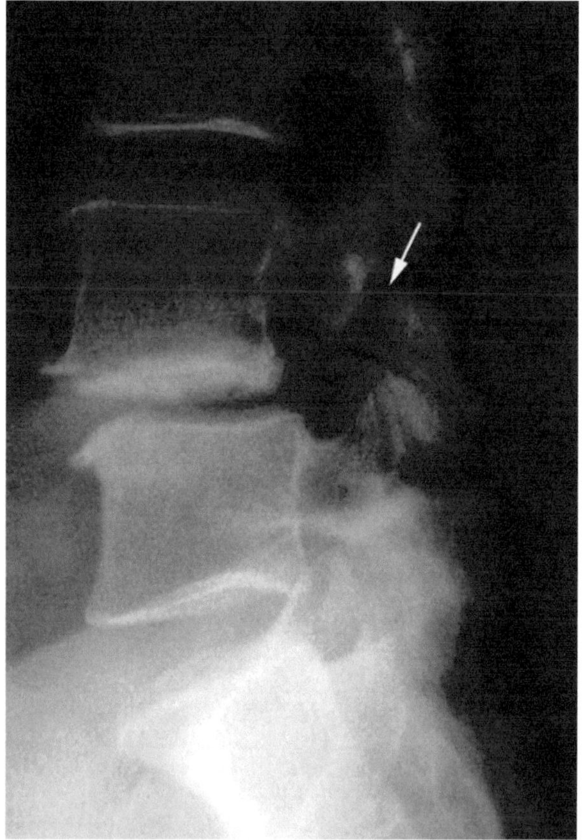

**Fig. 4.6** Type 2a isthmic spondylolisthesis. Lateral radiograph of the lumbar spine demonstrates bilateral L4 pars defects (arrow) with associated grade 1 L4/5 isthmic spondylolisthesis. The L4/5 disc is degenerate

## 4.6 Conservative Treatment

Conservative treatment is generally indicated as first-line therapy for patients with low-grade spondylolisthesis without neurologic deficits [31].

The clinical guidelines published by the North American Spine Society (NASS) in 2014 for the diagnosis and treatment of degenerative spondylolisthesis indicate that conservative treatment should be similar to the treatment used in degenerative lumbar stenosis [32]. Conservative management includes activity restriction, pain relief with the use of anti-inflammatory medications, and epidural steroid injections. Physical rehabilitation may include braces, physical therapy, ultrasound, electrical stimulation, and activity modification. Physical therapy can help reduce pain and strengthen the spinal musculature to restore range of motion and stabilize the spine [33–35].

In a prospective randomized trial of 29 patients (10 randomized to physiotherapy, 10 randomized to injections, and the remainder to controls), Koc et al. [36] demonstrated a significant improvement in pain in the groups treated with injections and physiotherapy at 6-month follow-up. In patients with predominant radiculopathy, short- and medium-term pain relief (3–36 months) can be seen with multiple X-ray-guided epidural transforaminal steroid injections [37–39].

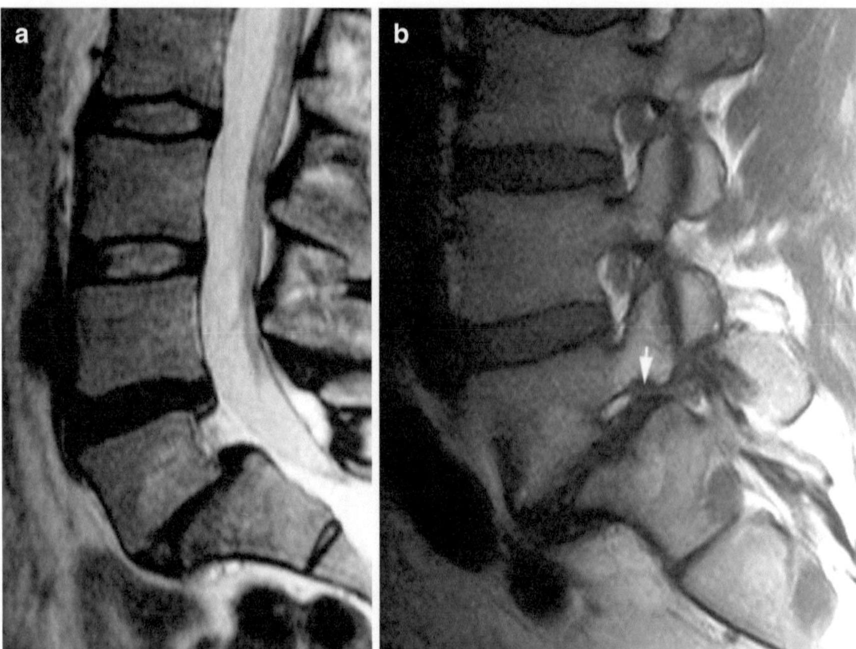

**Fig. 4.7** Type 2a isthmic spondylolisthesis. (**a**) Sagittal T2W F5E MRI shows L5/S1 isthmic spondylolisthesis with associated disc degeneration at the L4/5 level. (**b**) Parasagittal T1W SE MRI at the level of the pedicle shows compression of the exiting L5 nerve root (arrow) between the bulging L5/S1 disc and the undersurface of the L5 pedicle. Note the reduction of foraminal height due to the horizontal orientation of the foramen

## 4.7 Surgical Treatment

It is recommended to consider surgical management in those patients who have been refractory to conservative treatment [38]. It can be considered that conservative treatment has failed when after 3–6 months of follow-up they continue with symptoms that fail to subside with treatment [40–43].

### 4.7.1 Effectiveness of Surgical Vs. Nonsurgical Treatment of Degenerative Lumbar Spondylolisthesis

The SPORT (Spine Patient Outcomes Research Trial) study compared the effectiveness of surgical and nonsurgical treatment among participants with a confirmed diagnosis of degenerative spondylolisthesis (DS) with or without spinal stenosis who had claudication or radicular pain for at least 3 months. The study consisted of $n = 150$. Patients were randomly assigned to undergo medical treatment or surgical

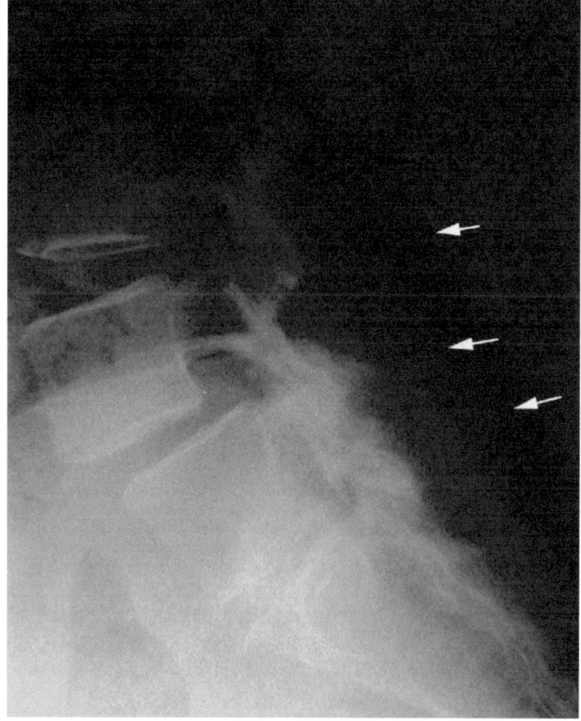

**Fig. 4.8** Lateral radiograph of the lower lumbar spine shows degenerative L4/5 spondylolisthesis above a transitional L5 vertebral body. Malalignment of the spinous processes with anterior slip of the L4 spinous process relative to L5 allows differentiation from isthmic spondylolisthesis

treatment. Nonsurgical interventions included physiotherapy, epidural steroid injections, nonsteroidal anti-inflammatory drugs, and opioids, while surgical intervention consisted of decompressive laminectomy with or without single-level bilateral fusion [44]. Surgical interventions had superior results at 3 months, 1 year, and 2 years, compared with those who underwent non-surgical intervention. Patients under 65 years of age were found to have greater treatment benefit in the surgery group than compared with older patients. The reoperation rate due to recurrent stricture or spondylolisthesis was 5% at 4 years.

## 4.8  Surgical Intervention Options for Degenerative Spondylolisthesis

### 4.8.1  Decompression Without Fusion

The goal of surgical intervention in patients with ED is to decompress the associated stenosis, that is, the narrowing of the spinal or foraminal canal to the level of pathology. Laminectomy for the treatment of ED has been reported to be associated with positive outcomes [45]. According to a meta-analysis of 11 studies, it was

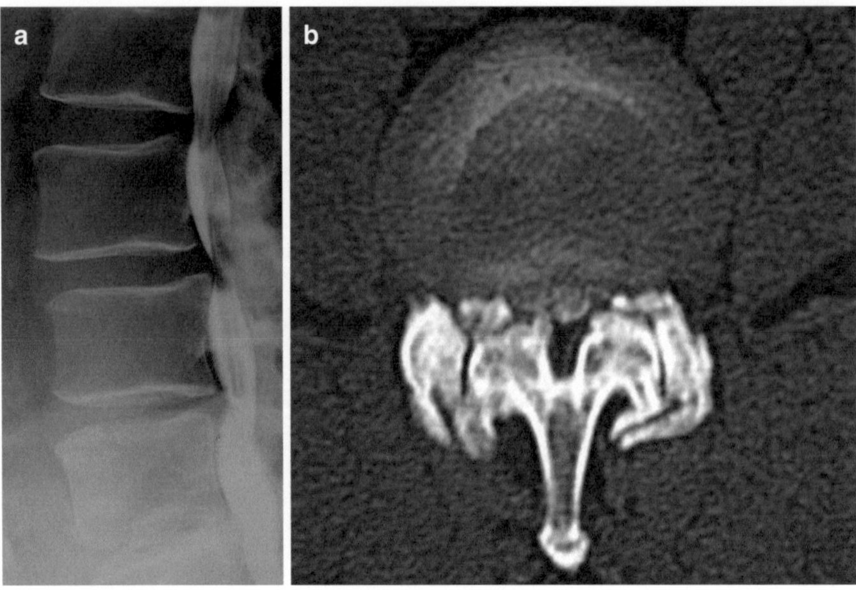

**Fig. 4.9** Degenerative L3/4 spondylolisthesis. (**a**) Lateral myelogram demonstrates mild L3/4 spondylolisthesis with associated central canal stenosis. (**b**) Axial CT myelogram through the L3/4 disc shows advanced facet osteoarthritis with a sagittal orientation of the facet joints

found that 69% of patients had a satisfactory outcome with laminectomy alone [46]. Thus similarly, Epstein [47] reported a series of 290 patients undergoing laminectomy for spondylolisthesis and found a success rate of 82%. Kristof and colleagues [48] reported a series of 49 patients who underwent laminectomy for patients with spondylolisthesis without hypermobility and found that the procedure was associated with excellent and good results in 73.5% of patients.

### 4.8.2 Decompression plus Fusion

Fusion decompression is currently the most widely used procedure for the surgical treatment of spondylolisthesis [45].

Herkowitz and Kurz, [49] found that patients who underwent laminectomy with arthrodesis had significantly less low back and lower leg pain and were therefore more likely to have a successful outcome. Martin et al. [50] performed a meta-analysis of 13 studies, consisting of $n = 578$, comparing the outcomes of patients undergoing fusion surgery vs. decompression alone and also instrumented versus non-instrumented fusion. The researchers found that patients who underwent fusion surgery, compared with decompression alone, were more likely to have successful clinical outcomes; the investigators also reported that the use of instrumented fusion reduced the risk of nonunion but had no impact on any other clinical outcomes.

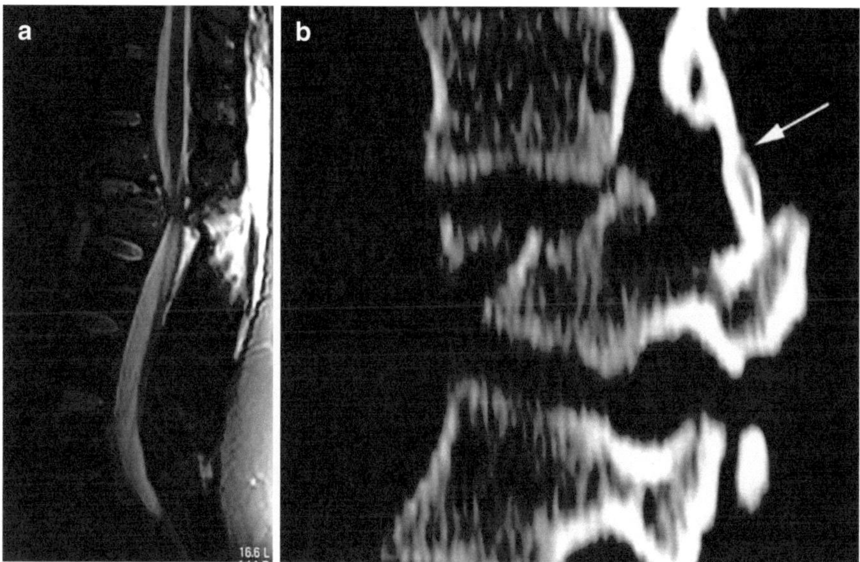


**Fig. 4.10** Traumatic L1/2 spondylolisthesis due to bifacet dislocation. (**a**) Sagittal CT MPR through the right facet level demonstrates L1/2 facet dislocation with fracture through the superior endplate of L1. Note that the pars interarticularis of L1 is intact (arrow). (**b**) Fat-suppressed sagittal T2W FSE MRI shows traumatic L1/2 spondylolisthesis with associated rupture of the L1/2 intervertebral disc and disruption of the posterior ligamentous complex

The role of fusion for low-grade spondylolisthesis has recently been debated. Forst and colleagues [51] randomized 247 patients to decompression alone and decompression plus fusion and found that the use of fusion was not associated with better outcomes; ODI scores at 2 years, 6-min walk test results, and recovery rates were found to be similar between the 2 groups, while length of stay, operative time, and blood loss were older in the fusion group. Ghogawala and colleagues [52] published their results of 66 patients who were randomized to decompression alone or decompression with fusion and found that patients in the fusion group had higher SF-36 scores at 2, 3, and 4 years, as well as a lower recovery rate compared to patients in the decompression alone group. More recently, Inose and colleagues [53] randomized patients with low-grade (<30%) L4-L5 spondylolisthesis to decompression alone, decompression and fusion, or decompression and stabilization and found no difference in visual analogue score (VAS) for the lower back pain and VAS for leg pain and Japanese Orthopedic Association (JOA) score among the three groups.

IM Austevoll et al. [54] conducted a multicenter, open-label study involving patients with symptomatic lumbar stenosis who had failed conservative treatment and who had single-level spondylolisthesis of 3 mm or more. Patients were randomized in a 1:1 ratio to undergo decompression surgery (decompression alone group) or decompression surgery with instrumented fusion (fusion group). Decompression alone was not inferior to decompression with instrumented fusion over a 2-year period, but reoperation could be seen to occur somewhat more often in the decompression-alone group than in the fusion group.

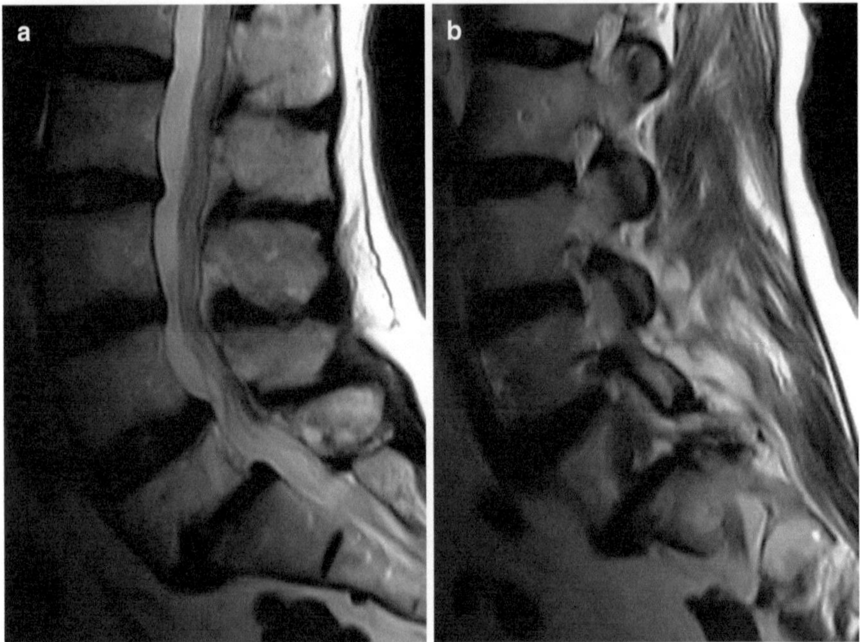

**Fig. 4.11** Pathological spondylolisthesis due to Paget's disease of L5. (**a**) Midline sagittal T2W FSE MRI shows typical features of chronic inactive Paget's disease of L5 with expansion of the vertebral body and Grade 1 L5/S1 spondylolisthesis. (**b**) Parasagittal T2W F5E MRI through the pedicle level shows elongation of the L5 pars interarticularis

### 4.8.3 Options of Surgical Fusion Treatment of Spondylolisthesis

The different treatment options for spondylolisthesis have been extensively studied to identify which offer better clinical results and a lower rate of complications and reoperations (Table 4.3), as the anterior approach for interbody fusion (ALIF) (Image 4.1) provides the best fusion rate due to the wide bone surface of the vertebral platforms compared to the one provided by posterior techniques. Indirect compression can be achieved with these techniques due to the ligamentotaxis effect exerted by the interbody cage. The muscular damage in this technique is minimal, complications, when they appear, tend to be more serious, the ureteral and intestinal injury, damage to the great vessels, and alterations in ejaculation in men are the most described [55].

Lateral lumbar interbody fusion (LLIF) is recognized as a less invasive surgical method and performed through an anterolateral transpsoas approach [56]. LLIF has been used as an alternative to conventional anterior approaches and can be used from the L1-L2 to L4-L5 segment. There are sub-variants to this technique called extreme lateral (XLIF) (Image 4.2) and oblique (OLIF) interbody fusion, where the

**Table 4.3** Advantages and complications on diferent surgical options for treatment of spondylolisthesis

|  | Benefits | Disadvantages |
|---|---|---|
| ALIF | • Less bleeding | • Lower lumbar segments only |
|  | • Big surface for cage placement | • Visceral or vessels damage |
|  | • Less muscular damage | • Retrograde ejaculation |
|  | • Better lordosis restoring | • Post-incisional hernias |
| LLIF | • Less bleeding | • Hip flexion pain |
|  | • Big surface for cage placement | • Visceral or vessels damage |
|  | • Less muscular damage | • Less lordosis restoring |
|  | • Fast surgical timing | • Post-incisional hernias |
|  | • Upper and lower segments |  |
| PLIF | • Only one approach | • Most dural tear incidence |
|  | • Almost no visceral or vessels damage | • Dural sac retraction |
|  | • All lumbar segments | • More bleeding |
|  |  | • More muscular damage |
|  |  | • Less surface for arthrodesis |
|  |  | • Less lordosis restoring |
|  |  | • Laminae and partial or complete facet resection |
| TLIF | • Only one approach | • Complete facet resection |
|  | • Minimal dural sac retraction | • Nerve root lesion |
|  | • Almost no visceral or vessels damage | • Dural tears |
|  | • All lumbar segments | • More bleeding |
|  |  | • More muscular damage |
|  |  | • Less surface for arthrodesis |
|  |  | • Less lordosis restoring |

site of entry of the interbody cage varies to a lateral and oblique position, respectively. These techniques present less bleeding and surgical time, shorter hospital stay, and lighter postoperative pain than the posterior approach. Among the complications reported are pain on flexion and extension of the hips due to manipulation of the iliac psoas, paresthesia, and motor alterations due to injury to the ilioinguinal, iliohypogastric, lateral femoral cutaneous, and genitofemoral nerves, and other less frequent injuries include the large vessels trauma and post-incisional hernias.

The PLIF and LLIF in degenerative spondylolisthesis were compared in a study published by Pawar et al. in 2015, [57] reported that the surgery time was similar between the groups, but the average blood loss was significantly lower in the LLIF than the group PLIF (438 vs 750 min, $p < 0.01$), the incidence of dural tear was lower with LLIF (0 vs 5, $p = 0.014$). In the LLIF group, foraminal height, intervertebral space height, and lumbar lordosis were restored. No permanent iatrogenic neurological deficits were reported in either group. The LLIF group significantly

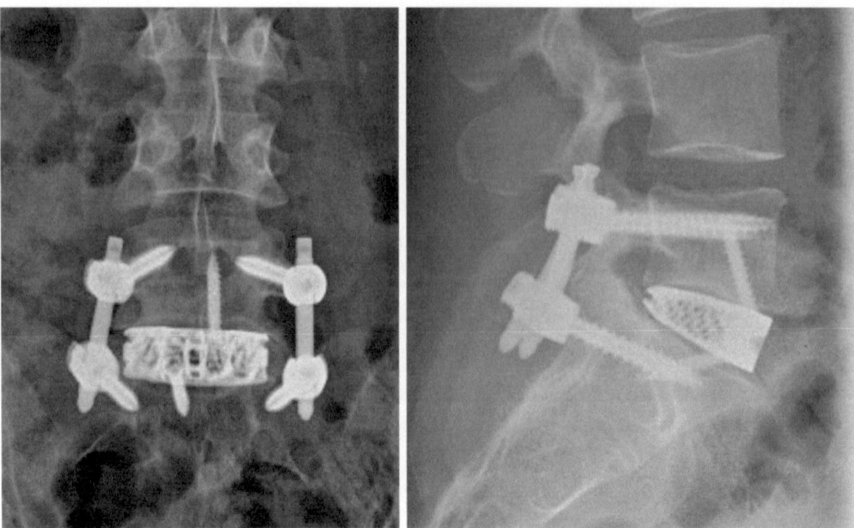

**Image 4.1** ALIF L5-S1 with pedicle screws

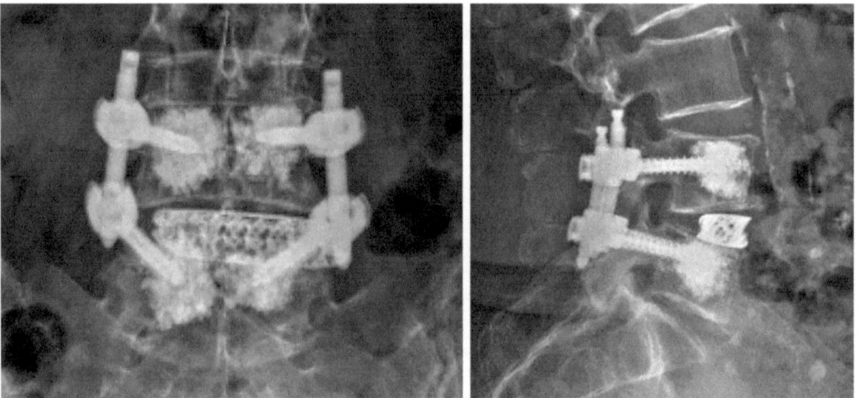

**Image 4.2** XLIF L4-L5 with cemented pedicle screws

decreased disability as measured by the Oswestry disability index, but without significant differences in other clinical outcome scores between groups.

In the comparison between LLIF and minimally invasive TLIF (Image 4.3) in the treatment of one or two levels of grade I-II of degenerative spondylolisthesis, it was found that blood loss was lower in the LLIF group than in TLIF. The average surgery time and length of hospital stays did not differ between groups. As a complication, there was a weakness in hip flexion, which was observed in the LLIF group in 31% of the patients and resolved within 6 months in all cases. The sensory or distal motor deficits reported were transient, and no significant difference was identified between the groups. The LLIF fusion rate was 100%, and the TLIF was 96%, one

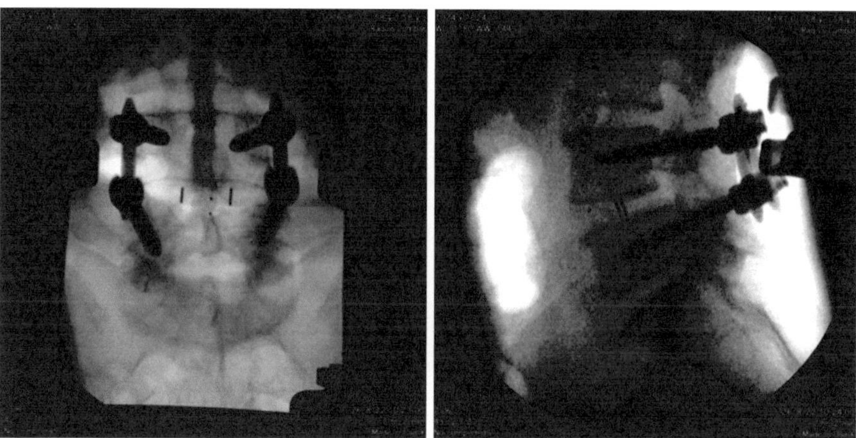

**Image 4.3**  Percutaneous L4-L5 TLIF

pseudarthrosis required reoperation and was the only one reported in the follow-up of the two groups. Pain, disability, and quality of life scores were significantly improved from baseline in both groups. Radiographically, the disc height improved significantly in both groups in all evaluations; however, there was a greater postoperative increase in the central area of the spinal canal in the TLIF, and the LLIF group presented subsidence at the two-year follow-up [55, 58].

The anterior and lateral approaches to the lumbar spine are more suitable for restoring sagittal balance. Through this kind of surgeries, bigger cages and with variable angles of lordosis can be implanted, sagittal balance parameters are very important for the outcome of the patients, Schwab FJ, et al. demonstrated that PT and PI-LL combined with SVA can predict patient disability and provide a guide for patient assessment for appropriate therapeutic decision making. Threshold values for severe disability (ODI > 40) included: PT 22° or more, SVA 47 mm or more, and PI − LL 11° or more [59].

Having so many options to achieve fusion, the main importance is that the fusion technique used by the surgeons in degenerative spondylolisthesis should be individualized to the clinical and imaging characteristics of each patient to have the best outcome possible.

# References


1. Metz LN, Deviren V. Low-grade spondylolisthesis. Neurosurg Clin N Am. 2007;18(2):237–48. https://doi.org/10.1016/j.nec.2007.02.010.
2. Beutler WJ, Fredrickson BE, Murtland A, et al. The natural history of spondylolysis and spondylolisthesis: 45-year follow-up evaluation. Spine. 2003;28(10):1027–35.
3. Rosenberg NJ. Degenerative spondylolisthesis. Pre-disposing factors. J Bone Joint Surg Am. 1975;57(4):467–74.

4. Vibert BT, Sliva CD, Herkowitz HN. Treatment of instability and spondylolisthesis: surgical versus nonsurgical treatment. Clin Orthop Relat Res. 2006;443:222–7.

5. Cauchoix J, Benoist M, Chassaing V. Degenerative spondylolisthesis. Clin Orthop. 1976;115:122–9.

6. Newman PH, Stone KH. The etiology of spondylolisthesis. J Bone Joint Surg Br. 1963;45(1):39–59.

7. Wiltse LL, Winter RB. Terminology and measurement of spondylolisthesis. J Bone Joint Surg Am. 1983;65(6):768–72.

8. Marchetti PG, Bartolozzi P. Classification of spondylolisthesis as a guideline for treatment. In: Brid-well KH, DeWald RL, editors. The textbook of spinal surgery. 2nd ed. Philadelphia: Lippincott-Raven; 1997. p. 1211–54.

9. Wiltse LL, Newman PH, Macnab I. Classification of spondylolysis and spondylolisthesis. Clin Orthop Relat Res. 1976;117:23–9.

10. Marchetti PG, Bartolozzi P. Spondylolisthesis: Modern trends in orthopaedic surgery. Bologna, Italy; 1999. p. 165–8.

11. During J, Goudfrooij H, Keesen W, et al. Toward standards for posture. Postural characteristics of the lower back system in normal and pathologic conditions. Spine. 1985;10(1):83–7.

12. Hanson DS, Bridwell KH, Rhee JM, et al. Correlation of pelvic incidence with low-and high-grade isthmic spondylolisthesis. Spine. 2002;27(18):2026–9.

13. Jackson RP, Phipps T, Hales C, et al. Pelvic lordosis and alignment in spondylolisthesis. Spine. 2003;28(2):151–60.

14. Labelle H, Roussouly P, Bertonnaud E, et al. The importance of spino-pelvic balance in L5-S1 developmental spondylolisthesis: a review of pertinent radiologic measurements. Spine. 2005;30(6S):S27–34.

15. Labelle H, Roussouly P, Bertonnaud E, et al. Spondylolisthesis, pelvic incidence, and spino-pelvic balance: a correlation study. Spine. 2004;29(18):2049–54.

16. Labelle H, Roussouly P, Chopin D. The importance of spino-pelvic balance after spinal instrumentation for high grade spondylolisthesis. Presented at the Scoliosis Research Society Annual Meeting, Quebec City, September, 2003.

17. Marty C, Boisaubert B, Descamps H, et al. The sagittal anatomy of the sacrum among young adults, infants, and spondylolisthesis patients. Eur Spine J. 2002;11(2):119–25.

18. Rajnics P, Templier A, Skalli W, et al. The association of sagittal spinal and pelvic parameters in asymptomatic persons and patients with isthmic spondylolisthesis. J Spinal Disord Tech. 2002;15(1):24–30.

19. Vaz G, Roussouly P, Bertonnaud E, et al. Sagittal morphology and equilibrium of pelvis and spine. Eur Spine J. 2002;11(1):80–7.

20. Whitesides TE Jr, Horton WC, Hutton WC, et al. Spondylolytic spondylolisthesis: a study of pelvic and lumbosacral parameters of possible etiologic effect in two genetically and geographically distinct groups with high occurrence. Spine. 2005;30(6S):S12–21.

21. Herbiniaux G. Traite sur divers accouchemens laborieux, et sur les polypes de la matrice [French]. Bruxelles, Belgium: J.L. DeBoubers; 1782.

22. Dietrich M, Kurowski P. The importance of mechanical factors in the etiology of spondylolysis. A model analysis of loads and stresses in human lumbar spine. Spine. 1985;10(6):532–42.

23. Farfan HF, Osteria V, Lamy C. The mechanical etiology of spondylolysis and spondylolisthesis. Clin Orthop Relat Res. 1976;117:40–55.

24. Troup JD. Mechanical factors in spondylolisthesis and spondylolysis. Clin Orthop Relat Res. 1976;117:59–67.

25. Millard L. The Scotty dog and his collar. J Ark Med Soc. 1976;72(8):339–40.

26. Standaert CJ, Herring S. Spondylolysis: a critical review. Br J Sports Med. 2000;34(6):415.

27. Libson E, Bloom RA, Dinari G. Symptomatic and asymptomatic spondylolysis and spondylolisthesis in young adults. Int Orthop. 1983;6(4):259–61.

28. Wiltse LL, Winter RB. Terminology and measurement of spondylolisthesis. J Bone Joint Surg. 1983;65A:768–72.

29. Danielson B, Frennerd K, Irstam L. Roentgenologic assessment of spondylolisthesis. I: A study of measurement variations. Acta Radiol. 1988;29:345–51.
30. Butt S, Saifuddin A. The imaging of lumbar spondylolisthesis. Clin Radiol. 2005;60:533–46.
31. Samuel Andre M, Moore Harold G, Cunningham Matthew E. Treatment for degenerative lumbar spondylolisthesis: current concepts and new evidence. Curr Rev Musculoskelet Med. 2017;10(4):521–9.
32. Matz Paul G, Meagher RJ, Lamer T, et al. Guideline summary review: an evidence-based clinical guideline for the diagnosis and treatment of degenerative lumbar spondylolisthesis. Spine J. 2016;16(3):439–48.
33. Marek S, Gunzburg R, Pope MH. Lumbar segmental instability. Philadelphia: Lippincott Williams & Wilkins; 1999.
34. Fritz JM, Erhard RE, Hagen BF. Segmental instability of the lumbar spine. Phys Ther. 1998;78(8):889–96.
35. Hall CM, Brody LT. Balance impairment. In: Therapeutic exercise: moving toward function. Philadelphia: L & W; 1999.
36. Koc Z, Ozcakir S, Sivrioglu K, et al. Effectiveness of physical therapy and epidural steroid injections in lumbar spinal stenosis. Spine (Phila Pa 1976). 2009;34(10):985–9.
37. Kreiner DS, Shaffer WO, Baisden JL, et al. North American Spine Society. An evidence-based clinical guideline for the diagnosis and treatment of degenerative lumbar spinal stenosis (update). Spine J. 2013;13(7):734–43.
38. Vad Vijay B, Bhat Atul L, Lutz Gregory E, et al. Transforaminal epidural steroid injections in lumbosacral radiculopathy: a prospective randomized study. Spine (Phila Pa 1976). 2002;27(1):11–6.
39. Dunn AS, Baylis S, Ryan D. Chiropractic management of mechanical low back pain secondary to multiple-level lumbar spondylolysis with spondylolisthesis in a United States Marine Corps veteran: a case report. J Chiropr Med. 2009;8(3):125–30.
40. Faldini C, Pagkrati S, Acri F, et al. Surgical treatment of symptomatic degenerative lumbar spondylolisthesis by decompression and instrumented fusion. J Orthop Traumatol. 2007;8(3):128–33.
41. Weinstein James N, Lurie Jon D, Tosteson Tor D, et al. Surgical compared with nonoperative treatment for lumbar degenerative spondylolisthesis. four-year results in the Spine Patient Outcomes Research Trial (SPORT) randomized and observational cohorts. J Bone Joint Surg Am. 2009;91(6):1295–304.
42. Fischgrund JS, Mackay M, Herkowitz HN, et al. Volvo Award winner in clinical studies. Degenerative lumbar spondylolisthesis with spinal stenosis: a prospective, randomized study comparing decompressive laminectomy and arthrodesis with and without spinal instrumentation. Spine (Phila Pa 1976) 1997. 1997;22(24):2807–12.
43. Fischgrund JS. The argument for instrumented decompressive posterolateral fusion for patients with degenerative spondylolisthesis and spinal stenosis. Spine (Phila Pa 1976). 2004;29(2):173–4.
44. Birkmeyer NJ, Weinstein JN, Tosteson AN, et al. Design of the Spine patient outcomes research trial (SPORT). Spine (Phila Pa 1976). 2002;27(12):1361–72.
45. Eismont FJ, Norton RP, Hirsch BP. Surgical management of lumbar degenerative spondylolisthesis. J Am Acad Orthop Surg. 2014;22(4):203–13.
46. Mardjetko SM, Connolly PJ, Shott S. Degenerative lumbar spondylolisthesis: a meta-analysis of literature 1970–1993. Spine (Phila Pa 1976). 1994;19(20):2256S.
47. Epstein NE. Decompression in the surgical management of degenerative spondylolisthesis: advantages of a conservative approach in 290 patients. J Spinal Disord. 1998;11(2):116–22. [discussion: 123]
48. Kristof RA, Aliashkevich AF, Schuster M, et al. Degenerative lumbar spondylolisthesis-induced radicular compression: nonfusion-related decompression in selected patients without hypermobility on flexion—extension radiographs. J Neurosurg Spine. 2002;97(3):281–6.

49. Herkowitz HN, Kurz LT. Degenerative lumbar spondylolisthesis with spinal stenosis. A prospective study comparing decompression with decompression and intertransverse process arthrodesis. J Bone Joint Surg Am. 1991;73(6):802–8.
50. Martin CR, Gruszczynski AT, Braunsfurth HA, et al. The surgical management of degenerative lumbar spondylolisthesis: a systematic review. Spine (Phila Pa 1976). 2007;32(16):1791–8.
51. Forsth P, O'lafsson G, Carlsson T, et al. A randomized, controlled trial of fusion surgery for lumbar spinal stenosis. N Engl J Med. 2016;374(15):1413–23.
52. Ghogawala Z, Dziura J, Butler WE, et al. Laminectomy plus fusion versus laminectomy alone for lumbar spondylolisthesis. N Engl J Med. 2016;374(15):1424–34.
53. Inose H, Kato T, Yuasa M, et al. Comparison of decompression, decompression plus fusion, and decompression plus stabilization for degenerative spondylolisthesis: a prospective, randomized study. Clin Spine Surg. 2018;31(7):E347–52.
54. Austevoll IM, Hermansen E, Fagerland MW, Storheim K, Brox JI, Solberg T, Rekeland F, Franssen E, Weber C, Brisby H, Grundnes O, Algaard KRH, Böker T, Banitalebi H, Indrekvam K, Hellum C, Investigators NORDSTEN-DS. Decompression with or without fusion in degenerative lumbar spondylolisthesis. N Engl J Med. 2021;385(6):526–38. https://doi.org/10.1056/NEJMoa2100990.
55. Mobbs RJ, Phan K, Malham G, Seex K, Rao PJ. Lumbar interbody fusion: techniques, indications and comparison of interbody fusion options including PLIF, TLIF, MI-TLIF, OLIF/ATP, LLIF and ALIF. J Spine Surg. 2015;3(1):2–18.
56. Bertagnoli R, Vazquez RJ. The AnteroLateral transPsoatic approach (ALPA): a new technique for implanting prosthetic disc-nucleus devices. J Spinal Disord Tech. 2003;16(4):398–404.
57. Pawar AY, Hughes AP, Sama AA, Girardi FP, Lebl DR, Cammisa FP. A comparative study of lateral lumbar interbody fusion and posterior lumbar interbody fusion in degenerative lumbar spondylolisthesis. Asian Spine J. 2015;9(5):668–74.
58. García-Ramos CL, et al. Lumbar degenerative spondylolisthesis II: treatment and controversies. Acta Ortop Mex. 2020;34(6):Nov.-Dic. 433-440.
59. Schwab FJ, Blondel B, Bess S, Hostin R, Shaffrey CI, Smith JS, Boachie-Adjei O, Burton DC, Akbarnia BA, Mundis GM, Ames CP, Kebaish K, Hart RA, Farcy JP, Lafage V, International Spine Study Group (ISSG). Radiographical spinopelvic parameters and disability in the setting of adult spinal deformity: a prospective multicenter analysis. Spine (Phila Pa 1976). 2013;38(13):E803–12. https://doi.org/10.1097/BRS.0b013e318292b7b9.

# Chapter 5
# Enhanced Recovery After Surgery (ERAS) Spine Pathways and the Role of Perioperative Checklists

Scott C. Robertson

## Contents



S. C. Robertson (✉)
Division of Neurosurgery, Quincy Medical Group, Quincy, USA

© The Author(s), under exclusive license to Springer Nature Switzerland AG 2024

C. Di Rocco (ed.), *Advances and Technical Standards in Neurosurgery*, Advances and Technical Standards in Neurosurgery 49, https://doi.org/10.1007/978-3-031-42398-7_5

## 5.1 Introduction

Enhanced recovery after surgery (ERAS) proposes a multimodal, evidence-based approach to perioperative care. ERAS pathways have been shown to help reduce complications, hospital length of stay (LOS), 30-day readmission rates, pain scores, and ultimately surgical costs, while improving patient satisfaction scores and outcomes in multiple surgical subspecialties [1–6]. Numerous specialties have implemented ERAS programs across the globe, providing a foundation for spine surgeons to begin the process themselves. Over the last few years, a significant number of papers have been addressing ERAS pathways for spinal surgery [7–19]. The majority have addressed the lumbar spine [9, 20–26]. The number of cervical ERAS pathways has been limited [27–29]. Many spine programs have begun the implementation of ERAS pathways, incorporating principles and interventions to various spine surgical procedures. Although differences in implementation across programs exist, there are a few common elements that promote a successful enhanced recovery approach [11, 16, 23, 25, 30–33]. All spinal ERAS pathways have three major elements, which are preoperative, perioperative, and postoperative phases. Within these phases some common elements include preoperative and intraoperative surgical checklists. Intraoperative checklist in addition to the "surgical time out" has been integrated into the workflow of most hospitals doing surgeries and have become a standard of care. The surgical checklist is designed to help reduce surgical errors and prevent wrong site/patient surgeries. Several surgical checklists have been developed throughout the years. Despite these safety protocols wrong site/level and other surgical errors continue to occur. Many cases of wrong level spine surgery (WLSS) still occur even when intraoperative imaging is performed [34, 35]. One survey reported that about 50% of spine surgeons have performed at least one WLSS during their career [36, 37]. Another survey reported that 36% of spine surgeons had performed at least one WLSS that was not recognized intraoperatively [38]. On a similar account, about 30% of spine surgery fellows have experienced wrong-site surgery [39]. From raw incidence rates, WLSS may seem rare, but these surveys show that the experience of WLSS is rather common among spine surgeons. WLSS is not yet a "never event." This may be due to poor quality of the intraoperative images, hindering subsequent level identification [34, 35, 38, 40]. Errors in interpretation of the imaging may also occur, including inconsistency in numbering vertebrae, inconsistency in landmark usage for level counting, and problems with numbering vertebrae due to lumbosacral transitional vertebrae (LSTV) and other anatomical variants [34, 38, 41–43]. This chapter will describe a framework for the development and implementation of ERAS pathway for patients undergoing spine surgery. In addition, we will propose preoperative imaging guidelines and a comprehensive spine surgical checklist to incorporate into the perioperative phase to help reduce further surgical errors and WLSS.

## 5.2    Spine ERAS Pathways

The spine ERAS pathway provides a guide for the patient's journey. ERAS pathways are generally divided into three phases: preoperative, perioperative, and postoperative. These phases can be subdivided into prehospital, preoperative, intraoperative, postoperative, and post-discharge phases (Table 5.1).

## 5.3    Prehospital and Preoperative Phase

The prehospital phase is to maximize the physical and functional status of the patient prior to surgical intervention as well as to engage and educate the patient about surgical expectations. The timeline for this portion of the ERAS is variable for each patient and can range from days to weeks.

**Table 5.1**  Spine ERAS phases

| Pre-hospital phase | Preoperative phase | Intraoperative phase | Postoperative phase | Post-discharge phase |
|---|---|---|---|---|
| Medical clearance Patient optimization Patient education Expectation setting Nutritional optimization and instructions Pain management plan Spine disability assessment testing Bone density study—Medical optimization Prehabilitation Orthotic fitting Preop surgical checklist Risk assessment and prediction tool (RAPT) Postop medications review | Limited fasting light meal up to 6 h Carbohydrate beverage up to 2 h preop Initiation of multimodal analgesia Chlorhexidine skin cleaning Preemptive anti-nausea medication Review procedure with patient/family Review radiology images and identify anatomical anomalies Antibiotics DVT prophylaxis | Opioid sparing/ multimodal anesthesia (TIVA) Spine surgical safety checklist Intra-operative 2nd radiology time out (2nd RTO) Exparel ESP field block Minimal invasive surgical techniques Nausea/vomiting prophylaxis Avoid catheters and drains Normthermia Normovolemia Local analgesia Limited muscle relaxant Vancomycin powder in wound | Early mobilization Early diet Discontinue IVF Discontinue drains and Foley Bowel regimen Multimodal analgesia Early PT/OT evaluation Discharge planning Patient education on wound care, activity, and medications Schedule follow-up | Minimal restriction of ADL Phone follow-up Scheduled follow-up visit Home health/ PT Reduction of multimodal analgesia Resource for questions, either written, hotline, digital app Outcome assessment – PROs Confirm compliance with instructions If not discharged home, facilities need a strict rehabilitation plan and knowledge of ERAS |

### 5.3.1  Patient Education

Once the patient has elected to proceed with surgery the educational process begins. The surgical procedure and expectations are reviewed with the patient. Surgical risk, benefits, and alternatives are explained as part of a typical informed consent. Several preoperative educational topics covered are reiterated during the perioperative and postoperative phases to reinforce the information. Group preoperative clinics to cover the educational topics can help save time in a busy clinic. Educational materials can be provided in a multimedia format with handouts, videos, and online resources, which can be accessed through smartphones. Patients scheduled for similar surgeries will meet with the surgeon, nurse, and other members of the team including anesthesia providers and physical therapist (PT).

The pathways include information about necessary appointments and consultations prior to surgery, postoperative expectations and disposition, pre-admission testing, perioperative eating and drinking, surgical site care, postoperative medications, physical restrictions, orthotic care, postoperative discharge needs, and appointments. Preoperative fitting and educational use of orthotic devices ensures compliance and reduces postoperative discharge time. Additional home needs including walkers, graspers, bedside commodes, and other supplies can be addressed during this visit. Home safety analysis and a detailed clinical assessment should always be interpreted in conjunction with supplemental assessment tools, including imaging, electrodiagnostic tools, and standardized disease-specific assessment tools. Some useful cervical assessment tools include the Myelopathy Disability Index, Japanese Orthopaedic Association Score, Short Form-36, and Neck Disability Index to help discussions on outcome expectations after surgery and determine postoperative rehabilitation planning [44–47]. Discussion with patient and family members about home care needs if living alone and potential for inpatient rehabilitation postoperatively. Determine if any home medical equipment will be needed for activities of daily living. Contacting case management for early review of insurance plans can determine the patient's eligibility for postoperative skilled care and rehabilitation benefits in patients with significant presurgical disabilities.

Additional education on smoking cessation and other high risk social behavior including alcohol consumption should be avoided both before and during the recovery period.

### 5.3.2  Medical Clearance and Optimization

Preoperative preparation should include smoking cessation and alcohol reduction. Smoking is a well-established, risk factor for non-union in spinal fusions. Smoking cessation can decrease risk of infection, perioperative respiratory problems, and wound complications. Weight loss in obese patients is encouraged. Holding antiplatelet and anticoagulation medications are needed prior to surgery. Obstructive sleep apnea management is important in cervical surgery.

Nutrition is a modifiable risk factor which can be optimized. Checking albumin is important since hypoalbuminemia is a predictor of complications. In addition, low pre-albumin, retinol-binding protein, and transferrin levels are associated with increased infection risk [48]. Diabetes is also associated with poor postoperative outcomes effecting wound healing and increased infections. Tight glycemic control prior to spinal surgery is recommended. Other things to consider are calcium and Vitamin D supplements in osteopenic patients and erythropoietin treatment in anemic patients prior to surgery. Bone density studies for surgical fusion cases requiring instrumentation provide useful information on bone quality. Newer osteoporotic instrumentation and cement augmentation may be needed.

Surgical site wound care including preoperative cleaning with antimicrobial solution (chlorohexidine gluconate) reduces bacterial skin flora and helps reduce wound infections.

### 5.3.3  Pain Management Plan

Screen for chronic opioid users who are analgesic tolerant and drug dependent. Chronic opioid users undergoing spinal surgery have been found to have worse outcomes compared to those who do not use opioids preoperatively. Opioid-tolerant patients experience greater acute pain and slower resolution of pain despite therapeutic doses [49, 50]. Pain is common and expected after surgery. Developing realistic expectations and a treatment plan is important. Inform patients of the possibility of dysphagia, incisional pain, cervical muscle tension, and persistent neurogenic pain. Postoperative prescriptions are placed for patients to pick up before surgery and have available when they get home. This prevents any delays in their medication regimen and assures the medications are available prior to the surgery.

### 5.3.4  Prehabilitation

Preoperative physical therapy or rehabilitation, also known as prehabilitation, is practiced accelerating the recovery process. Therapy prehabilitation is designed to build up muscle activity, promote the importance of physical activity along with providing equipment to improve independence where required. Cervical and lumbar range of motion exercises and strengthening may improve postoperative functional recovery. The patients begin early mobilization and exercising right after surgery thus preventing any delays waiting for physical therapy referrals. A postoperative plan for gradual increase in activity is reviewed and limitations. Many insurances require physical therapy evaluation and recommendations to be accepted to inpatient rehabilitation facilities. For patients who are going to require inpatient rehabilitation or skilled nursing facility postoperatively. Preop evaluations and submission for authorizations can begin before surgery which will reduce postoperative insurance authorization time and LOS. Even home health and home physical therapy request can be submitted preoperatively. Getting patients to care they need rehabilitation as soon as possible.

### 5.3.5    *Orthotic Care and Instructions*

When orthotic braces/collars are used fitting and care instructions are performed preoperatively. This allows for proper fitting while the patient is not in pain and can concentrate on the instructions. Patients and family members are instructed to bring the devices to surgery to prevent delays in postoperative mobilization of the patient. The nursing team and therapist should all be aware of proper fitting and use of orthotic devices.

### 5.3.6    *Preoperative Surgical Checklist*

Communication with the operating room team in advance to assure equipment and supplies are available for the procedure is essential. A basic spine preoperative checklist, which can be modified to individual surgical techniques, is provided in Fig. 5.1. Items among the checklist include surgical table, fixation frames, and equipment. Imaging including fluoroscopy, O-arm, and neuro-navigation if needed. In case of anatomical variation additional radiological studies and preoperative marker placement can assist in identifying the correct operative level. Recommendations for spine level identification are listed in Fig. 5.2, scheduling of neuromonitoring and other ancillary services. For surgical revision obtain old

1. OR Equipment, special needs, dural repair instruments

2. Surgical Implants and vendors

3. Ancillary services nerve monitoring, blood bank, pharmacy

4. Surgical supplies and medications

5. Radiology needs – fluoroscopy, O-arm, neuro-navigation, Preoperative marker placement to assist with localization and consensus agreement on ambiguous levels being labelled.

6. Outside records and operative reports if indicated

7. Anticoagulation stopped

**Fig. 5.1** Spine preoperative checklist

1. Preoperative Review and marking of anomalous anatomy (extra ribs, extra vertebrae, sacralized vertebrae, etc.)

2. Standardized counting method especially in thoracic area. Count from top and bottom with C2 as landmark and repeat as needed

3. Preoperative skin marker applied or injection of radio-opaque agent

4. Intraoperative confirmation of correct patient images

5. Intraoperative two-person confirmation of correct operative level/ laterality prior to bone removal, discectomy, or instrumentation

6. Utilization of intraoperative neuro-navigation imaging when available

7. Postoperative confirmation of correct surgical level and instrumentation before wound closure

**Fig. 5.2** Recommendations for spine level identification

operative reports and equipment for revision if needed. Any special medications from pharmacy or the blood bank should be conveyed. Contacting instrument companies for implants to be available. This preplanning will reduce surgical time and reduce omissions in the intraoperative pathway.

## 5.3.7 Discharge Planning

The risk assessment and prediction tool (RAPT) can determine if patient will be returning home or will require discharge to a secondary facility [51]. The expected hospital stay and discharge process are reviewed with the family. In addition, postoperative wound care, medications, and activities are reviewed and follow-up appointments discussed. These discussions prior to surgery will facilitate the patient and family's expectations postoperatively and prevent re-admissions.

## 5.4 Perioperative Phase

The perioperative phase focuses on the time of admission, the intraoperative period, and the immediate postoperative period. Having standardized perioperative protocols for elective surgery has been shown to reduce LOS and complications [52]. Preoperatively meet with the patient and family to review the surgical procedure and sign consent. Also, providing family with an estimate of surgical and recovery time will help reduce the anxiety while waiting.

Immediately prior to surgery communication with OR team members to confirm all equipment, medications, instruments and supplies are available from the spine preoperative checklist is essential. In addition, surgeons should review the anesthesia plan emphasizing a multimodal analgesia regimen with providers. In cases of complex cervical spine anatomy or in the presence of instability additional advanced airway adjuncts maybe required. An advanced airway cart with video-laryngoscope/bronchoscope and supplies should be made readily available. Blood pressure regulation is paramount to maintaining spinal cord perfusion in cases of severe spinal stenosis. Hypotension should be avoided which could lead to cord ischemia when the anterior spinal artery is compressed. Confirm all ancillary services including nursing, surgical technicians, radiology, pharmacy, and blood bank are prepared. Perioperative antibiotics, sequential compression devices (SCD), and prevention of hypothermia are a standard part of all surgeries.

### 5.4.1  Nutrition

Prolonged fasting is avoided because it has been proven to exert negative effects on the metabolism and musculature. The use of carbohydrate supplements has been found to be safe and reduce the physiologic stress that fasting has on the body. Limited fasting of light meal up to 6 hours preoperatively are the new guidelines with a carbohydrate beverage up to 2 h preoperative [53].

### 5.4.2  Analgesia

A multimodal analgesia regimen is used to help reduce postoperative pain and reduce opioid usage. Preemptive analgesia aims to prevent postoperative pain through a multimodal approach. Medications include regional anesthesia, nonsteroidal anti-inflammatory drugs (NSAIDS), opioids, anti-convulsants, and acetaminophen. Initially, acetaminophen and gabapentin were administered preoperatively. General anesthesia with endotracheal intubation to secure the airway with total intravenous anesthesia (TIVA) used intraoperatively with propofol, ketamine, ketorolac, lidocaine, antiemetics, and opioids and with permission inhaled agents. TIVA has been shown to reduce intraoperative blood loss in spine and other surgeries [54, 55]. Intraoperative erector spinae field blocks with liposomal bupivacaine can reduce postoperative back pain and facilitate early mobilization [56]. Intraoperative application of epidural duramorph and steroids can reduce pain and inflammation.

Some specific recommendations include Gabapentin 600 mg immediately preop, scopolamine patches for nausea for those with history of post-operative nausea, and IV acetaminophen 975 mg every 6 h for 24 h. Dexamethasone 6–10 mg IV is routinely used even in diabetic patients. Standard use of local anesthetics such as bupivacaine or extended release (Exparel) bupivacaine can be used at the time of closure of the wound. Intraoperative erector spinae field blocks with liposomal bupivacaine can reduce postoperative back pain allow and facilitate early mobilization. In posterior spinal approach cases, an additional deep layer injection along the facet joints and muscle layer will help reduce pain. Muscle relaxants like valium and cyclobenzaprine, ketamine, and ketorolac are also used as adjuncts for pain reduction. Judicious use of intravenous fluids (IVF) should be used to prevent fluid overload. In the immediate postoperative recovery, nursing should continue with multimodal pain management and limit opioid usage to reduce nausea, sedation, and prevent early mobilization of patient.

### 5.4.3  Surgery

Spinal surgery has a growing number of approaches, which may require alternative patient positioning and equipment. There are advantages and disadvantages to many of these approaches. In addition, newer minimally invasive techniques have been developed utilizing these approaches. The surgical approach selected will be determined based on the pathology and surgeon preference. In either case, a standardize surgical approach should be used which all team members are familiar with. The detailed surgical steps are beyond the scope of this chapter. Patients are positioned and padded appropriately to reduce secondary injuries and cautery pads applied. Individual items can be added or deleted to basic pathways depending on the surgical approach selected. Minimally invasive approaches can improve outcomes and reduce hospital stay, LOS, and narcotics usage. A surgical safety checklist is utilized in most operating rooms to help standardize the procedure and reduce complications and errors. However, wrong level surgery remains a problem despite standardized surgical checklist and "time outs". A Spine Surgical Safety Checklist (SSSC) is recommended which would include a second intraoperative 2—person "radiographic time out" (2nd RTO) performed prior to removal of bone, incision of disc, or placement of instrumentation (Table 5.2). Any change in neuromonitoring should be relayed to the surgeon immediately. All attempts to reduce surgical time, blood loss, and tissue trauma will improve outcomes. Having instruments and supplies readily available to address durotomies when they occur. Injection of wound with local anesthetic prior to wound closure is useful in managing postoperative pain and earlier patient mobilization. Application of vancomycin powder to reduce infections has been recommended. If excessive blood loss is expected tranexamic acid has been reported to reduce blood loss during surgery. Skin closure with medical glues provides a waterproof barrier, which can facilitate wound healing, reduce infections, and make wound care easier. Use of foley catheters should be limited and removed early. Alternative external urine collection devices should be utilized instead of foleys when medically indicated.

Neurologic status should be assessed in the operating room or immediately upon arrival to the postoperative care unit. Communication with the family to update them on completion of the surgery, patient disposition, and time in recovery is conveyed. Many hospitals have implemented electronic notifications through monitors,

**Table 5.2** Spine Surgical Safety Checklist (SSSC)

| Preoperative | Intraoperative | Postoperative |
| --- | --- | --- |
| 1. Confirm patient and procedure<br>2. Confirm patient preoperative imaging available<br>3. Identification of anomalous anatomy and confirmation of levels (i.e., transitional vertebrae, rib anomaly, extra vertebrae)<br>4. Consent for surgery confirming procedure to be performed. Including levels and laterality if indicated.<br>5. Diagnosis<br>6. Comorbidities<br>7. Lab, blood bank, and pathology notified of any needs<br>8. Special equipment needs (microscope, neuronavigation, C-arm, etc.)<br>9. Surgical plan and bailout surgical plan<br>10. Implants and biologics | 12. Preop antibiotics given, and antibiotic irrigation used intraoperatively<br>13. Neuro-monitoring assessment<br>14. Patient positioning w/ padding and bolstering. Bed controls operational<br>15. Confirmation of surgical levels and procedure with fluoroscopy<br>16. Intraoperative second 2-person "radiologic level confirmation time out" (2nd RTO) to confirm level/laterality and that relevant imaging matches the patient prior to discectomy or hardware placement.<br>17. Surgical decompression/stabilization, confirm final screw tightening<br>18. Secure hemostasis and minimize drain placement, secure drains and perform drain tug when utilized<br>19. Vancomycin powder application or additional antibiotic beads<br>20. Local anaesthetic infiltration, erector spinae field block<br>21. Final time out to confirm all indicated procedures completed and sponge counts correct<br>22. Final postoperative imaging and wound closure<br>23. Bed disposition (ICU, Med/Surg, Outpatient)<br>24. Specimens labelled correctly, sent off and received<br>25. Post-surgical debriefing | 26. Vital signs check<br>27. Neurological assessment<br>28. Postoperative multimodal pain management<br>29. Confirmation of specimens delivered<br>30. Physiotherapy plan initiated<br>31. Dietary plan initiated<br>32. Foleys removed, external urine collection systems applied if needed. |

pagers, or smart phones which can facilitate this. The importance of early mobilization, multimodal pain management, and resumption of activities of daily living (ADLs) is reiterated to the patient and family members.

## 5.5 Postoperative Phase

### 5.5.1 Nutrition

Early dietary intake encouraged and chewing gum has been found to reduce postoperative ileus and increase intestinal motility [57–60]. Regular use of stool softeners is ordered. Dysphagia from cervical surgery can be a problem so speech pathology referral, and appropriate dietary recommendations should be followed to reduce aspiration risk. Fluid overload should be voided. IVFs should be stopped once taking oral liquids or 4 h after surgery.

### 5.5.2 Respiratory Management

Early incentive spirometry is started in the postoperative area. Spirometry is recommended every hour when awake to reduce atelectasis. Patients are encouraged to continue regular spirometry for 3 days postoperatively. Early mobilization including walking and up to chair for meals will improve respiratory status. Identify any patients with sleep apnea or additional respiratory needs. Breathing treatments should be provided as needed. Close observation of the neck is essential to identify any wound swelling which could compromise the airway. Hematomas, particularly in anterior cervical approaches, can be a life-threatening complication which needs to be addressed emergently.

### 5.5.3 Wound Care

Wound checked and redressed daily. If medical glue is used on the wound ointments and soap should be avoided, which can cause early breakdown of the glue. Wound should be kept clean and dry. A standardized wound care protocol should be established for inpatients. These same wound care and bathing instructions should be reviewed and provided in a written form for discharge home. Specific care instructions for wound care and bathing should be provided to post-acute care facilities, including rehabilitation and skilled nursing facilities.

### 5.5.4 Mobility

Postoperative fear of movement is strongly associated with pain, disability, and physical recovery. Addressing the fear of movement and expectations after surgery will help prepare the patient for early mobilization in the peri-operative and postoperative phases. Early mobilization has significant benefits in the postoperative recovery [61]. A mobility plan with input from nursing and physical therapy should be developed to have better compliance. Postoperative mobility is encouraged 2 h after surgery including walking in halls, to the bathroom and up to chair for meals. Early discontinuation of all drains, IVF and SCDs will allow for easier mobilization of the patients. Ambulatory assist devices/ walkers should be provided early in the post-surgical phase and assessment of home needs re-evaluated. Orthotic care and usage should be reviewed after surgery and again before discharge.

### 5.5.5  *Analgesia*

Traditional postoperative patient controlled analgesic pumps using opioids is discouraged.

Multimodal analgesic will continue until discharge. Explain to patients that pain is normal and review treatments available to reduce pain. Regularly scheduled doses of acetaminophen, anti-inflammatories, gabapentin, anti-anxiolytics, and muscle relaxants can manage most pain. Opioids should be used sparingly for breakthrough pain. It is important for the nursing staff and patients to differentiate types of pain (incisional, muscle, and nerve) they are experiencing so the appropriate medications for treatment can be used. Cryotherapy in the form of ice packs or cooling devices can be used to help reduce neck pain and swelling. Early paracervical and periscapular muscle ROM encouraged to reduce muscle tension. Additional dexamethasone can be used 2–3 days postoperatively to reduce pain and swelling. Continuing a scheduled multimodal analgesic plan for the first week postoperatively can keep most pain under control. Postoperative access to medical providers for issues pertaining to pain or other questions is essential to reduce complications and prevent re-admissions.

### 5.5.6  *Physical Therapy/ Occupational Therapy (OT)*

Many patients with cervical myelopathy and hand weakness benefit from additional therapy services. PT and OT referrals are initiated day of surgery. Home needs including walkers, elevated toilet seats, grabbers, and accessibility needs are determined and provided prior to discharge. Case management evaluation for support services and discharge planning initiated. When the disposition of patients require inpatient rehabilitation services or skilled nursing facility postoperative care instructions should be shared with them. These facilities should continue the ERAS pathway with an emphasis on early mobilization, wound care, and multimodal analgesic to reduce pain. Scheduled surgical follow-ups should be kept.

### 5.5.7 Discharge Planning

Education including collar instructions, wound care, medications, activity level, and follow-up appointments are reviewed. In addition, numbers to contact for questions and postoperative appointments provided. These educational sessions can be held in a group setting for several patients when time and resources are limited. This information can be provided in a booklet the patient receives or through websites or smart phone applications. Many electronic medical records now have direct messaging to the surgeon and his staff.

## 5.6 Post-Discharge Phase

Patients will continue with home health if indicated. Physical therapy regimen either at home or as an outpatient is usually recommended for 4–6 weeks. Longer treatment may be needed for patient with significant cervical disease or cord injury. Each patient should be contacted the next day after discharge by phone and then seen in the office for a 2-week wound check. Close monitoring of symptoms or changes in health should be conveyed to the surgeon's office and seek assistance if needed. Dedicated nursing hotline for questions should be established at the hospital or surgeon's office. Patients are encouraged to resume daily activities with minimal restrictions. Outcome assessment can be determined using the same preoperative cervical assessment tools used. Smart phones can be used to send photos of the wound for evaluation. Some mobile applications can track data including VAS, vital signs, and provide alerts to patients and physicians [31]. The educational discharge information may also be provided in an electronic format they can retrieve from their phone or computer. The use of e-health is very promising, allows for personalized 24-hour monitoring, and does not force postoperative problems onto the general practitioner or external emergency services. Additional, electronic tools and programs at home can facilitate the tracking of patient medications, activities, and provide reminders.

## 5.7 Discussion

The traditional approach to surgical spine care emphasized the surgery and did not address some of the pre and postoperative issues. No standardized pathways existed which allowed for inconsistent care. Traditional approaches called for overnight fasting and minimal perioperative analgesic management. Spine patients were given controlled analgesia using IV morphine and hydromorphone and oral narcotics. No intraoperative checklists were used to avoid complications and errors of omissions during surgery. Despite recent implementation of general surgical checklist over the last decade, wrong level spine surgery and "never" events continued to occur. Wrong-level spine surgery is multifactorial and even with intraoperative imaging errors occur. Issues with intraoperative imaging include the lack of getting intraoperative imaging, mistaken identification of the correct patient and date of imaging, poor image quality, misinterpretation of the images, anatomical variations, or failure to reconfirm the level with intraoperative imaging after exposure has occurred. Recent studies have shown 72% of wrong-site surgery occurred due to lack of a "time-out" and in one study 60% of wrong-level surgery occurred in surgeons who did not perform intraoperative imaging [62, 63].

A second intraoperative 2-person confirmation of level/laterality radiology "time out" will reduce wrong level surgery. Standardized method of counting vertebrae and recognition of lumbosacral transitional vertebrae and anomalous ribs is imperative to identifying the correct levels. There is a general consensus on C2 being used as a reference landmark in most cervical surgeries. Thoracic localization often requires localization from both above and below the proposed surgical level for more accuracy. A comprehensive wall mounted surgical safety checklist in the OR was shown to improve compliance [64]. Spine surgical safety checklist has been shown to reduce intraoperative time by anticipating the needs of the staff and preventing delays [65].

Complications were seen when Foley catheters and IVFs were continued for days significantly limiting mobility and increasing infection risk. Alternative urine collection devices are available which reduce hospital-acquired UTIs. Traditional bed rest after spine surgery with limited mobility, consumption of meals in bed, and limited access to bathroom resulted in additional pressure on back incisions, deep venous thrombosis, prolonged atelectasis leading to pneumonia. Current literature supports early mobilization and the risk reduction benefit. One of the biggest hurdles is overcoming the culture to keep the patients in bed and reducing activity in fear of falls. A team approach between nursing staff and physical therapy is necessary for early mobilization of the patients. Incentive spirometry and sleep apnea machines were not routinely used. Recent studies have showed all these issues have resulted in more complications, LOS, readmissions, and costs. Arnold et al. [66]. found the complications with the largest effect on LOS in ACDF surgery was pulmonary, urinary, and cardiac complications. Many of these could have been avoided with earlier intervention and prevention protocols.

Immobility was often encouraged with no set physical therapy instructions or direction for the nursing staff. Patients requiring additional inpatient rehabilitation services were not often identified until a few days postoperatively leading to delays in referrals and extended LOS. Opioid-related adverse drug events have been shown to occur in over 13% of patients undergoing surgery [49]. These adverse events lead to 55% longer LOS, 47% higher cost of care, 36% increased risk of 30-day readmission, and 3.4 times higher risk of inpatient mortality.

The use of spinal ERAS pathways has been shown to improve pain scores and patient satisfaction surveys while reducing complications, hospital LOS, 30-day readmissions, and hospital cost [9, 50, 51]. Soffin et al. [28] investigated ERAS for anterior cervical discectomy and fusion ($n = 25$) and cervical disc arthroplasty

($n = 8$). Compliance was 85.6%, with patients receiving 18 of 19 ERAS elements. LOS was 416 minutes on average and minimal complications were reported, with no patient requiring readmission in 90 days.

Decreased length of index hospital stay, complications, and readmissions show the economic benefit of ERAS regimens [28, 31, 33, 53]. Another benefit of ERAS for spine surgery is related to total cost savings, which accompany streamlined and less invasive methods. Wang et al. [26, 67] reported savings of $3442 or 15.2% per procedure with the application of ERAS methods, including endoscopic decompression versus traditional TLIF, the anesthetic technique, and liposomal bupivacaine in an acute care setting. In addition, Staartjes et al. [16] showed a reduction in nursing cost of 46.8% associated with ERAS protocol reduction in LOS. Operation time after the ERAS protocol was also decreased, showing further means of potential cost saving. Mathieson et al. [50] reported that patients undergoing spine surgery who received an ERAS preoperative regimen of NSAIDs, acetaminophen, and gabapentin with incorporation of intraoperative intravenous ondansetron and ketamine and a postoperative NSAID course reported greater and earlier mobilization, less opioid use, and decreased nausea and sedation early postoperatively. In addition, LOS was reduced by 2 days for the ERAS intervention group compared with the pre-ERAS cohort.

Utilization of Surgical Safety Checklist and specialty-specific spine modifications have been shown to significantly reduce complications and wrong site surgery [65, 68, 69]. Implementation and adherence appear to be the greatest barriers in adopting these checklists. Institutions must have safety culture environment in place with strong leadership to champion these programs [64, 70]. Spine surgical safety checklist with a focus on reducing WLSS can reduce surgical errors [71, 72].

Minimally invasive surgical techniques represent a logical integration in the ERAS protocol because it has been shown to improve patient satisfaction and pain scores, minimize complications, and shorten recovery time [73–76]. Moreover, additions such as liposomal bupivacaine as a erector spinae field block or direct injection into the incision site have been shown to provide patients with extended local analgesia after spine surgery compared with standard preparations of bupivacaine without impairing healing [26, 56]. Incorporation of ERAS methods in spine surgery may also increase potential for transition to outpatient procedures [77–80]. Alternatively, some protocols used short-acting opioids such as sufentanil to reduce opioid load. Opioid-free anesthesia relies on nonopioid analgesic agents such as propofol, ketamine, and dexmedetomidine and local anesthetic agents to carry out analgesia and anesthesia. Opioid use disorders in spine surgery are also associated with higher complication rates, extended hospitalization, and higher total costs [81]. Nonopioid drugs may achieve intraoperative anesthesia, with reduced postoperative nausea, pain, ileus, and LOS.

Variation in spine surgery and patient populations may differ sufficiently to warrant multiple ERAS protocols depending on indication and intervention. Based on the surgical approach elected to treat spine care pathways may need to be customized and outcomes assessed separately. In comparative studies for treatment of multilevel cervical spondylosis and myelopathy an anterior approach had fewer

**Fig. 5.3** Spine ERAS
Healthcare Team

| Laboratory | Office Staff | Mental Health |
|---|---|---|
| Pharmacy | Surgeon | Dietary |
| Anesthesia | **Patient/ Family** | Physical Therapy |
| Radiology | Nurses | Social Worker |
| Primary Care Physician | Medical Device Representatives | Home Care |

complications, lower morbidity, and better outcome assessment scores compared to posterior cervical fusions [82]. Establishing a modified posterior cervical ERAS pathway may help overcome the short comings of this approach. Modifications to current lumbar spine pathways to cover anterior, oblique, lateral, transforaminal, and posterior surgical approaches may need to be developed.

The current spinel ERAS pathways require a multifaceted team approach to patient care (Fig. 5.3). For the pathways to be effective, it requires the compliance and engagement of all parties, including the patients, surgeon, anesthesia team, nursing staff, and all other providers in each department of the pathway. Maximal benefits are unlikely if there is noncompliance or poor adoption of the pathways. One of the pillars of spinal ERAS is to make the patient proactive in their surgical care. Education provided before, during, and after the surgery is essential for patient compliance in their recovery process and to improve outcomes.

Implementation of spinal ERAS pathways may need to overcome certain barriers. It is always difficult to fight against conservatism and resistance to the adoption of new procedures or innovations, and ERAS is no exception. Resistance can be found at any level and concerns all stakeholders, from the administrative levels to the healthcare staff. Basic surgical routines such as use of drains and foley catheters, the use of a collar or brace, the timing of discharge, the use of opioids, activity level, transport home in a personal car and driving, and so on can vary greatly and significantly influence the LOS. Collaboration and collegial unification of procedures and protocols of care is an essential step in the development of ERAS. Adherence and implementation of surgical checklists is paramount to reducing complications. Optimizing the fluidity of the patient pathway is a prerequisite, as is the appropriate postoperative follow-up. The entirety of care is extended and improved even if the physical stay is shortened.

Spine surgery represents a typically invasive intervention with a protracted recovery phase that often requires rehabilitation and intensive postoperative pain management. Given the benefits of ERAS to decrease complications and improve patient-reported physiologic and psychological states, its incorporation into spine surgery represents a natural transition. In addition, anticipated increases in annual cases of spine surgery from an aging population portends increasing volume of spine surgery. Quantitative quality measures such as patient-reported outcomes have emerged as an objective and increasingly used metric to evaluate surgical success by way of measuring postoperative pain, functional ability, and quality of life after spine surgery. Standardization of ERAS for spine surgery may benefit such patient-reported outcomes, enhance surgeon and patient decision making, and optimize the rehabilitative course. Opportunities for improved outcomes and decreased complication rates also make spine surgery an appropriate setting for ERAS development.

## 5.8  Conclusion

The literature is growing showing the benefits of spinal ERAS pathways. The primary principles of these ERAS pathways include patient education, multimodal pain management, early mobilization, and surgical techniques to reduce blood loss and reduce tissue destruction. The adoption of these pathways can be easily incorporated into most surgical practices. A spine specific surgical checklist is a key component of the intraoperative phase. A second intraoperative time radiological out to confirm correct operative level and side will reduce WLSS. Because of the recent introduction of ERAS to neurosurgery, a consensus has not yet been reached for evidence-based recommendations of cervical ERAS pathways. Lumbar ERAS pathways are further along in development. Additional electronic tools are available to improve communication and compliance and should be adopted into spine surgery practices. This chapter provides a framework for spine ERAS pathways to build upon. In the future, we predict multiple evidence-based approach specific spine ERAS pathways based on approach will be available.

## References


1. Liu JY, Wick EC. Enhanced recovery after surgery and effects on quality metrics. Surg Clin North Am. 2018;98(6):1119–27. https://doi.org/10.1016/j.suc.2018.07.001.
2. Ljungqvist O, Jonathan E. Rhoads lecture 2011: insulin resistance and enhanced recovery after surgery. JPEN J Parenter Enteral Nutr. 2012;36(4):389–98. https://doi.org/10.1177/0148607112445580.
3. Saidian A, Nix JW. Enhanced recovery after surgery: urology. Surg Clin North Am. 2018;98(6):1265–74. https://doi.org/10.1016/j.suc.2018.07.012.
4. Smith HJ, Leath CA III, Straughn JM Jr. Enhanced recovery after surgery in surgical specialties: gynecologic oncology. Surg Clin North Am. 98(6):1275–85. https://doi.org/10.1016/j.suc.2018.07.013.
5. Tiernan JP, Liska D. Enhanced recovery after surgery: recent developments in colorectal surgery. Surg Clin North Am. 2018;98(6):1241–9. https://doi.org/10.1016/j.suc.2018.07.010.

6. Zhu S, Qian W, Jiang C, Ye C, et al. Enhanced recovery after surgery for hip and knee arthroplasty: a systematic review and meta-analysis. Postgrad Med J. 93(1106):736–42. https://doi.org/10.1136/postgradmedj-2017-134991.
7. Ali ZS, Ma TS, Ozturk AK, et al. Pre-optimization of spinal surgery patients: development of a neurosurgical enhanced recovery after surgery (ERAS) protocol. Clin Neurol Neurosurg. 2018;164:142–53. https://doi.org/10.1016/j.clineuro.2017.12.003.
8. Angus M, Jackson K, Smurthwaite G, et al. The implementation of enhanced recovery after surgery (ERAS) in complex spinal surgery. J Spine Surg. 2019;5:116–23. https://doi.org/10.21037/jss.2019.01.07.
9. Brusko GD, Kolcun JP, Heger JA, et al. Reductions in length of stay, narcotics use, and pain following implementation of an enhanced recovery after surgery program for 1- to 3-level lumbar fusion surgery. Neurosurg Focus. 2019;46:E4. https://doi.org/10.3171/2019.1.FOCUS18692.
10. Carr DA, Saigal R, Zhang F, et al. Enhanced perioperative care and decreased cost and length of stay after elective major spinal surgery. Neurosurg Focus. 2019;46:E5. https://doi.org/10.3171/2019.1.FOCUS18630.
11. Dietz N, Sharma M, Adams S, et al. Enhanced recovery after surgery (ERAS) for spine surgery: systematic review. World Neurosurg. 2019;130:415–26. https://doi.org/10.1016/j.wneu.2019.06.181.
12. Elsarrag M, Soldozy S, Patel P, et al. Enhanced recovery after spine surgery: a systematic review. Neurosurg Focus. 2019;46:E3. https://doi.org/10.3171/2019.1.FOCUS18700.
13. Fleege C, Arabmotlagh M, Almajali A, et al. Pre- and postoperative fast-track treatment concepts in spinal surgery: patient information and patient cooperation. Orthopade (Ger). 2014;43(12):1062–4., 1066–9. https://doi.org/10.1007/s00132-014-3040-5.
14. Muhly WT, Sankar WN, Ryan K, et al. Rapid recovery pathway after spinal fusion for idiopathic scoliosis. Pediatrics. 2016;137(4):e20151568. https://doi.org/10.1542/peds.2015-1568.
15. Rao RR, Hayes M, Lewis C, et al. Mapping the road to recovery: shorter stays and satisfied patients in posterior spinal fusion. J Pediatr Orthop. 2017;37(8):e536–42. https://doi.org/10.1097/BPO.0000000000000773.
16. Staartjes VE, de Wisplelaere MP, Schroder ML. Improving recovery after elective degenerative spine surgery: 5-year experience with an enhanced recovery after surgery (ERAS) protocol. Neurosurg Focus. 2019;46(4):E.7. https://doi.org/10.3171/2019.1.FOCUS18646.
17. Venkata HK, van Dellen JR. A perspective on the use of an enhanced recovery program in open, non-instrumented day surgery for degenerative lumbar and cervical spinal conditions. J Neurosurg Sci. 2018;62(3):245–54. https://doi.org/10.23736/S0390-5616.16.03695-X.
18. Wainwright TW, Immins T, Middleton RG. Enhanced recovery after surgery (ERAS) and its applicability for major spine surgery. Best Pract Res Clin Anaesthesiol. 2016;30(1):91–102. https://doi.org/10.1016/j.bpa.2015.11.001.
19. Zhang CH, Yan BS, Xu BS, et al. Study on feasibility of enhanced recovery after surgery combined with mobile microendoscopic discectomy-transforaminal lumbar interbody fusion in the treatment of lumbar spondylolisthesis. Zhonghua Yi Xue Za Zhi (Chinese). 2017;97(23):1790–5. https://doi.org/10.3760/cma.j.issn.0376-2491.2017.23.007.
20. Bradywood A, Farrokhi F, Williams B, et al. Reduction of inpatient hospital length of stay in lumbar fusion patients with implementation of an evidence-based clinical care pathway. Spine. 2017;42(3):169–76. https://doi.org/10.1097/BRS.0000000000001703.
21. Cheung WY, Arvinte D, Wong YW, et al. Reduced acute care costs with the ERAS® minimally invasive transforaminal lumbar interbody fusion compared with conventional minimally invasive transforaminal lumbar interbody fusion. Neurosurgery. 2018;83(4):827–34. https://doi.org/10.1093/neuros/nyx400.
22. Dai B, Gao P, Dong QR, et al. Clinical study of the application of enhanced recovery after surgery in cervical spondylotic myelopathy. Zhongguo Gu Shang (Chinese). 2018;31(8):740–5. https://doi.org/10.3969/j.issn.1003-0034.2018.08.011.
23. Smith J, Probst S, Calandra C, et al. Enhanced recovery after surgery (ERAS) program for lumbar spine fusion. Perioper Med (Lond). 2019;8:4.

24. Soffin EM, Wetmore DS, Beckman JD, et al. Opioid-free anesthesia within an enhanced recovery after surgery pathway for minimally invasive lumbar spine surgery: a retrospective matched cohort study. Neurosurg Focus. 2019;46:E8. https://doi.org/10.3171/2019.1.FOCUS18645.
25. Soffin EM, Vaishnav AS, Wetmore D, et al. Design and implementation of an enhanced recovery after surgery (ERAS) program for minimally invasive lumbar decompression spine surgery: initial experience. Spine (Phila Pa 1976). 2019;44(9):E561–70. https://doi.org/10.1097/BRS.0000000000002905.
26. Wang MY, Chang PY, Grossman J. Development of an enhanced recovery after surgery (ERAS) approach for lumbar spinal fusion. J Neurosurg Spine. 2017;26(4):411–8. https://doi.org/10.3171/2016.9.SPINE16375.
27. Li J, Li H, Xv ZK, et al. Enhanced recovery care versus traditional care following laminoplasty: a retrospective case-cohort study. Medicine (Baltimore). 2018;97:e13195. https://doi.org/10.1097/MD.0000000000013195.
28. Soffin EM, Wetmore DS, Barber LA, et al. An enhanced recovery after surgery pathway: association with rapid discharge and minimal complications after anterior cervical spine surgery. Neurosurg Focus. 2019;46:E9. https://doi.org/10.3171/2019.1.FOCUS18643.
29. Robertson SC. Enhance recovery after surgery (ERAS) spine care pathways for cervical spondylotic myelopathy and OPLL. In: Zileli, Parthiban, editors. WFNS Spine Committee Book: Cervical Spondylotic Myelopathy and OPLL; Chap 25, pp46-58. Springer Publishing, 2021.
30. Chakravarthy VB, Yokoi H, Coughlin DJ, et al. Development and implementation of a comprehensive spine surgery enhanced recovery after surgery protocol: the Cleveland Clinic experience. Neurosurg Focus. 2019;46:E11. https://doi.org/10.3171/2019.1.FOCUS1957.
31. Debono B, Corniola MV, Pietoon R, et al. Benefits of enhanced recovery after surgery for fusion on degenerative spine surgery: impact on outcome, length of stay, and patient satisfaction. Neurosurg Focus. 2019;46:E6. https://doi.org/10.3171/2019.1Focus18669.
32. Grasu RM, Cata JP, Dang AQ, et al. Implementation of an Enhanced Recovery After Spine Surgery program at a large cancer center: a preliminary analysis. J Neurosurg Spine. 2018;29(5):588–98. https://doi.org/10.3171/2018.4.SPINE171317.
33. Nazarenko AG, Konovalov NA, Krutko AV, et al. Postoperative applications of the fast track technology in patients with herniated intervertebral discs of the lumbosacral spine. Zh Vopr Neirokhir Im N N Burdenko (Russian). 2016;80(4):5–12. https://doi.org/10.17116/neiro20168045-12.17.
34. Watts BV, et al. Wrong site spine surgery in the veterans administration. Clin Spine Surg. 2019;32:454–7.
35. Hsiang J. Wrong-level surgery: a unique problem in spine surgery. Surg Neurol Int. 2011;2:47.
36. Mody MG, et al. The prevalence of wrong level surgery among spine surgeons. Spine. 2008;33:194–8.
37. Mayer JE, et al. Analysis of the techniques for thoracic- and lumbar-level localization during posterior spine surgery and the occurrence of wrong-level surgery: results from a national survey. Spine J. 2014;14:741–8.
38. Mesfin A, Canham C, Okafor L. Prevention training of wrong-site spine surgery. J Surg Educ. 2015;72:680–4.
39. Paull DE, et al. Errors upstream and downstream to the Universal Protocol associated with wrong surgery events in the Veterans Health Administration. Am J Surg. 2015;210:6–13.
40. Hadjipavlou AG, Marshall RW. Wrong site surgery. Bone Jt J. 2013;95-B:434–5.
41. James MA, Seiler JG, Harrast JJ, Emery SE, Hurwitz S. The occurrence of wrong-site surgery self-reported by candidates for certification by the American Board of Orthopaedic Surgery. J Bone Joint Surg Am. 2012;94:e2(1-12).
42. Goodkin R, Laska LL. Wrong disc space level surgery: medicolegal implications. Surg Neurol. 2004;61:323–41. discussion 341-342
43. Mannoji C, et al. Radiograms obtained during anterior cervical decompression and fusion can mislead surgeons into performing surgery at the wrong level. Case Rep Orthop. 2014;2014:398457.

44. Al-Tamimi YZ, Guilfoyle M, Seeley H, et al. Measurement of long-term outcome in patients with cervical spondylotic myelopathy treated surgically. Eur Spine J. 22(11):2552–7. Published online 2013 Aug 30. https://doi.org/10.1007/s00586-013-2965-4.

45. Cheung WY, Arvinte D, Wong YW, et al. Neurological recovery after surgical decompression in patients with cervical spondylotic myelopathy - a prospective study. Int Orthop. 2008;32(2):273–8. https://doi.org/10.1007/s00264-006-0315-4.

46. Kalsi-Ryan S, Singh A, Massicotte EM, et al. Ancillary outcome measures for assessment of individuals with cervical spondylotic myelopathy. Spine (Phila Pa 1976). 2013;38(22 Suppl 1):S111–S22. https://doi.org/10.1097/BRS.0b013e3182a7f499.

47. Salvi FJ, Jones JC, Weigert BJ. The assessment of cervical myelopathy. Spine J. 2006;6(6 Suppl):182S–9S.

48. Dos Santos JC, Soares EC, Fihlo HRC, et al. Nutritional risk factors for postoperative complications in Brazilian elderly patients undergoing major elective surgery. Nutrition. 2003;19:321–6.

49. Martini ML, Nistal DA, Deustch BC, et al. Characterizing the risk and outcome profiles of lumbar fusion procedures in patients with opioid use disorders: a step toward improving enhanced recovery protocols for a unique patient population. Neurosurg Focus. 2019;46:E12. https://doi.org/10.3171/2019.1.FOCUS18630.

50. Mathiesen O, Dahl B, Thomsen BA, et al. A comprehensive multimodal pain treatment reduces opioid consumption after multilevel spine surgery. Eur Spine J. 2013;22:2089–96. https://doi.org/10.1007/s00586-013-2826-1.

51. Slover J, Mullaly K, Karia R, et al. The use of the risk assessment and prediction tool in surgical patients in a bundled payment program. Int J Surg. 2017;38:119–22. https://doi.org/10.1016/j.ijsu.2016.12.038.

52. Sivaganesan A, Wick JB, Chotai S, et al. Perioperative protocol for elective spine surgery is associated with reduced length of stay and complications. J Am Acad Orthop Surg. 2019;27(5):183–9. https://doi.org/10.5435/JAAOS-D-17-00274.

53. Apelbaum J, Agarkar M, Connis RT, et al. Practice guidelines for preoperative fasting and the use of pharmacologic agents to reduce the risk of pulmonary aspiration: application to healthy patients undergoing elective procedures an updated report by the American Society of Anesthesiologists Task Force on Preoperative Fasting and the Use of Pharmacologic Agents to Reduce the Risk of Pulmonary Aspiration. Anesthesiology. 2017;126:376–93.

54. Shamloul M, Abd-Elgaleel A, Askar I. Total intravenous anaesthesia versus volatile induction and maintenance anaesthesia for controlled hypotension in lumbar spine fixation surgery: comparative clinical study. Egypt J Hosp Med. 2018;73(4):6555–61. https://doi.org/10.21608/ejhm.2018.15416.

55. Moffatt DC, McQuitty RA, Wright AE, Kamucheka TS, Haider AL, Chaaban MR. Evaluating the role of anesthesia on intraoperative blood loss and visibility during endoscopic sinus surgery: a meta-analysis. Am J Rhinol Allergy. 2021;35(5):674–84. https://doi.org/10.1177/1945892421989155. Epub 2021 Jan 21. PMID: 33478255

56. Greenbaum AB, et al. Erector spinae fascial plane blocks with liposomal bupivacaine improve enhanced recovery parameters compared with thoracic epidural anesthesia. J Am Coll Surg. 2019;229(4):S173.

57. Charoenkwan K, Matovinovic E. Early versus delayed oral fluids and food for reducing complications after major abdominal gynecologic surgery. Cochrane Database Syst Rev. 2014;2014(12):CD004508. https://doi.org/10.1002/14651858.CD004508.pub4.

58. Fujii T, Morita H, Sutoh T, et al. Benefit of oral feeding as early as one day after elective surgery for colorectal cancer: oral feeding on first versus second postoperative day. Int Surg. 2014;99(3):211–5. https://doi.org/10.9738/INTSURG-D-13-00146.1.

59. Hoshi T, Yamashita S, Tanaka M, et al. Early oral intake after arthroscopic surgery under spinal anesthesia. J Anesth. 1999;13(4):205–8. https://doi.org/10.1007/s005400050058.

60. Xiaorong Y, Ye L, Zhao L, et al. Early versus delayed postoperative oral hydration after general anesthesia: a prospective randomized trial. Int J Clin Exp. 2014;7(10):3491–6.

61. Epstein NE. A review article on the benefits of early mobilization following spinal surgery and other medical/surgical procedures. Surg Neurol Int. 2014;5(Suppl 3):S66–73. https://doi.org/10.4103/2152-7806.130674.
62. Stahel PF, Mehler PS, Clarke TJ, Varncll J. The 5th anniversary of the 'universal protocol': pitfalls and pearls revisited. Patient Saf Surg. 2009;3:14.
63. El-Ghandour NMF, Aguirre AO, Goel A, Kandeel H, Ali TM, Chaurasia B, Elmorsy S, Abdel Aziz MS, Soliman MAR. Neurosurgical wrong surgical site in lower-middle- or low-income countries (LMICs): a survey study. World Neurosurg. 2021;152:e235–40. https://doi.org/10.1016/j.wneu.2021.05.079. Epub 2021 May 28
64. Cushley C, Knight T, Murray H, Kidd L. Writing's on the wall: improving the WHO Surgical Safety Checklist. BMJ Open Qual. 2021;10(1):e001086. https://doi.org/10.1136/bmjoq-2020-001086. PMID: 33452183; PMCID: PMC7813408
65. Suresh V, Ushakumari PR, Pillai CM, Kutty RK, Prabhakar RB, Peethambaran A. Implementation and adherence to a speciality-specific checklist for neurosurgery and its influence on patient safety. Indian J Anaesth. 2021;65(2):108–14. https://doi.org/10.4103/ija.IJA_419_20. Epub 2021 Feb 10. PMID: 33776084; PMCID: PMC7983834
66. Arnold PM, Rice LR, Anderson KK, et al. Factors affecting hospital length of stay following anterior cervical discectomy and fusion. Evid Based Spine Care J. 2011;2(3):11–8. https://doi.org/10.1055/s-0030-1267108.
67. Wang MY, Chang HK, Grossman J. Reduced acute care costs with the ERAS® minimally invasive transforaminal lumbar interbody fusion compared with conventional minimally invasive transforaminal lumbar interbody fusion. Neurosurgery. 2018;83:827–34. https://doi.org/10.1093/neuros/nyx400.
68. Papadakis M, Meiwandi A, Grzybowski A. The WHO safer surgery checklist time out procedure revisited: strategies to optimise compliance and safety. Int J Surg. 2019;69:19–22. https://doi.org/10.1016/j.ijsu.2019.07.006. Epub 2019 Jul 13
69. Treadwell JR, Lucas S, Tsou AY. Surgical checklists: a systematic review of impacts and implementation. BMJ Qual Saf. 2014;23(4):299–318. https://doi.org/10.1136/bmjqs-2012-001797. Epub 2013 Aug 6. PMID: 23922403; PMCID: PMC3963558
70. Weinger MB. Time out! Rethinking surgical safety: more than just a checklist. BMJ Qual Saf. 2021;30(8):613–7. https://doi.org/10.1136/bmjqs-2020-012600. Epub 2021 Mar 23
71. Kulkarni AG, Patel JY, Asati S, Mewara N. "Spine Surgery Checklist": a Step towards Perfection through Protocols. Asian Spine J. 2022;16(1):38–46. https://doi.org/10.31616/asj.2020.0432. Epub 2021 May 21. PMID: 34015208; PMCID: PMC8873991
72. Vitale M, Minkara A, Matsumoto H, Albert T, Anderson R, Angevine P, Buckland A, Cho S, Cunningham M, Errico T, Fischer C, Kim HJ, Lehman R Jr, Lonner B, Passias P, Protopsaltis T, Schwab F, Lenke L. Building consensus: development of best practice guidelines on wrong level surgery in spinal deformity. Spine Deform. 2018;6(2):121–9. https://doi.org/10.1016/j.jspd.2017.08.005. Epub 2017 Oct 18
73. Fletcher ND, Shourbaji N, Mitchell PM, et al. Clinical and economic implications of early discharge following posterior spinal fusion for adolescent idiopathic scoliosis. J Child Orthop. 2019;46(4):257–2632014. https://doi.org/10.3171/2019.1.FOCUS18700.
74. Gornitzky AL, Flynn JM, Muhly WT, et al. A rapid recovery pathway for adolescent idiopathic scoliosis that improves pain control and reduces time to inpatient recovery after posterior spinal fusion. Spine Deform. 2016;4(4):288–95. https://doi.org/10.1016/j.jspd.2016.01.001.
75. Lee L, Feldman LS. Enhanced recovery after surgery: economic impact and value. Surg Clin North Am. 2018;98(6):1137–48. https://doi.org/10.1016/j.suc.2018.07.003.
76. Lee L, Mata J, Ghitulescu GA, et al. Cost-effectiveness of enhanced recovery versus conventional perioperative management for colorectal surgery. Ann Surg. 2015;262(6):1026–33. https://doi.org/10.1097/SLA.0000000000001019.
77. Sanders AE, Andras LM, Sousa T, et al. Accelerated discharge protocol for posterior spinal fusion patients with adolescent idiopathic scoliosis decreases hospital postoperative charges 22%. Spine (Phila Pa 1976). 2017;42(2):92–7. https://doi.org/10.1097/BRS.0000000000001666.

78. Goldstein CL, Macwan K, Sundararajan K, et al. Perioperative outcomes and adverse events of minimally invasive versus open posterior lumbar fusion: meta-analysis and systematic review. J Neurosurg Spine. 2016;24(3):416–27. https://doi.org/10.3171/2015.2.SPINE14973.
79. Lu VM, Kerezoudis P, Gilder HE, et al. Minimally invasive surgery versus open surgery spinal fusion for spondylolisthesis: a systematic review and meta-analysis. Spine (Phila Pa 1976). 2017;42(3):E177–85. https://doi.org/10.1097/BRS.0000000000001731.
80. Phan K, Mobbs RJ. Minimally invasive versus open laminectomy for lumbar stenosis: a systematic review and meta-analysis. Spine (Phila Pa 1976). 2016;41(2):E91–E100. https://doi.org/10.1097/BRS.0000000000001161.
81. Kessler ER, Shah M, Gruschkus SK. Cost and quality implications of opioid-based postsurgical pain control using administrative claims data from a large health system: opioid-related adverse events and their impact on clinical and economic outcomes. Pharmacotherapy. 2013;33(4):383–91. https://doi.org/10.1002/phar.1223.
82. Shamj MF, Cook C, Pietrobon R, et al. Impact of surgical approach on complications and resource utilization of cervical spine fusion: a nationwide perspective to the surgical treatment of diffuse cervical spondylosis. Spine J. 2009;9(1):31–8. https://doi.org/10.1016/j.spinee.2008.07.005.

# Chapter 6
# Myelomeningocele: Long-Term Neurosurgical Management


**E. Marcati, G. Meccariello, L. Mastino, M. Picano, P. D. Giorgi, and G. Talamonti**


## Contents




E. Marcati · G. Meccariello · L. Mastino · M. Picano · G. Talamonti (✉)
Department of Neurosurgery, ASST Niguarda Hospital, Milan, Italy

P. D. Giorgi
Department of Orthopedics, ASST Niguarda Hospital, Milan, Italy



© The Author(s), under exclusive license to Springer Nature Switzerland AG 2024

C. Di Rocco (ed.), *Advances and Technical Standards in Neurosurgery*, Advances and Technical Standards in Neurosurgery 49, https://doi.org/10.1007/978-3-031-42398-7_6

## 6.1    Introduction

Open spina bifida or myelomeningocele (MMC) is the most challenging and complex birth defect of the central nervous system compatible with life [1].

A failure in the dorsal fusion of the nascent neural tube during embryonic life is responsible for this abnormal spinal cord development.

The standard surgical strategy consists in the early anatomical reconstruction of the defect after birth. Even if there is no consensus about the timing of MMC repair, surgery within the first 48–72 h is often recommended to prevent cerebrospinal fluid (CSF) infection, further neurological deterioration, and to reduce the risk of shunt malfunction; indeed, an additional risk of shunt occlusion due to the increase of proteins and debris in the CSF when MMC repair is performed later has been described [1].

The MMC repair is only the first step in the treatment pathway for these patients. Hydrocephalus, Chiari malformation Type 2 (CM II), tethered cord syndrome (TCS), and scoliosis are the most common problems they will face during the rest of their life. Other conditions that may greatly impact on the long-term outcome and quality of life are latex allergy, alimentary disturbances, progressively worsening bladder and bowel syndromes, psychological and cognitive complications related to the neurological deficits, and/or urological and sexual dysfunctions.

In the last decades, prenatal MMC repair is gaining acceptance, since it decreases the rates of CM II and hydrocephalus [2–5]. Nevertheless, some concerns are being addressed and perplexities remain in the scientific community. Apart from the maternal risks and the preterm delivery [3, 6], the postnatal "better" neurological outcome is not clearly demonstrated [7]. There is a higher need of postnatal repair for wound dehiscence and cerebrospinal fluid leakage [4, 8–12], secondary tethered cord syndrome (TCS) seems to have higher incidence and earlier occurrence [10, 13], and high postnatal mortality has been recently reported [4, 5].

Regardless of the technique used for MMC repair, these patients will require medical and neurosurgical care for all their life.

## 6.2    Hydrocephalus

Hydrocephalus is one of the most common comorbidities associated with MMC, representing a significant adverse prognostic factor in terms of intellectual development and survival [14, 15]. Its incidence following postnatal closure of the MMC defect ranges from 63% to 91% [16–19], whereas it affects only 40% of prenatally treated patients [3, 9]. However, Chakraborty et al. [20] recently reported that the incidence of hydrocephalus in MMC children operated after delivery has dropped to 50% due to better general management and patient selection. In high-income country, advances in prenatal diagnosis have resulted in a decrease in children with high-level lesions whose pregnancy is often interrupted. Consequently, there is a decrease in MMC children with hydrocephalus, since higher the level of lesion, higher is the risk of hydrocephalus.

Several mechanisms have been advocated to explain and classify MMC-related hydrocephalus. Raimondi et al. postulated that the overcrowded posterior cranial fossa, due to the development of the nervous and vascular structures in an inadequate osseous container, could cause a "constrictive hydrocephalus" in MMC [16].

In 1989, McLone and Knepper [21] proposed their unified theory to explain hydrocephalus and CM II. The continuous loss of CSF through the spinal defect causes an insufficient mesenchymal induction during the embryonic life, resulting in a hypoplastic posterior cranial fossa, caudal descent of the hindbrain, and secondary hydrocephalus.

Probably, the hydrocephalus in MMC is related to both CSF obstruction and reduced reabsorption. The CM II could lead to the occlusion of the IV ventricle's outlets, affecting the CSF circulation at the cervico-medullary junction. Additionally, the typical hindbrain herniation present in CM II can hinder the CSF flow at the aqueduct level. On the other hand, the overcrowded posterior cranial fossa may generate an increased resistance to the cerebral venous outflow with reduction in the CSF reabsorption [14–16, 21].

### 6.2.1 Timing of Shunt Surgery

According to the neurosurgical aphorism that "the ideal shunt is no shunt", in the last years, efforts have been done to identify MMC patients who really need CSF diversion [20]. Indeed, ventriculomegaly is a common finding but is not necessarily progressive and may stabilise without any intervention [14, 22, 23].

Therefore, the decision for shunt placement must depend on both severity and progression of ventricular dilation.

The timing for shunting still represents a not definitely settled question. The hydrocephalus may be already present at birth, but it often develops within a few weeks. Several authors advocate shunt insertion at the same time of MMC closure. Hubballah reported no significant increase in the infection risk when coincident MMC closure and shunt placement is performed [24]. Indeed, by reducing the likelihood of CSF leak, shunt placement could help wound healing, protect the brain from the effects of hydrocephalus, and reduce hospital stay [25, 26].

In 1995, Pang suggested that, after surgery, in MMC newborns a particular catabolic response takes place, related to the surgical stress, the general anaesthesia, and the blood transfusion. During this period, anabolic processes are reduced, including wound healing and resistance to infections. This phenomenon, together with the immature immune system of newborns, the CSF exposure to organisms from the open sac, transient bacteraemia during surgical manipulation for back closure, and unrecognised urinary tract infections were suggested as risk factors of simultaneous MMC repair and shunt treatment [27]. Furthermore, careful dural and muscular closure should result in a dry wound even in cases of gross hydrocephalus [15].

Indeed, except for few selected cases, shunt placement may be postponed without significant risks. It has been reported that one-week interval between MMC repair and shunt placement represents a safe period for both wound healing and risks of shunt infection/obstruction [1].

In 2008, Chakraborty published his experience, demonstrating a significant reduction in the VPS placement rate (51.9%) avoiding early treatment in asymptomatic patients even in case of some degree of ventricular dilation [20]. Namely, the incidence of hydrocephalus requiring VPS is coming close to the rates reported following prenatal MMC repair [28].

### 6.2.2  Shunt Failure

Shunt failure is generally caused by either shunt malfunction or shunt infection. The need for shunt placement in MMC has been found to correlate with a negative effect on long-term outcome. Indeed, the main determinants of reduced longevity and IQ are device infections rather than a valve per se [29].

In paediatric patients without MMC, the average failure rate ranges 23–33% [30]. Considering the whole lifetime, 84% of all patients with hydrocephalus require at least one VPS revision [31]. Shunt-related complications seem to be higher in patients with MMC and long-term follow-up [32]. Bowman and co-workers reported 95% of shunt failure rate with 20–25 years of follow-up. The most common cause of shunt malfunction in MMC patients is infection, and it occurs mainly in the first year of placement [33]. Anyway, the risk of shunt malfunction persists all lifelong.

Clinical manifestations of shunt malfunction in patients with MMC may be extremely variable and ambiguous, making the diagnosis quite difficult [1, 15, 34]. Beside classical symptoms and signs of increased intracranial pressure (ICP), because of the specific pathophysiology of MMC, shunt malfunction might increase the ventricular pressure without progressive ventriculomegaly, could mimic CM II and tethered cord imbalance, or could result in syringomyelia [1, 35]. Therefore, facing a deterioration in neurological performances in MMC-children with hydrocephalus, it is always imperative to first assess shunt function [1]. The MMC-related hydrocephalus is typically chronic, and these patients develop a greater ability to compensate high ICP, so that signs and symptoms of shunt failure can be very sneaky. It is quite common to find a slight decrease in school performances, hyperactivity, and emotional disturbances as the only symptoms of shunt malfunction. Clinical manifestations can even develop with unchanged or slit ventricles. On the other hand, asymptomatic shunt malfunction can also occur. Shunt independence may be theoretically possible. It has been reported in 3.2% of children with non-tumoral hydrocephalus, 22% of them affected by MMC [36]. About 50% of MMC patients older than 7 years has a nonfunctioning shunt, clearly documented on X-rays (i.e. tubing fractures, disconnections, or obstruction) and remains totally asymptomatic with unchanged ventricular size [37]. In these circumstances, it is reasonable to avoid shunt revision and propose a strictly clinical observation [1, 36].

However, all signs and symptoms of shunt failure must be carefully investigated in order to avoid a dramatic evolution. When compensatory mechanisms are exhausted, sudden death due to respiratory or cardiac arrest may occur. Because of the presence of CM II, children with MMC would be more exposed to these events [15, 38, 39]. Hydrocephalus would destabilise the equilibrium of CM II, which would be the ultimate cause of sudden death [1, 35].

In 2010, Tennant and co-workers found a reduced 20-years survival rate in children affected by both spina bifida and hydrocephalus, going from 86.7% without hydrocephalus to 50% with [40].

We have developed an algorithm for surgical indication in asymptomatic MMC-patients with non-functioning VPS (Fig. 6.1). Patients with recent (less than 1 year) shunt placement or revision undergo shunt replacement regardless of their asymptomatic status. Conversely, all asymptomatic patients without shunt surgery during the last year are carefully and periodically investigated by the neurosurgeon and the paediatric neuropsychologist and neuroimaging is repeated. The availability of a baseline imaging study obtained when the VPS was working correctly is of paramount importance, since it represents the basis for comparison in these patients who frequently present with wide and anomalous ventricles. Meanwhile, we have aggressive indications for shunt revision in patients who are symptomatic, even if

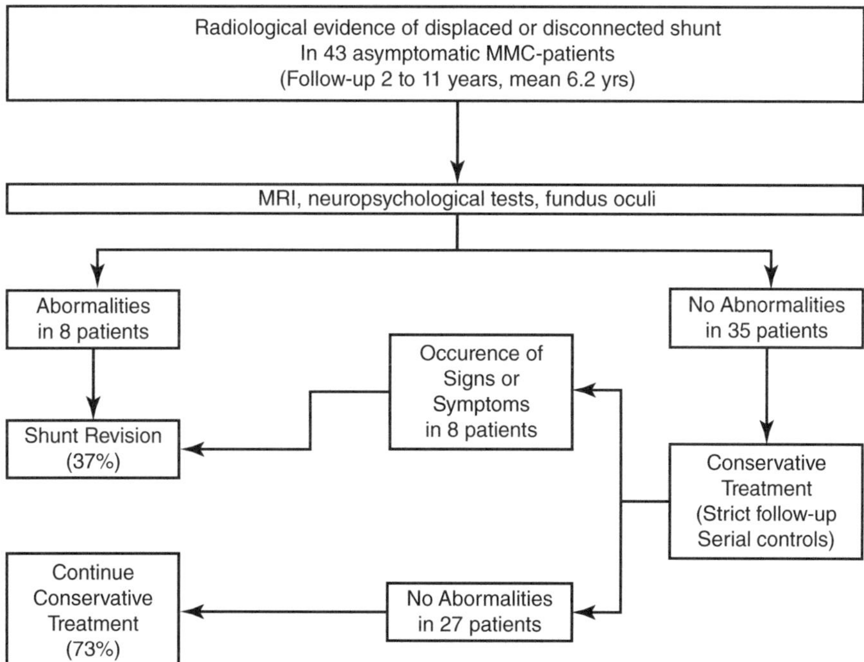


**Fig. 6.1** Algorithm for the management of asymptomatic patients with disconnected or displaced ventriculoperitoneal shunts. To be enrolled in this protocol, no surgery must have been required within the last year

the symptoms are mild or unusual. In our experience, death and severe morbidity usually represent consequences of delayed shunt malfunction recognition, while shunt revision is a relatively safe procedure (~0.5% of both mortality and morbidity rates in our series) [1].

### 6.2.3 Endoscopic Third Ventriculostomy

Endoscopic third ventriculostomy (ETV) has been proposed as an alternative CSF diversion technique in MMC [41]. However, the ETV success rate is quite low in all infants below 1 year of age, but even worse in MMC-children. Jones and Kwok's series [42] of 25 patients affected by MMC-related hydrocephalus reported successful ETV in 1 of 11 newborns despite initial good fenestration of the floor of the third ventricle. MMC is a dysraphism, thus a malformation of the midline that may pose serious problem to perform ETV (Fig. 6.2). Mori et al. identified on preoperative MRI and CT scans the presence of several anatomical features hampering the success of the procedure: a huge massa intermedia (63.2%), sloping of the third ventricle floor (30%), a narrow anteroposterior length of the third ventricle floor (20%), and a narrow prepontine cistern with crowding of the posterior fossa (38.1%) [43]. Pavez and co-workers reported abnormal findings, including the inability to recognise any mammillary bodies, the presence of septations, atypical veins in the floor of the third ventricle, floor umbilications, and arachnoid adherences [44]. Other authors confirmed the lack, in MMC-related hydrocephalus, of a suitable anatomical conformation for performing an endoscopic procedure [1, 16, 45, 46].

Hydrocephalus in MMC can evolve over time [1, 41]. Gradually, the continuous extrathecal CSF drainage and progressive maturation of the subarachnoid space reduce the intracranial pressure, leading to a cranial bone overgrowth and a further overcrowding of posterior cranial fossa. This will worsen the aqueductal stenosis

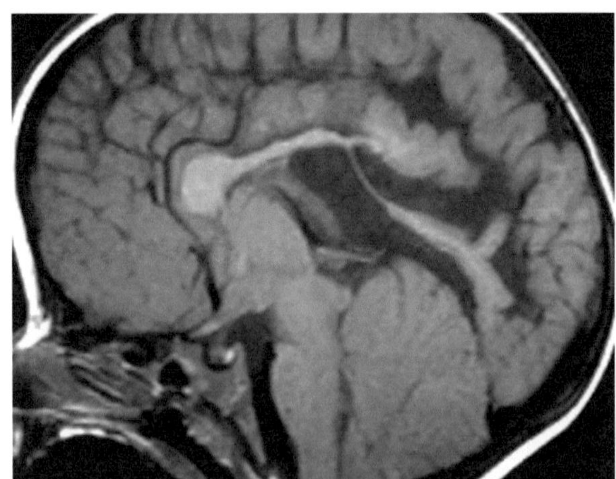

**Fig. 6.2** MRI, T1 weighted image, sagittal view obtained in a 3-year-old MMC child. A huge *massa intermedia* precludes any endoscopic third ventriculostomy. Other malformations are evident on the *corpus callosum,* the parieto-occipital cortex, the brainstem, and the cerebellum

and transform the hydrocephalus primarily in an obstructive type. In this setting, ETV may become an effective and suitable treatment [16, 17, 47]. In 1996, Teo and Jones [41] published a large series of patients treated with ETV affected by MMC-related hydrocephalus. They reported an overall success rate of 72%, with a significant difference between children with less than 6 months (12.5%) and over 6 months (80%), and if the ETV was performed as a primary procedure (29%) or at the time of shunt malfunction (84%). On the other hand, progressive hydrocephalus due to shunt malfunction without related MMC had a long-term success in 13/14 cases.

In our practice, ETV is no longer offered as a first-line treatment for newborns with MMC, but instead as a second option after VP shunt failure [1]. Anyway, in our series, the rate of MMC-patients who become shunt-free after ETV is 61.2% that is lower than patients with obstructive but higher than patients with post-infective or post-haemorrhagic hydrocephalus [47].

In MMC patients, neuroendoscopy remains invaluable for performing other manoeuvres than ETV, such as aqueductoplasty, stenting, pellucidotomy, and freeing the catheter tip from the choroid plexus, and/or retrieving catheter fragments from the ventricles [1].


## 6.3 Arnold-Chiari Malformation and Brainstem Dysfunction

In the current classification, Arnold-Chiari malformation or Chiari Malformation type II is defined as the descent of cerebellar tonsils, brainstem, and fourth ventricle through the foramen magnum (FM) and occurs almost exclusively in patients with MMC [48].

In 1883, Cleland first reported the distortion of the "inferior vermiform process, which extends up so far that what appears to be the pyramid touches the corpora quadrigemina, whereas the uvula looks backwards and the laminated tubercle hangs down from an exaggerated velum posticum, as an appendix ¾ of an inch in length, lying in the fourth ventricle" [49]. Later, in 1891, Hans Chiari described three different malformations [50], and in 1896, he classified four different types, including CM type II, which was defined as hindbrain herniation typically present in patients affected by MMC [48]. In 1894, Arnold reported a case of MMC associated with the downward dislocation of the fourth ventricle [51]; therefore, later in 1907, the nomenclature of CMII was changed in Arnold-Chiari malformation. Several authors then proposed new criteria up to the current classification of CM in 6 types [52]. Beside hindbrain herniations, a wide range of supratentorial and infratentorial anomalies and skull malformations with varying degrees of severity are found in CM II. The cerebellar vermis, displaced below the FM, can even reach the thoracic spine. The cerebellum is typically hypoplastic, the cisterna magna is often absent, and a "cerebellar inversion" is quite common, with an upward herniation of the cerebellum over the tentorium. These classical features produce the typical ultrasonographic "banana signs". Other characteristic aspects of CM II are a small posterior cranial fossa that appears "overcrowded", a low insertion of the tentorium, a dorsal medullary "kink" in the cervical spine due to the dorsal displacement of the brainstem. In the supratentorial compartment, fusion of the colliculi, a large massa intermedia, agenesis of the corpus callosum, and ventricular anomalies are common. Colpocephaly, consisting in a consistent enlargement of the occipital horns compared with the frontal ones, is typical. Finally, skull malformations, such as Lückenschädel or lacunar skull and shortening of the clivus, are also frequently described in CM II [48].

## 6.3.1  Pathophysiological Mechanisms

Different mechanisms have been proposed, failing to explain all the typical features of CM II. Then, in 1989, McLone and Knepper proposed a unifying theory involving both the neuroectodermal and the mesenchymal growth deficiency [21]. According to the authors, during the embryonic and foetal life, the open neural tube drains the whole CSF interfering with the normal neurocele occlusion. A proper occlusion is required to ensure ventricles expansion and maturation and essential for the neural and calvarian development. Consequently, the loss of ventricle distension seen in CM II causes a reduced development of the posterior cranial fossa, causing the dislocation of cerebellum and brainstem, respectively, cephalad and caudad.

Finally, hydrocephalus would be the consequence of the crowded posterior cranial fossa and the occlusion of CFS outflow at the foramina of Luschka and Magendie. This hypothesis is also corroborated by the evidence that intrauterine closure reduces the incidence and severity of CM II [53].

## 6.3.2  Clinical Features

Several authors consider the CM II syndrome as the main factor determining the quality of life, survival, and independence of individuals with MMC [1, 54].

Clinical manifestations of CM II are various and complex and, in this scenario, hydrocephalus plays a critical role; indeed, the increased ICP could exacerbate brainstem compression and downward dislocation turning a radiographic CM II into a symptomatic one. It is well known that shunt placement could completely reverse the CM II syndrome [1, 35, 48, 54, 55].

Signs and symptoms of brainstem and cranial nerves dysfunction have been explained with different theories, including cranial nerves traction, particularly on the vagus nerve, vascular impairment determining brainstem ischaemia, infarction, necrosis, primary dysgenesis, and hypoplasia of cranial nerve nuclei [56].

However, symptoms of CM II are commonly described as more severe and rapidly progressive in neonates, often manifesting with a "stereotyped pattern" [57, 58]. Dysphagia usually appears as the first sign, followed by stridor, apnea, and finally quadriparesis and opisthotonos [48, 57].

Neurogenic dysphagia is usually related to glossopharyngeal and vagus nerve dysfunction and manifests with swallowing impairment causing aspiration with pneumonitis, absence of gag reflex, choking, nasal regurgitation, and poor feeding, leading to weight loss and malnutrition [48, 54]. Stridor is due to airway obstruction. It is initially inspiratory and evolves subsequently becoming generalised. It is usually related to bilateral vocal cord abductor paresis or plegia due to vagus nerve traction or brainstem compression and generally resolves spontaneously or after shunt placement or cervical decompression [56, 59]. Prolonged expiratory apnea with cyanosis (PEAC) is a total cessation of expiratory effort that appears generally during frightened or painful experiences, causing cyanosis, bradycardia, can lead to death, and does not relief by mechanical ventilation. PEAC seems to be related to both reversible factors, such as caudal displacement of the brainstem and mechanical compression of the medulla, and irreversible factors, such as developmental immaturity of the respiratory centres, hypoplasia or aplasia of bulbar cranial nerve nuclei, or ischaemic and haemorrhagic events in the brainstem [59, 60].

In older children, symptoms of CM II tend to be subtler and are rarely life threatening. Clinical manifestations of cervical myelopathy are predominant with a slowly progressive muscular weakness, spasticity, loss in dexterity, and gait disturbances [1]. As in CM I, occipital headache may be present as the sole symptom. Clinical manifestations of syringomyelia should always be carefully investigated [1, 48, 54].

Even if virtually present in all children affected by MMC, CM II is described as clinically relevant in only 20–30% of cases [1, 35, 61, 62].

Considering that most symptoms are not present at birth, some authors advocated neuronal destruction due to compressive forces as the main cause of brainstem dysfunction rather than primary dysgenesis. Accordingly, they proposed an early and aggressive surgical treatment with cranio-cervical decompression (CCD) even in cases of moderate symptoms and controlled hydrocephalus [57, 61]. On the other hand, other authors, supporting the idea of an intrinsic hindbrain dysgenesis, recommended VPS placement or revision as the first line of treatment [1, 35]. Patients who do not respond to VPS should be promptly managed by CCD in order to avoid further brainstem damages [54, 63].

In our series, CM II was documented by MRI in 99% of patients. Despite some symptoms, such as swallowing disturbances, were relatively frequent, clear symptomatology was reported in one-third of patients: those with serious symptoms (especially if newborns) underwent immediate treatment. Conversely, those with mild and not progressive symptoms (especially if teens or adults) were strictly followed. The patients who eventually required surgery for CM II syndrome were 11.4%. In all cases, treatment started with shunt placement/revision or external ventricular drainage (EVD). Even patients without evidence of shunt malfunction first underwent EVD. One-half of patients improved with CSF drainage, whereas the other half had to be managed by CCD [1, 35]. There was a clear relationship between age and the need for CCD: newborns and infants younger than 3 years of age were more likely to require CCD.

In newborns, the mortality rate after CCD has been reported to decrease from 70% to 15–20% when an urgent surgical treatment is performed [48]. Although the prognosis remained poor for intrinsic abnormalities of the brainstem, the CCD could provide time for its maturation. Older patients usually improved with CCD, suggesting that, in these population with more mature brainstem, a major role was played by compressive pathogenesis [1].

### *6.3.3 Surgical Technique*

From an operative point of view, some authors prefer the term "posterior cervical decompression" instead of "foramen magnum decompression". Indeed, in CM II, the FM is often large and the torcular is usually low-lying, making the suboccipital craniectomy risky and sometimes unnecessary.

A midline incision from the FM to the lowest level of cerebellar descent is suggested. Caution should be taken in exposing the C1 posterior ring, which is frequently incomplete in infants [48]. In contrast to CM I, in CM II, we prefer osteodural decompression over bone decompression alone, regardless of age. In all cases, we extend the decompression up to the free cord caudal to the tonsils. When the tonsils arrive below C2, we generally perform an "open door" laminoplasty using a graft from the occiput to maintain the door open. Particular care is taken to

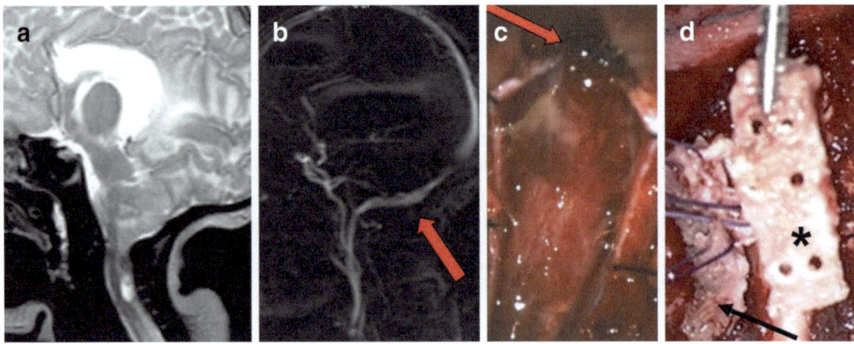

**Fig. 6.3** This 10-day-old child underwent MMC repair on the first day of life. During the following days, CM II syndrome progressively developed with worsening tirage and hypertonus. On fourth day of life, she was first managed with external ventricular drainage, which provided transitory improvement. (**a**) MRI, T2-weighted image, sagittal view showing a severe CM II. The posterior fossa was very small, while the third ventricle was enlarged despite drainage. A catheter point was evident in the upper part of the ventricle. (**b**) Angio-MRI, venous phase, sagittal view showing a very low-lying torcular (red arrow). (**c**) Intraoperative image showing hamartomatous tonsils up to C4 level. The red arrow points at the haemostatic clip tangential to the torcular, which was just at the level of the foramen magnum. (**d**) Intraoperative image showing our technique for "open door" laminoplasty. The laminotomy was performed on the right side, the laminae were fractured on the contralateral side, and then luxated toward the left (black arrow). An autologous bone graft from the occiput (asterisk) was fixed using absorbable wires to keep the door open

preserve the articular processes (Fig. 6.3). In our series, one newborn died after CCD, who had a completely distorted bulbar anatomy at the autopsy [1]. Stormy postoperative courses were the rule in younger infants who often required tracheostomy and jejunostomy. Teens and adults had smoother courses. Anyway, all patients improved. The jejunostomy could eventually be removed in all cases, whereas the tracheostomy could be closed in all cases but one. There was no case of kyphosis during the follow-up, but five patients died due to late shunt malfunction. Indeed, we believe that mortality in MMC-patients is mainly dependent on the relatively acute CM II decompensation triggered by the shunt malfunction, rather than by the shunt malfunction itself. Therefore, the importance of careful follow-up and aggressive management of possible shunt malfunction cannot be overemphasised in these patients.

## 6.4  Hydrosyringomyelia and Subarachnoid Cysts

Hydromyelia is an enlargement of the central canal covered with an ependymal layer, while syringomyelia is an intramedullary cavity covered by a gliotic lining. Being hardly distinguishable, these conditions are usually referred as hydrosyringomyelia [64]. Found in 40–80% of patients with MMC, it become symptomatic just in 2–5% of patients [64, 65].

La Marca et al. categorised syringes as holocord or segmental and distended or not. In case of segmental syringes, they were further divided in "high-level" and "low-level", according to the involved spinal segment [66].

The classical hydrosyringomyelic syndrome with a "cape like" dissociated sensory loss, loss of pain and thermal sensation, and preservation of proprioception is not common in MMC-patients [64, 66]. In fact, clinical presentation may include sensory loss, pain, weakness, gait abnormality, scoliosis, and bladder and/or bowel dysfunctions.

When syringes are asymptomatic, small, with no signs of growth, most authors agree on an initial conservative treatment with clinical and radiological follow-up [1].

If they appear large and/or progressively growing and/or the patient presents clinical signs of lower or upper limb function impairment and/or upcoming urological dysfunction, surgical treatment is generally considered.

The development of hydrosyringomyelia can be linked to the progression of other associated conditions, to always consider first. For instance, progressive hydrocephalus, Chiari II malformation, and TCS may, respectively, require shunt revision, decompression, and tethered cord release.

In our experience, most syringomyelic cysts in MMC-patients are completely asymptomatic and remain not progressive, regardless their diameter. Patients requiring treatment are a few. There may be syringomyelic cysts, which are related to altered CSF dynamics at the foramen magnum. In these rare cases, the cervical level is invariably affected, CM II acts like a CM I, and deserve the same treatment. The other progressive cysts requiring treatment in MMC-patients are mainly dorsal or lumbar and require drainage.

In 1997, La Marca et al. proposed a complex algorithm to plan the correct sequence of surgical treatments based on six imaging groups and three symptoms' groups. Regardless the extension of the hydrosyringomyelic cavity, segmental or holocord, the ventricular-peritoneal shunt revision was always considered the first procedure to attempt [66].

After shunt revision or in the absence of other associated conditions, if the symptoms persist or the cavity tends to increase in size, then hydrosyringomyelia can be treated with a syringo-subarachnoid (SSAs), syringo-pleural (SPLs), or syringo-peritoneal shunt (SPEs).

Vernet et al. compared SSAs to SPLs. They observed better results in patients treated with SPLs as compared to SSAs, possibly for the presence of a perimedullary arachnoiditis and a larger pressure gradient between the respective cavities (syrinx-pleural space vs syrinx-subarachnoid space) [67].

Instead, the choice between a SPL and SPE shunting depends on the proximity between the laminotomy and the pleural entry point. Furthermore, in SPLs, there is the advantage to avoid a change in the patient's position during the procedure.

A more recent study concluded that all the three modalities present similar results in terms of clinical improvement and deterioration after placement, but SPEs have the higher rate of malfunction. Therefore, they confirmed that the SPLs may be the best choice, showing the higher clinical improvement and the lowest reoperation rate [68].

In our experience, when the cyst arrives to the most caudal cord portion, favourable results may be obtained with a wide marsupialisation. This represents a sort of "terminal ventriculostomy" and can be easily accomplished when the cyst reaches the placode area.

In addition to the syringomyelic cysts, MMC patients frequently also present medullary arachnoid cysts. In the vast majority of cases, these cysts are asymptomatic and not progressive even though the MRI shows that the cord is indented. Otherwise, the cysts may develop around the spinal cord due to the presence of arachnoid adhesions. In rarest cases, these cysts may remain isolated and may progressively increase worsening their clinical picture with spinal cord compression. In this scenario, surgical treatment consists of fenestration or drainage of the cyst. In our experience, only one patient required cyst fenestration.

## 6.5 Tethered Cord Syndrome

The tethered cord is characterised by the attachment ("tethering") of the spinal cord to the posterior dural sac, at the level of the MMC repair. Despite MRI almost invariably shows some degree of cord/dura attachment, most MMC-patients do not present a true TCS. In the literature, the incidence of TCS ranges from less than 10% up to 30% [69]. Two peaks of age are generally reported: between 2 and 4 and between 8 and 10 years [69, 70]. Pouratian et al. described a single and longer peak between 5 and 9 years [71]. A smaller group of patients (4–14%) can develop TCS in adulthood [72]. However, it is not so uncommon for TCS to present in childhood but be treated in adulthood.

### 6.5.1  Pathophysiological Mechanisms

During the initial MMC closure, various expedients have been proposed to limit neural adhesions to the dural sac, for example to perform the placode's free lateral edges re-approximation by pial microsutures (neurulation) (Fig. 6.4). This procedure is commonly recommended for its ability to minimise scar adhesions [1, 73]. It probably does not prevent the subsequent occurrence of TCS, but limits scar and adhesions thus making easier and safer the possible future detethering procedure.

A tight dural closure has been indicated as a possible cause of TCS [73, 74]. Indeed, Pang et al. suggested to perform duraplasty and obtain an adequately large dural sac [75]. Eibach et al. suggested reducing the placode by removing the

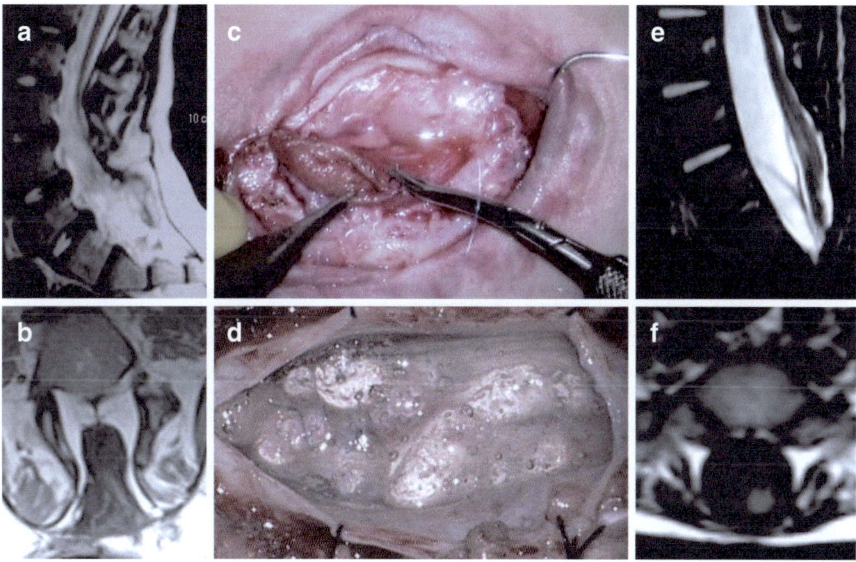

**Fig. 6.4**  (**a**, **b**): MRI, T1-weighted image, sagittal (**a**) and axial (**b**) views obtained in a patient whose neural plaque was replaced inside the dural sac without any neural tube reconstruction. Extended cord/sac adhesions are evident. (**c**) Intraoperative picture showing the reconstruction of the neural tube (neurulation) with pial microsutures during the initial MMC repair. (**d**) Following neurulation, the intradural space is perfused using a gel of hyaluronic acid to prevent adhesions. (**e**, **f**): T2-weighted image, sagittal view (**e**) and T1-weighted image, axial view (**f**) obtained in a patient who was managed with neurulation and hyaluronic acid. Limited adhesions are evident and the neural tube is well bathed into the CSF

non-functioning neural tissue with the help of intraoperative monitoring [74]. We achieved encouraging results with intradural perfusion of a gel of hyaluronic acid, which should have the potential to prevent adhesions [1, 76] (Fig. 6.4d). Many dural grafting materials with different adhesions effects have been proposed (muscle fascia, bovine pericardium, Silastic, Goretex, MEDPOR, and homologous amniotic membrane), but there is no evidence of the superiority of any of them in preventing TCS or its recurrence [77, 78]. Despite such efforts to prevent neural adhesions, secondary TCS remains a problem after MMC repair.

It is believed that a dysmorphic placode and/or the absence of CSF around the placode itself may favour scar and adhesions. This would lead to a stretch-induced neurological condition: the normal spinal cord movements would be restricted causing the lower part of the spinal cord to stretch with a potential secondary injury [79]. In addition, the elongation of the spine related to growth spurts would cause potential traction on the MMC scar with the possible development of TCS for a mechanical, vascular, and/or metabolic cord injury [70].

Indeed, TCS cannot be related only to the mechanical stretch. Yamada et al. have demonstrated ischaemia and mitochondrial anoxia in an animal model, consistent with the usual slow progression of TCS [80]. This vascular injury seems to occur especially in the grey matter [81]. Moreover, current studies reported cellular and molecular alterations in MMC placodes with significantly higher levels of glial fibrillary acidic protein and vimentin-immunoreactivity compared to normal placodes [81, 82]. Cohrs et al. study included 12 patients who underwent untethering after MMC repair and identified specific pro-inflammatory, such as chemokines and cytokines, and proapoptotic mediators [81].

### 6.5.2 Clinical Features and Diagnosis

Possible signs and symptoms of TCS are a constellation: increased weakness with development of new neurological deficit, hypertonia, clonic movements, gait worsening, progressively worsening scoliosis, orthopaedic anomalies (i.e. foot deformity), severe pain at the level of the scar, worsening of urinary function, and so on [1, 79].

In MMC patients, the gait worsening may be related to different causes, for example, leg weakness and clubfoot. Therefore, the evaluation of children's strength requires an experienced neurological observer to investigate all major muscle groups. Back or leg pain may be not specific but frequently have dermatomal distribution and accompany spasticity. Urological dysfunctions are also difficult to be recognised as TCS-related, since all these patients present urinary impairment since the birth. The occurrence or worsening of recurrent urinary infections and sensory impairment may help the diagnosis. The neuro-urologists play a crucial role.

In MMC patients, shunt dysfunction may mimic a TCS that leaded David McLone to suggest: "check the shunt first" [1].

Several authors have discussed the use of various imaging techniques to help TCS diagnosis, such as prone MRI and ultrasonography studies of the spinal cord motion, but their practical utility remains unproved [83, 84]. Phase MRI of the longitudinal cord motions has offered some promise for predicting clinical tethering [70].

Standard MRI still is the primary imaging procedure to evaluate the anatomical features of a tethered cord. A low position of the conus medullaris does not imply a TCS, because all MMC-patients have low-lying conus/cord. Even the presence of more or less extended cord-sac adhesions is not diagnostic being present in the vast majority of patients. However, the MRI remains crucial allowing the identification of possible associated lesions such as syringomyelia, split cord, lipomas, or dermoids (Fig. 6.5). Caldarelli et al. proposed a radiological scale based on the MRI appearance of tethered cord and identified four different levels of tethering (Table 6.1) [85].

Other instrumental examinations may help in the diagnosis of TCS. For example, an electromyography that shows recent denervation potentials may be highly suggestive of TCS. Nevertheless, the diagnosis of TCS is still mainly based on clinical criteria.

### 6.5.3 Surgery

Surgical indication for detethering should be tailored to the patient's condition and quality of life. In our series, 25% of patients presented symptoms of possible TCS during the follow-up [1]. However, when we excluded cases of mimicked TCS (for

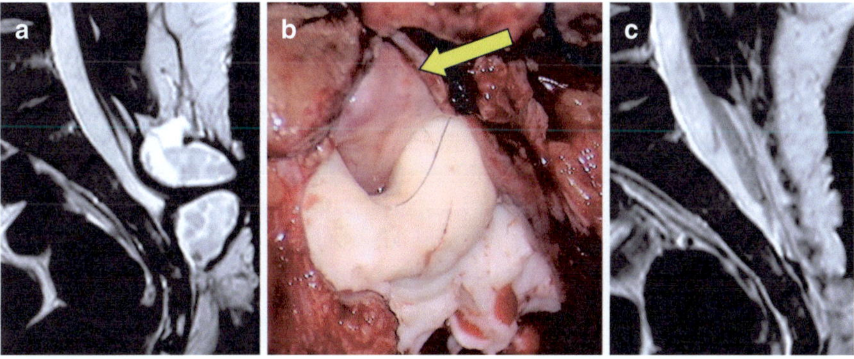

**Fig. 6.5** This 12-year-old girl was followed as outpatient after MMC-repair in the neonatal period. During the following years, she first complained of progressively worsening scar and feet pain. (**a**) MRI, T2-weighted image, sagittal view showing an iatrogenic inclusion dermoid. (**b**) Intraoperative picture showing the neural tube (yellow arrow) and the typical dermoid tissue consisting of fat, sebum, skin debris. A hair is evident. (**c**) MRI, T2-weighted image, sagittal view showing no residual dermoid and the reconstructed neural tube surrounded by CSF

**Table 6.1** Radiologic classification of tethered cord

| | |
|---|---|
| Grade I | Low-lying conus adherent to lumbar scar<br>Conus medullaris enveloped by subarachnoid space<br>No evidence of adhesion along the spinal cord |
| Grade II | Grade I +<br>Evidence of hydromyelia or focal dilatation of the central canal OR large adhesion of the placode to lumbar scar without evidence of adhesion along the spinal cord |
| Grade III | Large adhesion of the placode to lumbar scar with evidence of abnormal tissue (lipoma, dermoid)<br>Evidence of adhesion (ventral and dorsal) along the spinal cord<br>Dural sac incomplete or absent<br>Hydro/syringomyelia |
| Grade IV | Grade III +<br>Severe scoliosis/kyphosis aggravating the spinal tethering |

example due to hydrocephalus), cases of not progressive symptoms, and cases where the symptom did not affect the quality of life, there remained just 12% of patients with indication to detethering. Unfortunately, detethering can prevent further worsening but has poor effect on the already present deteriorations. Therefore, we generally have more aggressive indications in walking patients, because these have more to lose. Paraplegic patients are detethered only when the TCS alters their quality of life, such as in the case of untreatable pain or hypertonus, progressive scoliosis, and so on.

Several authors suggested that, for the best outcome, patients should be treated within 5 years of the clinical onset [86]. Phuong et al. reported that 60% of patients with delayed TCS treatment experienced further worsening, and 89% required other orthopaedic and/or urologic procedures [87].

A midline vertical incision is generally used, even if the original incision was transverse [79]. Laminectomy of the lowest intact lamina is generally performed to expose the unopened dura first. Afterwards, the normal spinal cord rostral to the malformation is exposed and arachnoid dissection starts on both sides progressing downward. The use of electrophysiological intraoperative monitoring is invaluable to determine the level of intact neurological functions and to minimise additional injuries. The ventral roots are progressively exposed. The usual intra-operative finding is a dense scar tissue between the posterior aspect of the spinal cord (neural placode) and the overlying dura [79], especially in case of silk sutures for dural repair [1]. In our experience, the scar and adhesions are always asymmetric, with one side easier to release than the other (Fig. 6.6). To avoid damaging the placode, it should be released in all directions, according to the grading system proposed by Kirollos and Van Hille (Table 6.2) [88].

Hudgins et al. suggested to leave the adherent dura over the neural tissue, while our group proposed to carefully isolate the neural plaque and to repair the neural tube (neurulation) by pial sutures as for the initial MMC repair [1, 79].

Once the cord is completely untethered, it should be inspected in search of other possible pathological entities, such as dermoid tumours, thickened filum, and lipomas. Afterwards, the dura is closed in a watertight fashion. In general, the dural sac

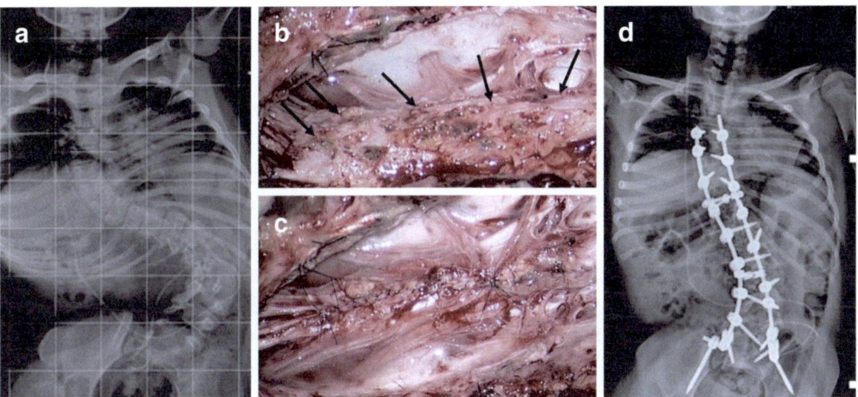

**Fig. 6.6** This 10-year-old boy was referred to us because of respiratory distress and severe pain. He had been operated on in a low-income country and was never followed up on. (**a**) Preoperative posteroanterior (PA) standing X-ray showing severe scoliosis. (**b**) Intraoperative picture showing a phase of the detethering procedure, preliminary to orthopaedic correction. The ventral roots are exposed on the less compromised side. Asymmetrical scar adhesions are evident (arrows). (**c**) Intraoperative picture showing a later phase of the detethering procedure: the ventral roots are exposed on both sides and the neural tube has been reconstructed using pial microsutures. (**d**) Postoperative PA standing X-ray showing the orthopaedic correction

**Table 6.2** Classification of cord untethering in case of intradural adhesion

| Grade I | Release of intradural elements circumferentially from dura and from vertical traction + spacious dural sac |
|---|---|
| Grade II | Significant untethering but persistent tethering of nerve roots to < ¼ circumference of dura |
| Grade III | Incomplete mobilisation of cord and/or nerve roots adherent through fibrous tissue to > ¼ circumference of dura |

is relatively wide, and no dural graft is necessary. The muscle layer is re-approximated, if possible myofascial flaps are fashioned to cover the repaired dural sac. Unlike the first intervention, usually there are no main problems with skin suture.

### 6.5.4 Complications and Outcome

The most common postoperative complications include superficial wound dehiscence, wound infections, and CSF subcutaneous pseudomeningocele. As a result, central nervous system infections may occur at a rate ranging from 10% to 35% of all cases [69, 70].

To prevent CSF leakage, the patient should be maintained on flat and prone bed rest for 3–4 days with or without lumbar drainage and then slowly mobilised [69].

Foster et al. demonstrated an association between detethering and positive change in height-for-age percentile, especially in children from 5 to 18 years old [89].

More generally, after detethering, most of the actual studies report an overall clinical improvement, ranging between 75% and 90% of cases [90, 91]. Early diagnosis is considered the most important good prognostic factor [91].

The possibility of retethering remains a significant long-term complication, and a regular clinical and radiological follow-up is generally recommended. In our experience, 10% of detethered MMC-patients require further detethering procedures. Moreover, the rate of successful detethering decreases with each subsequent procedure, parallel to an increased risk of neurological and wound complications. In repeatedly operated patients, a dense arachnoiditis may be encountered and be difficult to untangle [92].

## 6.6  Scoliosis

Scoliosis is the most frequent deformity in spina bifida, affecting up to 50% of patients with MMC [93]. In this population, spinal deformities occur early and in half of the cases surgical treatment is indicated [94].

Related to the etiopathogenesis, vertebral deformities are classified as congenital and developmental. Congenital include scoliosis with vertebral malformation due to failure of formation or segmentation and kyphosis due to dysplastic posterior elements. Developmental scoliosis is classified as neurological or as secondary to hip deformity or pelvic obliquity. Combined upper and lower motor neuron lesions lead to flaccid and spastic neurological scoliosis that often coexist MMC [94].

Incidence in neurological scoliosis is highest in non-ambulatory patients and relates to the level of the neurological and anatomical (last intact laminar arch) lesion [95].

The progressive nature of these curves is caused by the lack of trunk muscles and posterior bone elements. Spinal muscles are displaced anteriorly to the vertical axis, creating a strong bending moment. In addition, in the sitting position, the arm of the bending moment is increased by gravity leading to further worsening of the deformity.

The progression of the curves cannot be easily predicted and is influenced by different factors, being the tethered cord the first, present in 25–30% of the cases.

Morphologically, it appears as a long C-shaped curve often associated to pelvic obliquity. The sitting imbalance represents a valid quality of life parameter in MMC with scoliosis. The trunk imbalance causes ischium or sacrum pressure ulcerations and worsens autonomy. Patients need to use their hands as support of the trunk and can be unable to perform basic daily living activities, becoming functionally like a quadriplegic. Moreover, the rib to pelvic impingement can cause an extremely invalidating pain and respiratory impairment may occur [96].

### 6.6.1 Conservative Treatment

Orthotic treatment with the brace may arrest scoliosis progression with a curve under 40° and provides support for the sitting position [97].

The soft "static" control braces are well tolerated compared to rigid "active" braces usually used in idiopathic scoliosis. Conservative management is not effective in severe deformities. In most cases, the orthosis is a bride measure to surgery in younger patients [98].

### 6.6.2 Surgical Indications and Planning

Surgery is considered as the definitive treatment, but it is complicated by the anatomic abnormalities and comorbidities of MMC. In literature, there is no consensus about indications and best surgical strategy. Surgical treatment is suggested for scoliosis over 50° [99].

Certainly, curve degree alone cannot be the only indication. Sitting imbalance, cardiopulmonary impairment, pain (rib to pelvis impingement), and pressure sores are additional indications for surgery. The main aim is to correct the deformity improving sitting balance, quality of life, and vital functions. On the other hand, pressure skin ulcerations can be worsened by spinal correction if rigid residual pelvic obliquity persists or in case of reduction of lumbar lordosis. Controversies about surgical treatment include the high rate of complications, the functional loss, and no evidence-based studies of benefits especially in terms of quality of life [100].

Khoshbin et al. concluded that the spinal surgery for scoliosis secondary to spina bifida corrects coronal deformity and stops progression of the curve, but has no clear effect on health-related quality of life [101].

Multidisciplinary discussions with families and caregivers need to be well balanced.

Careful preoperative evaluation is always necessary. The skin in the area of the surgery must be assessed for scarring as large corrections, and spinal instrumentation can make closure difficult. The gait and method of active transfers should be observed to determine the consequences of the loss of lumbosacral motion following fixation. Diminished hip extension will be further compromised if the lumbar lordosis is surgically reduced and ambulation will become more difficult. The radiographic assessment should include full spine views in standing position for ambulatory patient and sitting for non-ambulatory, thus eliminating the affect of hip contractures on the spinal alignment. The dynamic (side bends or traction) views are used to test the flexibility of the spinal deformity. A computed tomography scan is helpful to analyse the three-dimensional anatomy and plan the spinopelvic fixation.

When scoliosis is secondary to TCS, the tethered cord release alone could sometimes arrest the progression of the deformity but never improve it. Magnitude of the curve (over 40°) and age (Risser 0-2) seem to be related with the probability of scoliosis progression despite detethering [102].

Surgical treatment of these scoliosis is probably the most challenging type of spinal surgery. The posterior elements are dysplastic, offering a poor mass for fusion. Timing of surgery depends on the decision of using growth preserving techniques or definitive surgery. In the treatment of early onset scoliosis (<10 years), consequences of definitive fusion may include shortened lung growth and the "crankshaft phenomenon" (continued anterior spinal growth and posterior tether resulting in a rotational deformity) [103].

The growth-friendly systems offer another option for the treatment of severe (>70°) early onset deformities. The benefits of additional trunk growth must be balanced against the need of repeated surgeries and the high risk of mechanical complication of these devices [104].

### 6.6.3   Definitive Surgery

Current posterior segmental instrumentation allows significant deformity correction with solid fixation reducing the postoperative immobilisation. Attempts to save mobile lumbar segments, especially the lumbosacral junction, are needed in ambulatory patients even in the presence of pelvic obliquity. In the MMC scoliosis, these long curves will require long posterior fixation obtained through increased segmental anchors. Usually in non-ambulatory status with associated pelvic obliquity (>20°), the fusion should be extended to the pelvis. Although the well-known benefit of correction and fusion surgery, the role and timing of tethered cord release is less clear. Combined tethered cord release and posterior fusion procedures could be effective to correct spinal deformity and to prevent neurological worsening. In scoliosis with TCS, the tight cord must first be released before the spine is distracted to avoid catastrophic neurological deterioration [105].

In order to avoid high risk of posterior implant failure, some authors suggest associating an anterior surgery to address fusion especially across levels with marginal posterior elements. Anterior additional surgery has lowered the rates of nonunion [106].

Mazur et al. reported a pseudarthrosis rate of 33% in posterior surgery versus 11% in the group treated with a combined anterior and posterior approach [107].

Actually, circumferential fusion is considered the best choice to avoid mechanical complications and improving sitting balance. Advancements in the surgical technique have had a significant impact on the results of deformity correction. Moreover, the introduction of new minimally invasive techniques has improved clinical results and reduced the rate of complications, making definitive surgery more accessible even in the more fragile myelomeningocele patients.

### 6.6.4 Surgical Pearls

Considering the high potential benefits and harms of surgery, nowadays there is a strong need to identify better and innovative strategies. The anterior fusions have undergone a dramatic evolution over the last 20 years. The minimally invasive lateral approach is recommended in order to reduce morbidity, blood loss, and postoperative hospital stay compared to traditional open anterior approach [108].

In the 2021, Giorgi et al. suggested a new two-stage surgical pathway with minimally invasive anterior fusion for severe MMC scoliosis (main curve >70°, pelvic obliquity >20°). In the first single stage, a detethering procedure was followed by corrective surgery with posterior fusion. A hybrid construct extended to the pelvis with bilateral double rods at the side of the dysraphism was used (Fig. 6.7a). In the delayed second stage, a minimally invasive anterior fusion at level of the spinal dysraphism close to the apex of the curve was performed (Fig. 6.7b, c). This

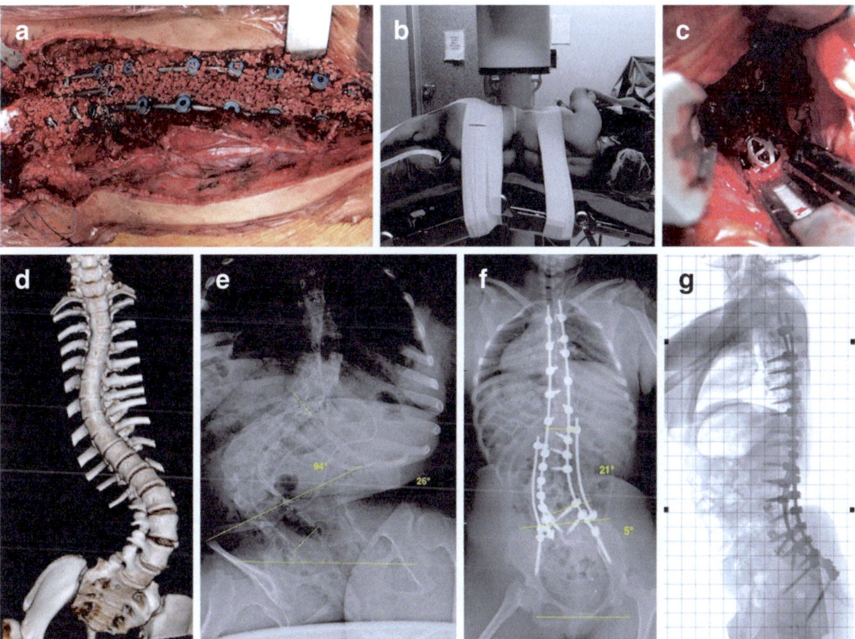

**Fig. 6.7** Single curve scoliosis in myelomeningocele with tethered cord syndrome. (**a**) First posterior stage: following neurosurgical detethering, the orthopaedic stage consists of instrumented posterior spinal fusion. (**b, c**) Second anterior stage: minimally invasive antero-lateral surgery. Patient positioning (**b**); operative photo of interbody fusion with Harm's mesh at L3-L4 disc space (**c**). (**d**) Initial 3D CT-scan to study spinopelvic deformity. (**e**) Preoperative PA weight-bearing X-rays showing 94° scoliosis deformity and 26° pelvic obliquity. (**f**) Postoperative PA weight-bearing X-rays after first posterior corrective surgery that shows good correction of scoliosis and pelvic obliquity. (**g**) Postoperative lateral weight-bearing X-rays after anterior delayed surgery showing 3 lumbar Harm's meshes positioning

innovative surgical pathway allowed to minimise complications providing good fusion rates without loss of correction and implant failure (Fig. 6.7d–g) [109].

Miladi et al. in 2014 presented a novel posterior minimally invasive fusionless surgery for neuromuscular scoliosis: the bipolar technique [110].

This procedure is based on the concept of global derotation with scoliosis reduction in traction acting at the extremities of the curve. The aim is to obtain a progressive balanced correction of the scoliosis and pelvic obliquity prior to the insertion of the rod without any excessive forces on the two anchor sites. Proximally, a short posterior midline incision at the cervicothoracic junction is performed. The interspinous ligaments must be preserved. A solid "claw" with hooks (supralaminar and pedicle hook affixed to four adjacent vertebrae) are then placed. Distally a short posterior longitudinal midline skin incision is made at the lumbosacral junction. The lateral aspect of paravertebral muscle is exposed bilaterally through a paramedian approach, as described by Wiltse. The distal anchor is performed with an iliosacral screw. Bone exposure must be minimal, and no graft is used to avoid bony fusion. The proximal and distal fixation points are then connected in moderate distraction with a rod passed through the paravertebral muscle to complete the correction of the deformity. Biomechanically, a bridge system suspended in traction from two extremities is created. This minimally invasive posterior procedure was found to be safe in critical cases such as MMC and effective in maintaining scoliosis correction reducing complications (Fig. 6.8) [111].

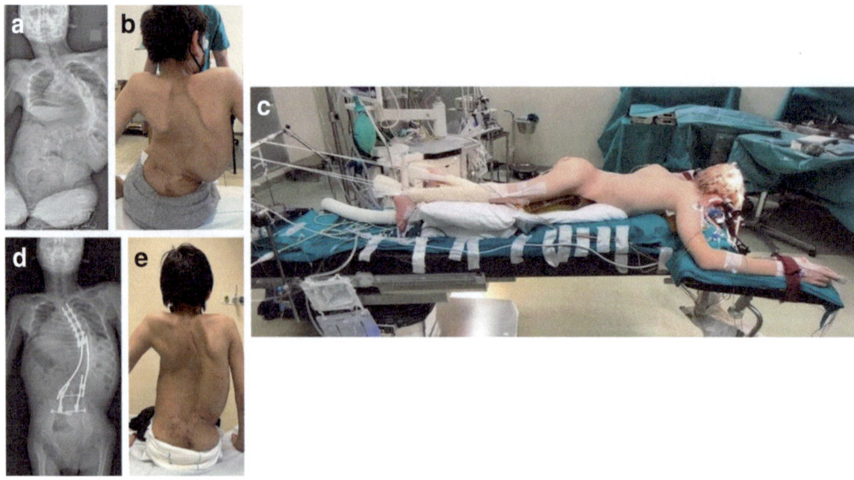

**Fig. 6.8** Single curve scoliosis in myelomeningocele without tethered cord syndrome. (**a, b**) Preoperative PA standing X-ray (**a**) and patient image (**b**) showing spinopelvic deformity. (**c**) Patient positioning with a bridge system suspended in traction from 2 extremities. (**d, e**): Postoperative PA standing X-ray (**d**) and patient image (**e**) showing balanced correction of the spinopelvic deformity after posterior bipolar minimally invasive technique

# References


1. Talamonti G, D'Aliberti G, Collice M. Myelomeningocele: long-term neurosurgical treatment and follow-up in 202 patients. J Neurosurg Pediatr. 2007;107(5):368–86.
2. Adzick NS. Fetal myelomeningocele: natural history, pathophysiology, and in-utero intervention. In Seminars in fetal and neonatal medicine 2010 (15, 1, pp. 9-14). WB Saunders.
3. Adzick NS, Thom EA, Spong CY, Brock JW III, Burrows PK, Johnson MP, Howell LJ, Farrell JA, Dabrowiak ME, Sutton LN, Gupta N. A randomized trial of prenatal versus postnatal repair of myelomeningocele. N Engl J Med. 2011;364(11):993–1004.
4. Pontell ME, Yengo-Kahn AM, Taylor E, Kane M, Newton JM, Bennett KA, Wellons JC, Braun SA. Intrauterine closure of myelomeningocele defects with primary linear repair versus bipedicle fasciocutaneous flaps: a post-MOMS cohort study with long-term follow-up. J Neurosurg Pediatr. 2022;31(2):143–50.
5. Cortes MS, Chmait RH, Lapa DA, Belfort MA, Carreras E, Miller JL, Samaha RB, Gonzalez GS, Gielchinsky Y, Yamamoto M, Persico N. Experience of 300 cases of prenatal fetoscopic open spina bifida repair: report of the International Fetoscopic Neural Tube Defect Repair Consortium. Am J Obstet Gynecol. 2021;225(6):678-e1.
6. Verweij EJ, de Vries MC, Oldekamp EJ, Eggink AJ, Oepkes D, Slaghekke F, Spoor JK, Deprest JA, Miller JL, Baschat AA, DeKoninck PL. Fetoscopic myelomeningocele closure: is the scientific evidence enough to challenge the gold standard for prenatal surgery? Prenat Diagn. 2021;41(8):949–56.
7. Sival DA, Patuszka A, Koszutski T, Heep A, Verbeek RJ. Neurologic outcome comparison between fetal open-, endoscopic-and neonatal-intervention techniques in spina bifida aperta. Diagnostics. 2023;13(2):251.
8. Zamłyński J, Olejek A, Koszutski T, Ziomek G, Horzelska E, Gajewska-Kucharek A, Maruniak-Chudek I, Herman-Sucharska I, Kluczewska E, Horak S, Bodzek P. Comparison of prenatal and postnatal treatments of spina bifida in Poland–a non-randomized, single-center study. J Matern Fetal Neonatal Med. 2014;27(14):1409–17.
9. Pedreira DA, Zanon N, Nishikuni K, de Sá RA, Acacio GL, Chmait RH, Kontopoulos EV, Quintero RA. Endoscopic surgery for the antenatal treatment of myelomeningocele: the CECAM trial. Am J Obstet Gynecol. 2016;214(1):111–e1.
10. Jackson EM, Schwartz DM, Sestokas AK, Zarnow DM, Adzick NS, Johnson MP, Heuer GG, Sutton LN. Intraoperative neurophysiological monitoring in patients undergoing tethered cord surgery after fetal myelomeningocele repair. J Neurosurg Pediatr. 2014;13(4):355–61.
11. Graf K, Kohl T, Neubauer BA, Dey F, Faas D, Wanis FA, Reinges MH, Uhl E, Kolodziej MA. Percutaneous minimally invasive fetoscopic surgery for spina bifida aperta. Part III: neurosurgical intervention in the first postnatal year. Ultrasound Obstet Gynecol. 2016;47(2):158–61.
12. Sacco A, Ushakov F, Thompson D, Peebles D, Pandya P, De Coppi P, Wimalasundera R, Attilakos G, David AL, Deprest J. Fetal surgery for open spina bifida. Obstet Gynaecol. 2019;21(4):271.
13. Flanders TM, Franco AJ, Lincul KL, Pierce SR, Oliver ER, Moldenhauer JS, Adzick NS, Heuer GG. Tethered cord release in patients after open fetal myelomeningocele closure: intraoperative neuromonitoring data and patient outcomes. Childs Nerv Syst. 2022;16:1–8.
14. Cavalheiro S, da Costa MD, Barbosa MM, Dastoli PA, Mendonça JN, Cavalheiro D, Moron AF. Hydrocephalus in myelomeningocele. Childs Nerv Syst. 2021;37(11):3407–15.
15. Marlin AE. Management of hydrocephalus in the patient with myelomeningocele: an argument against third ventriculostomy. Neurosurg Focus. 2004;16(2):1–3.
16. Tamburrini G, Frassanito P, Iakovaki K, Pignotti F, Rendeli C, Murolo D, Di Rocco C. Myelomeningocele: the management of the associated hydrocephalus. Childs Nerv Syst. 2013;29:1569–79.

17. Di Rocco C, Cinalli G, Massimi L, Spennato P, Cianciulli E, Tamburrini G. Endoscopic third ventriculostomy in the treatment of hydrocephalus in pediatric patients. Adv Tech Stand Neurosurg. 2006:119–219.
18. Wakhlu A, Ansari NA. The prediction of postoperative hydrocephalus in patients with spina bifida. Childs Nerv Syst. 2004;20:104–6.
19. McCarthy DJ, Sheinberg DL, Luther E, McCrea HJ. Myelomeningocele-associated hydrocephalus: nationwide analysis and systematic review. Neurosurg Focus. 2019;47(4):E5.
20. Chakraborty A, Crimmins D, Hayward R, Thompson D. Toward reducing shunt placement rates in patients with myelomeningocele. J Neurosurg Pediatr. 2008;1(5):361–5.
21. McLone DG, Knepper PA. The cause of Chiari II malformation: a unified theory. Pediatr Neurosurg. 1989;15(1):1–2.
22. Elgamal EA. Natural history of hydrocephalus in children with spinal open neural tube defect. Surg Neurol Int. 2012;3:112.
23. Sutton LN. Fetal surgery for neural tube defects. Best Pract Res Clin Obstet Gynaecol. 2008;22(1):175–88.
24. Hubballah MY, Hoffman HJ. Early repair of myelomeningocele and simultaneous insertion of ventriculoperitoneal shunt: technique and results. Neurosurgery. 1987;20(1):21–3.
25. Machado HR, Santos de Oliveira R. Simultaneous repair of myelomeningocele and shunt insertion. Childs Nerv Syst. 2004;20:107–9.
26. Miller PD, Pollack IF, Pang D, Albright AL. Comparison of simultaneous versus delayed ventriculoperitoneal shunt insertion in children undergoing myelomeningocele repair. J Child Neurol. 1996;11(5):370–2.
27. Pang D. Surgical complications of open spinal dysraphism. Neurosurg Clin N Am. 1995;6(2):243–57.
28. Beuriat PA, Poirot I, Hameury F, Demede D, Sweeney KJ, Szathmari A, Di Rocco F, Mottolese C. Low level myelomeningoceles: do they need prenatal surgery? Childs Nerv Syst. 2019;35:957–63.
29. McLone DG, Czyzewski D, Raimondi AJ, Sommers RC. Central nervous system infections as a limiting factor in the intelligence of children with myelomeningocele. Pediatrics. 1982;70(3):338–42.
30. Riva-Cambrin J, Kestle JR, Holubkov R, Butler J, Kulkarni AV, Drake J, Whitehead WE, Wellons JC, Shannon CN, Tamber MS, Limbrick DD. Risk factors for shunt malfunction in pediatric hydrocephalus: a multicenter prospective cohort study. J Neurosurg Pediatr. 2016;17(4):382–90.
31. Stone JJ, Walker CT, Jacobson M, Phillips V, Silberstein HJ. Revision rate of pediatric ventriculoperitoneal shunts after 15 years. J Neurosurg Pediatr. 2013;11(1):15–9.
32. Tuli S, Drake J, Lamberti-Pasculli M. Long-term outcome of hydrocephalus management in myelomeningoceles. Childs Nerv Syst. 2003;19:286–91.
33. Bowman RM, McLone DG, Grant JA, Tomita T, Ito JA. Spina bifida outcome: a 25-year prospective. Pediatr Neurosurg. 2001;34(3):114–20.
34. Hall P, Lindseth R, Campbell R, Kalsbeck JE, Desousa A. Scoliosis and hydrocephalus in myelocele patients: the effects of ventricular shunting. J Neurosurg. 1979;50(2):174–8.
35. Talamonti G, Marcati E, Mastino L, Meccariello G, Picano M, D'Aliberti G. Surgical management of Chiari malformation type II. Childs Nerv Syst. 2020;36:1621–34.
36. Iannelli A, Rea G, Di Rocco C. CSF shunt removal in children with hydrocephalus. Acta Neurochir. 2005;147:503–7.
37. Humphrey RP. Spinal dysraphism. In: Wilkins RH, Rengachary SS, editors. Neurosurgery. New York: McGraw-Hill; 1985. p. 2041–52.
38. Staal MJ, Meihuizen-de Regt MJ, Hess J. Sudden death in hydrocephalic spina bifida aperta patients. Pediatr Neurosurg. 1987;13(1):13–8.
39. Iskandar BJ, Tubbs S, Mapstone TB, Grabb PA, Bartolucci AA, Oakes WJ. Death in shunted hydrocephalic children in the 1990s. Pediatr Neurosurg. 1998;28(4):173–6.

40. Tennant PW, Pearce MS, Bythell M, Rankin J. 20-year survival of children born with congenital anomalies: a population-based study. Lancet. 2010;375(9715):649–56.
41. Teo C, Jones R. Management of hydrocephalus by endoscopic third ventriculostomy in patients with myelomeningocele. Pediatr Neurosurg. 1996;25(2):57–63.
42. Jones RF, Kwok BC, Stening WA, Vonau M. Third ventriculostomy for hydrocephalus associated with spinal dysraphism: indications and contraindications. Eur J Pediatr Surg. 1996;6(S 1):5–6.
43. Mori H, Oi S, Nonaka Y, Tamogami R, Muroi A. Ventricular anatomy of hydrocephalus associated with myeloschisis and endoscopic third ventriculostomy. Childs Nerv Syst. 2008;24:717–22.
44. Pavez A, Salazar C, Rivera R, Contreras J, Orellana A, Guzman C, Iribarren O, Hernandez H, Elzo J, Moraga D. Description of endoscopic ventricular anatomy in myelomeningocele. Minim Invasive Neurosurg. 2006;49(03):161–7.
45. Peretta P, Ragazzi P, Galarza M, Genitori L, Giordano F, Mussa F, Cinalli G. Complications and pitfalls of neuroendoscopic surgery in children. J Neurosurg Pediatr. 2006;105(3):187–93.
46. Jenkinson MD, Hayhurst C, Al-Jumaily M, Kandasamy J, Clark S, Mallucci CL. The role of endoscopic third ventriculostomy in adult patients with hydrocephalus. J Neurosurg. 2009;110(5):861–6.
47. Talamonti G, Nichelatti M, Picano M, Marcati E, D'Aliberti G, Cenzato M. Endoscopic third ventriculostomy in cases of ventriculoperitoneal shunt malfunction: does shunt duration play a role? World Neurosurg. 2019;127:e799–808.
48. Stevenson KL. Chiari type II malformation: past, present, and future. Neurosurg Focus. 2004;16(2):1–7.
49. Cleland. Contribution to the study of spina bifida, encephalocele, and anencephalus. J Anat Physiol. 1883;17(3):257–92.
50. Chiari HA. Ueber veränderungen des kleinhirns infolge von hydrocephalie des grosshirns1. DMW-Deutsche Medizinische Wochenschrift. 1891;17(42):1172–5.
51. Arnold J. Myelocytes, Transposition von Gewebskeimen und Sympodie. Beitr Pathol Anat. 1894;16:1–28.
52. Shah AH, Dhar A, Elsanafiry MS, Goel A. Chiari malformation: has the dilemma ended? J Craniovertebr Junction Spine. 2017;8(4):297.
53. Tulipan N. Intrauterine closure of myelomeningocele: an update. Neurosurg Focus. 2004;16(2):1–4.
54. McLone DG, Dias MS. The Chiari II malformation: cause and impact. Childs Nerv Syst. 2003;19:540–50.
55. Talamonti G, Zella S. Surgical treatment of CM2 and syringomyelia in a series of 231 myelomeningocele patients. Neurol Sci. 2011;32:331–3.
56. Charney EB, Rorke LB, Sutton LN, Schut L. Management of Chiari II complications in infants with myelomeningocele. J Pediatr. 1987;111(3):364–71.
57. Pollack IF, Pang D, Albright AL, Krieger D. Outcome following hindbrain decompression of symptomatic Chiari malformations in children previously treated with myelomeningocele closure and shunts. J Neurosurg. 1992;77(6):881–8.
58. Mastino L, Mai R, Cenzato M, D'Aliberti G, Talamonti G. Movement disorder as unusual manifestation of Chiari malformation type II in a newborn. J Pediatr Neurol. 2021;19(06):414–8.
59. Cochrane DD, Adderley R, White CP, Norman M, Steinbok P. Apnea in patients with myelomeningocele. Pediatr Neurosurg. 1990;16(4–5):232–9.
60. Zafar A, Hussain N. Prolonged expiratory apnoea with cyanosis in Arnold Chiari II malformation. JRSM Open. 2017;8(3):2054270416669303.
61. Vandertop WP, Asai A, Hoffman HJ, Drake JM, Humphreys RP, Rutka JT, Becker LE. Surgical decompression for symptomatic Chiari II malformation in neonates with myelomeningocele. J Neurosurg. 1992;77(4):541–4.

62. Park TS, Hoffman HJ, Hendrick BE, Humphreys RP. Experience with surgical decompression of the Arnold-Chiari malformation in young infants with myelomeningocele. Neurosurgery. 1983;13(2):147–52.

63. Kim I, Hopson B, Aban I, Rizk EB, Dias MS, Bowman R, Ackerman LL, Partington MD, Castillo H, Castillo J, Peterson PR. Decompression for Chiari malformation type II in individuals with myelomeningocele in the National Spina Bifida Patient Registry. J Neurosurg Pediatr. 2018;22(6):652–8.

64. Dias MS. Neurosurgical management of myelomeningocele (spina bifida). Pediatr Rev. 2005;26(2):50–60.

65. Piatt JH. Syringomyelia complicating myelomeningocele: review of the evidence. J Neurosurg Pediatr. 2004;100(2):101–9.

66. La Marca F, Herman M, Grant JA, McLone DG. Presentation and management of hydromyelia in children with Chiari type-II malformation. Pediatr Neurosurg. 1997;26(2):57–67.

67. Vernet O, Farmer JP, Montes JL. Comparison of syringopleural and syringosubarachnoid shunting in the treatment of syringomyelia in children. J Neurosurg. 1996;84(4):624–8.

68. Rothrock RJ, Lu VM, Levi AD. Syrinx shunts for syringomyelia: a systematic review and meta-analysis of syringosubarachnoid, syringoperitoneal, and syringopleural shunting. J Neurosurg Spine. 2021;35(4):535–45.

69. Caldarelli M, Boscarelli A, Massimi L. Recurrent tethered cord: radiological investigation and management. Childs Nerv Syst. 2013;29:1601–9.

70. Ferreira Furtado LM, Val Filho JA, Dantas F, de Sousa CM. Tethered cord syndrome after myelomeningocele repair: a literature update. Cureus. 2020;12:10.

71. Pouratian N, Elias WJ, Jane JA, Phillips LH. Electrophysiologically guided untethering of secondary tethered spinal cord syndrome. Neurosurg Focus. 2010;29(1):E3.

72. George TM, Fagan LH. Adult tethered cord syndrome in patients with postrepair myelomeningocele: an evidence-based outcome study. J Neurosurg. 2005;102(2):150–6.

73. Mattogno PP, Massimi L, Tamburrini G, Frassanito P, Di Rocco C, Caldarelli M. Myelomeningocele Repair: Surgical Management Based on a 30-Year Experience. Acta Neurochir Suppl. 2017;124:143–8.

74. Eibach S, Moes G, Hou YJ, Zovickian J, Pang D. New surgical paradigm for open neural tube defects. Childs Nerv Syst. 2021;37:529–38.

75. Pang D, Zovickian J, Oviedo A. Long-term outcome of total and near-total resection of spinal cord lipomas and radical reconstruction of the neural placode: part I—surgical technique. Neurosurgery. 2009;65(3):511–29.

76. Talamonti G, D'Aliberti G, Nichelatti M, Debernardi A, Picano M, Redaelli T. Asymptomatic lipomas of the medullary conus: surgical treatment versus conservative management. J Neurosurg Pediatr. 2014;14(3):245–54.

77. Mehta VA, Bettegowda C, Ahmadi SA, Berenberg P, Thomale UW, Haberl EJ, Jallo GI, Ahn ES. Spinal cord tethering following myelomeningocele repair. J Neurosurg Pediatr. 2010;6(5):498–505.

78. Marton E, Giordan E, Gioffrè G, Canova G, Paolin A, Mazzucco MG, Longatti P. Homologous cryopreserved amniotic membrane in the repair of myelomeningocele: preliminary experience. Acta Neurochir. 2018;160:1625–31.

79. Hudgins RJ, Gilreath CL. Tethered spinal cord following repair of myelomeningocele. Neurosurg Focus. 2004;16(2):1–4.

80. Yamada S, Won DJ, Pezeshkpour G, Yamada BS, Yamada SM, Siddiqi J, Zouros A, Colohan AR. Pathophysiology of tethered cord syndrome and similar complex disorders. Neurosurg Focus. 2007;23(2):1.

81. Cohrs G, Drucks B, Sürie JP, Vokuhl C, Synowitz M, Held-Feindt J, Knerlich-Lukoschus F. Expression profiles of pro-inflammatory and pro-apoptotic mediators in secondary tethered cord syndrome after myelomeningocele repair surgery. Childs Nerv Syst. 2019;35:315–28.

82. Kowitzke B, Cohrs G, Leuschner I, Koch A, Synowitz M, Mehdorn HM, Held-Feindt J, Knerlich-Lukoschus F. Cellular profiles and molecular mediators of lesion cascades

in the placode in human open spinal neural tube defects. J Neuropathol Exp Neurol. 2016;75(9):827–42.

83. Vernet O, O'Gorman AM, Farmer JP, McPhillips M, Montes JL. Use of the prone position in the MRI evaluation of spinal cord retethering. Pediatr Neurosurg. 1996;25(6):286–94.

84. Brezner A, Kay B. Spinal cord ultrasonography in children with myelomeningocele. Dev Med Child Neurol. 1999;41(7):450–5.

85. Caldarelli M, Di Rocco C, Colosimo C, Fariello G, Di Gennaro M. Surgical treatment of late neurological deterioration in children with myelodysplasia. Acta Neurochir. 1995;137:199–206.

86. Hertzler DA, DePowell JJ, Stevenson CB, Mangano FT. Tethered cord syndrome: a review of the literature from embryology to adult presentation. Neurosurg Focus. 2010;29(1):E1.

87. Phuong LK, Schoeberl KA, Raffel C. Natural history of tethered cord in patients with meningomyelocele. Neurosurgery. 2002;50(5):989–95.

88. Kirollos RW, Van Hille PT. Evaluation of surgery for the tethered cord syndrome using a new grading system. Br J Neurosurg. 1996;10(3):253–60.

89. Foster KA, Lam S, Lin Y, Greene S. Putative height acceleration following tethered cord release in children. J Neurosurg Pediatr. 2014;14(6):626–34.

90. Bowman RM, Mohan A, Ito J, Seibly JM, McLone DG. Tethered cord release: a long-term study in 114 patients. J Neurosurg Pediatr. 2009;3(3):181–7.

91. Herman JM, McLone DG, Storrs BB, Dauser RC. Analysis of 153 patients with myelomeningocele or spinal lipoma reoperated upon for a tethered cord. Pediatr Neurosurg. 1993;19(5):243–9.

92. Aldave G, Hansen D, Hwang SW, Moreno A, Briceño V, Jea A. Spinal column shortening for tethered cord syndrome associated with myelomeningocele, lumbosacral lipoma, and lipomyelomeningocele in children and young adults. J Neurosurg Pediatr. 2017;19(6):703–10.

93. Westcott MA, Dynes MC, Remer EM, Donaldson JS, Dias LS. Congenital and acquired orthopedic abnormalities in patients with myelomeningocele. Radiographics. 1992;12(6):1155–73.

94. Piggott HA. The natural history of scoliosis in myelodysplasia. J Bone Joint Surg Br. 1980;62(1):54–8.

95. Trivedi J, Thomson JD, Slakey JB, Banta JV, Jones PW. Clinical and radiographic predictors of scoliosis in patients with myelomeningocele. JBJS. 2002;84(8):1389–94.

96. Bartnicki B, Synder M, Kujawa J, Stańczak K, Sibiński M. Siting stability in skeletally mature patients with scoliosis and myelomeningocele. Ortop Traumatol Rehabil. 2012;14(4):383–9.

97. Müller EB, Nordwall A. Brace treatment of scoliosis in children with myelomeningocele. Spine. 1994;19(2):151–5.

98. Letts M, Rathbone D, Yamashita T, Nichol B, Keeler A. Soft Boston orthosis in management of neuromuscular scoliosis: a preliminary report. J Pediatr Orthop. 1992;12(4):470–4.

99. Noonan K. Myelomeningocele. In: Morrissy R, Weinstein SL, editors. Lovell and Winter's pediatric orthopaedics. Philadelphia: Lippincott Williams & Wilkins; 2006. p. 605–47.

100. Wright JG. Hip and spine surgery is of questionable value in spina bifida: an evidence-based review. Clin Orthop Relat Res. 2011;469:1258–64.

101. Khoshbin A, Vivas L, Law PW, Stephens D, Davis AM, Howard A, Jarvis JG, Wright JG. The long-term outcome of patients treated operatively and non-operatively for scoliosis deformity secondary to spina bifida. Bone Joint J. 2014;96(9):1244–51.

102. McGirt MJ, Mehta V, Garces-Ambrossi G, Gottfried O, Solakoglu C, Gokaslan ZL, Samdani A, Jallo GI. Pediatric tethered cord syndrome: response of scoliosis to untethering procedures. J Neurosurg Pediatr. 2009;4(3):270–4.

103. Redding GJ, Mayer OH. Structure-respiration function relationships before and after surgical treatment of early-onset scoliosis. Clin Orthop Relat Res. 2011;469:1330–4.

104. Watanabe K, Uno K, Suzuki T, Kawakami N, Tsuji T, Yanagida H, Ito M, Hirano T, Yamazaki K, Minami S, Kotani T. Risk factors for complications associated with growing-rod surgery for early-onset scoliosis. Spine. 2013;38(8):E464–8.

105. Mehta VA, Gottfried ON, McGirt MJ, Gokaslan ZL, Ahn ES, Jallo GI. Safety and efficacy of concurrent pediatric spinal cord untethering and deformity correction. Clin Spine Surg. 2011;24(6):401–5.
106. Murans G, Gustavsson B, Saraste H. One-stage major spine deformity correction surgery: comparison between groups with and without additional neurosurgical intervention, with more than 24 months of follow-up. J Neurosurg Spine. 2010;13(6):666–71.
107. Mazur J, Menelaus MB, Dickens DR, Doig WG. Efficacy of surgical management for scoliosis in myelomeningocele: correction of deformity and alteration of functional status. J Pediatr Orthop. 1986;6(5):568–75.
108. Uribe JS, Dakwar E, Cardona RF, Vale FL. Minimally invasive lateral retropleural thoracolumbar approach: cadaveric feasibility study and report of 4 clinical cases. Operative. Neurosurgery. 2011;68(suppl_1):ons32-9.
109. Giorgi PD, Schirò GR, Capitani P, D'Aliberti GA, Talamonti G. Surgical pathway proposal for severe paralytic scoliosis in adolescents with myelomeningocele. Childs Nerv Syst. 2021;37:2279–87.
110. Miladi L, Mousny M. A novel technique for treatment of progressive scoliosis in young children using a 3-hook and 2-screw construct (H3S2) on a single sub-muscular growing rod: surgical technique. Eur Spine J. 2014;23:432–7.
111. Gaume M, Vergari C, Khouri N, Skalli W, Glorion C, Miladi L. Minimally invasive surgery for neuromuscular scoliosis: results and complications at a minimal follow-up of 5 years. Spine. 2021;46(24):1696–704.

# Chapter 7
# The Anterior Interhemispheric Transcallosal Approach to the Ventricles: How We Do It

Lydia J. Bernhardt and Alan R. Cohen

## Contents



## 7.1 Introduction

Intraventricular tumors of the lateral and third ventricles are relatively rare, accounting for 1–2% of all primary brain tumors in most large series [1–4]. They can be uniquely challenging to approach due to their deep location, propensity to become large before they are discovered, and association with hydrocephalus [5, 6]. The surgeon's goal is to develop a route to these deep lesions that will cause the least morbidity, provide adequate working space, and achieve a complete resection. This must be performed with minimal manipulation of the neural structures encircling the ventricles, avoiding functional cortical areas, and acquiring early control of feeding vessels [7, 8].


L. J. Bernhardt (✉) · A. R. Cohen (✉)
The Johns Hopkins University School of Medicine, Baltimore, MD, USA
e-mail: ljb@jhmi.edu; alan.cohen@jhmi.edu



© The Author(s), under exclusive license to Springer Nature
Switzerland AG 2024
C. Di Rocco (ed.), *Advances and Technical Standards in Neurosurgery*,
Advances and Technical Standards in Neurosurgery 49,
https://doi.org/10.1007/978-3-031-42398-7_7

We often use the anterior interhemispheric or transcallosal route for lesions in the lateral ventricular bodies, anterior horns, and atrium, as well as some third ventricular tumors. In this chapter, we provide an overview of the history of the transcallosal approach, relevant surgical anatomy, our patient selection including a discussion of the advantages and limitations of the transcallosal approach compared to the transcortical approaches, a stepwise description of the technical details of the approach and tumor resection and some thoughts on complication avoidance.

## 7.2  History

The interhemispheric transcallosal route to the lateral ventricles was pioneered by Walter Dandy, who in 1921, described the posterior transcallosal approach with division of the splenium for removal of pineal tumors [9]. He followed this by reporting a series of third ventricle tumors in 1933 [3]. Busch performed the first interforniceal approach in 1944 for a malignant glioma [10]. Some of the initial reports on transcallosal surgery closer to its current form were published in the 1970s [11–14], including a landmark article from Shucart and Stein, who in 1972 published their experience with 25 intraventricular tumors, including the transcallosal approach [15]. Since that time others have reported their experiences [16, 17]. Recent reports have focused on technical highlights and refinements. In 1996, Yasargil emphasized the importance of preserving the posterior half of the corpus callosum. He also proposed a trans-precuneal approach for trigonal lesions [18]. In 1988, Wen et al. presented an anatomical study of the choroidal fissure and of the supra- and subchoroidal surgical routes [19]. In 2001, Rosenfeld et al. described a limited anterior forniceal splitting technique for the management of hypothalamic hamartomas [20].

## 7.3  Pathological Entities

The differential diagnosis of tumors in the lateral and third ventricles depends on the age of the patient, location of the tumor, and radiological characteristics [1, 21]. Tumors found in the lateral ventricle of children younger than 5 years of age are often choroid plexus tumors, whereas in older children they tended to be gliomas. Choroid plexus tumors are often quite vascular and demonstrate a tumor blush on magnetic resonance (MR) imaging and angiography (Fig. 7.1). On MR imaging, they may show heterogeneous signal characteristics caused by necrosis and calcification and are iso- to hypodense on T1-weighted images relative to the white matter. Children with tuberous sclerosis may develop giant cell astrocytomas, which are often seen near the foramen of Monro. Astrocytoma may be found in all parts of the ventricle and frequently may sometimes arise from the thalamus, where they can

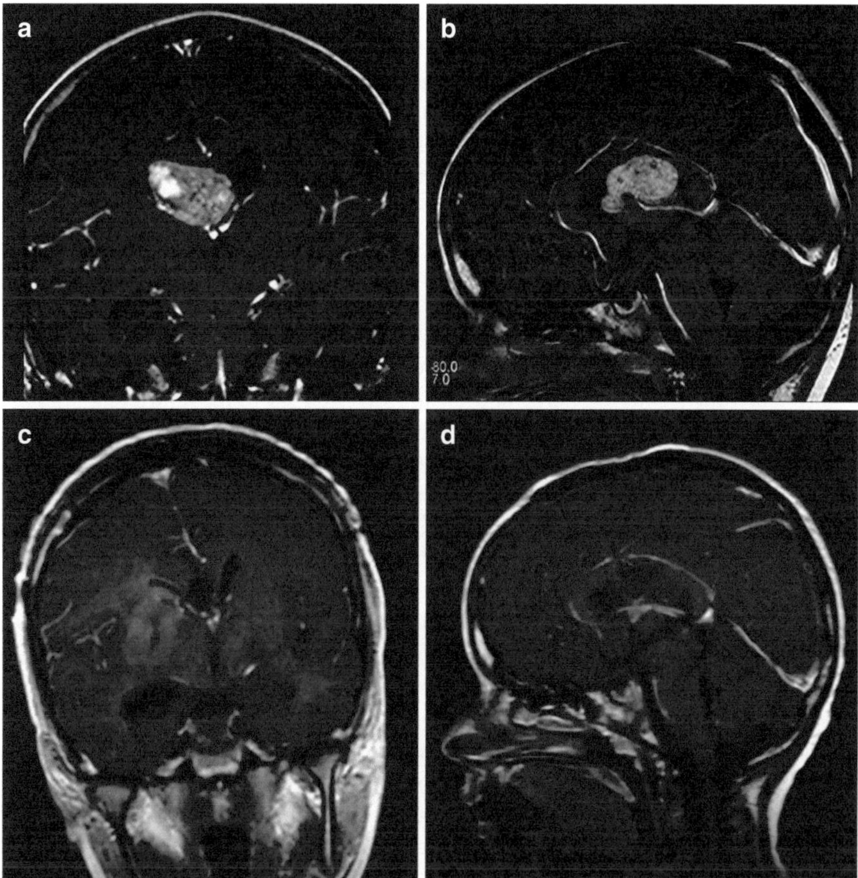

**Fig. 7.1** (**a**, **b**) Subependymal giant cell astrocytoma centered in the right lateral ventricle in an eleven-year-old boy, approachable via anterior interhemispheric transcallosal approach, MRI T1 with contrast, coronal, and sagittal views. (**c**, **d**) Postoperative T1 with contrast, coronal, and sagittal views, of the same patient

appear to infiltrate. Ependymomas, when supratentorial, can be intraventricular as well as intraparenchymal [2, 4, 6, 8, 22, 23].

In adults older than 30 years of age, tumors in the atrium and trigone are often meningiomas. They are isointense to brain on T1-weighted images and brightly enhance with gadolinium administration. The most common hypo- or isointense, nonenhancing tumor in the body of the lateral ventricle is the subependymoma, often occurring near the foramen of Monro. Outside the trigone, tumors in older patients are often either a primary neoplasm or a metastasis. Homogeneous intraventricular homogeneous masses that engulf the choroid glomus on computed tomography (CT) and have a significant choroidal artery supply on angiography, are often benign. Central neurocytomas, which occur mostly in older children or adults in the second to fourth decade of life, tend to adhere to the septum pellucidum and are primarily solid with some cystic regions, containing calcifications and signal voids that represent tumor vessels [24–26].

Other nonneoplastic processes such as cysts, sarcoidosis, xanthogranulomas, arteriovenous malformations, cavernous hemangiomas, and cysticercosis lesions are found in the lateral ventricle with varying frequency [21].

## 7.4 Approach Selection

The anterior transcallosal route is an excellent approach for lesions in the lateral ventricular body, anterior horn, and atrium, as well as third ventricular tumors. Tumors that arise from the posterior trigone, temporal horn, or superior frontal horn may be best managed by transcortical approaches.

There are several benefits of the transcallosal route over the transcortical route. Traditionally, the transcallosal route provides access to the lateral ventricles while sparing cerebral tissue and minimizing the risk of porencephalic cyst formation, subdural hygroma formation, and postoperative epilepsy (although recently some groups have reported decreased seizure rates in the transcortical vs the transcallosal approach [27, 28]). The anatomy is relatively constant. The distance to the third ventricle is shorter than via the transcortical approach, providing a more direct line of vision to the depths of the anterior third ventricle. The transcallosal approach can be used with small or large ventricular size and is a superior approach if the ventricles are small [29, 30]. Use of the transcortical approach in the absence of hydrocephalus requires disruption of a fairly large amount of cortex and white matter, and the maintenance of retraction can be difficult. If departure from the initial plane of entry is required, the transcortical route can significantly limit the surgeon's mobility. Transcallosal approaches are also useful if the transcortical alternative requires an excessive corticotomy or a long route through the white matter. Some tumors that may preferably be approached through the corpus callosum include ependymomas, subependymomas, intraventricular meningiomas, colloid cysts, hypothalamic hamartomas, cavernomas, and intraventricular metastases.

If the ventricles are enlarged, access to the foramen of Monro and the third ventricle can be accomplished with either the transcortical or transcallosal technique. Advantages of the transcortical-transventricular exposure are that there is less chance of compromising essential draining veins going to the sagittal sinus and less chance of injuring the pericallosal arteries. Subcortical lesions, such as neuroectodermal tumors, are best managed via transcortical access because of their infiltrative nature [31].

One of the potential contraindications if a mid- or posterior callosotomy is planned is crossed dominance, a condition in which the hemisphere controlling the dominant hand is contralateral to the hemisphere mediating language and speech. Crossed dominance can occur when there is evidence of extracallosal dysfunction, particularly following cerebral injury (due to surgery, trauma, or infection) during childhood and resulting in relocation of function. These patients may be at risk for writing and speech-related deficits following callosal sectioning [32]. Transcallosal surgery may also be contraindicated if the splenium of the corpus callosum is sectioned in the presence of a homonymous hemianopia in the dominant hemisphere, causing alexia [33].

## 7.5   Preoperative Planning

Patients usually come to medical attention with a CT scan and subsequently undergo MR imaging with and without contrast, with navigation aids. CT angiography, MR angiography, or traditional cerebral angiography may be useful in identifying major feeding vessels in vascular lesions such as meningioma, choroid plexus tumors, and central neurocytoma. If the lesion is thought to be prohibitively vascular, preoperative embolization may aid resection.

Patients with intraventricular tumors may have subtle cognitive disabilities such as memory, perception, and fine motor skill deficits that may or may not be related to hydrocephalus or mass effect of the lesion. A neuropsychological evaluation for cognitive deficits can be an important part of the preoperative assessment, as injury to the fornices causing memory deficits is a concern during the transcallosal approach. Preoperative visual testing with a neuroophthalmological examination is offered to any patient with a visual complaint.

## 7.6   Relevant Surgical Anatomy

The lateral ventricles are paired C-shaped structures that wrap around the ipsilateral thalamus. Each ventricle is divided into five sections: anterior horn, body, temporal horn, atrium, and occipital horn. Each of these five sections has a roof, a floor, and a medial and lateral wall. The walls of the lateral ventricles are formed by the thalamus, septum pellucidum, corpus callosum and its radiations, caudate nucleus, and the fornix. The caudate nucleus is an almond-shaped structure that forms the lateral wall of the body, anterior lateral wall of the atrium, and roof of the temporal horn. The fornix starts as the fimbria of the hippocampi in the medial temporal horn and runs along the thalamus in the anterior wall of the atrium. After giving off commissural fibers, it continues in the inferior medial wall of the body. Finally, it forms the superior and anterior borders of the foramen of Monro [6, 34].

The thalamus, which is in the center of the lateral ventricles, is seen in the floor of the body, interior wall of the atrium, and medial roof of the temporal horn. The choroidal fissure is an important surgical landmark defined by the groove between the thalamus and the fornix where the tela choroidea gives rise to the choroid plexus. The septum pellucidum is a thin, often diaphanous wall, which separates the frontal horns and body in the midline. The genu of the internal capsule lies in the lateral wall between the caudate and thalamus at the level of the foramen of Monro. The remainder of the lateral ventricular surfaces is formed by the corpus callosum and its radiations [34].

The corpus callosum (CC), which is made up of 300 million axons, forms the largest part of the ventricular walls and contributes to the wall of each of the five parts of the lateral ventricle. The corpus callosum has two anterior parts, the rostrum and genu; a central part, the body, and a posterior part, the splenium. The rostrum is situated below and forms the floor of the frontal horn. The genu gives rise to a large fiber tract, the forceps minor, which forms the anterior wall of the frontal horn as it sweeps obliquely forward and lateral to connect the frontal lobes. The genu and the body of the corpus callosum form the roof of both the frontal horn and the body of the lateral ventricle. The splenium gives rise to a large tract, the forceps major, which forms a prominence, called the bulb, in the upper part of the medial wall of the atrium and occipital horn as it sweeps posteriorly to connect the occipital lobes. Another fiber tract, the tapetum, which arises in the posterior part of the body and splenium of the corpus callosum, sweeps laterally and inferiorly to form the roof and lateral wall of the atrium and the temporal and occipital horns. The tapetum separates the fibers of the optic radiations from the temporal horn.

Diffusion tensor imaging-based tractography using fractional anisotropy has allowed more detailed functional mapping of specific tracts through the callosum. In a tractography study by Hofer and Frahm, the anterior 1/6th of the CC, deemed Region 1, contains fibers projecting into the prefrontal region (Fig. 7.2). The rest of the anterior half of the CC, Region 2, contains fibers projecting to premotor and supplementary motor cortical areas. Region 3 was defined as the posterior half minus the posterior third and comprises fibers projecting into the primary motor cortex. Region 4, the posterior third minus the posterior fourth, houses the crossing of primary sensory fibers. Region 5, the posterior fourth, is where callosal parietal, temporal, and occipital fibers cross the CC [35].

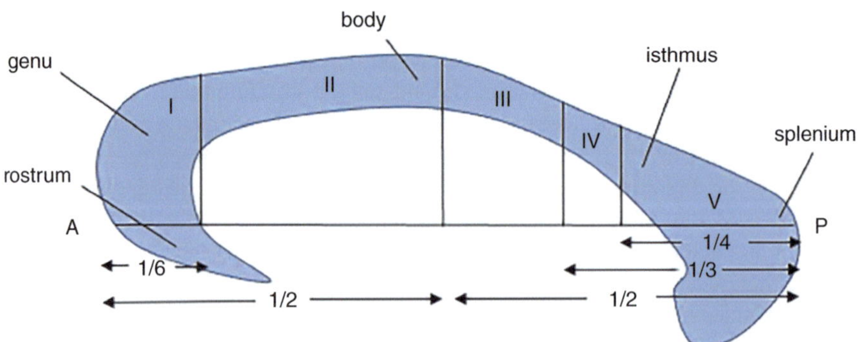


**Fig. 7.2** Anatomy of the corpus callosum. Adapted from Hofer and Frahm 2006 [35]. Region I: prefrontal; region II: premotor and supplementary motor; region III: motor; region IV: sensory; region V: parietal, temporal, and occipital. A: anterior; P: posterior

The primary arteries to the choroid plexus are the anterior and posterior choroidal arteries, branches of which provide the vascular supply to tumors in this region. Understanding the course of the arteries helps the surgeon choose an approach for each lesion and thus permits early control, when possible, of the feeding vessels [6].

The anterior choroidal artery arises from the internal carotid artery, distal to the posterior communicating artery. It leaves the anterior incisural space and enters the lateral ventricle through the choroidal fissure, coursing posteriorly to lie near the lateral posterior choroidal artery. The anterior choroidal artery generally supplies the choroid plexus in the temporal horn and atrium. Because the choroidal arteries pass through the choroidal fissure, opening this fissure early will facilitate proximal control of the feeding vessels [36].

The posterior choroidal arteries are grouped into lateral and medial divisions. The lateral posterior choroidal artery is comprised of one to six branches, which arise in the ambient and quadrigeminal cisterns from the posterior cerebral artery (PCA). These branches then pierce the ventricle and pass around the pulvinar and through the choroidal fissure at the level of the crus of the fornix to supply the choroid plexus in the posterior temporal horn, atrium, and body of the ventricles. The medial posterior choroidal arteries arise as one to three branches from the PCA in the interpeduncular and crural cisterns. These arteries circumnavigate the midbrain and move to the pineal gland to enter the roof of the third ventricle. This vessel then passes in the velum interpositum, between the thalami, adjacent to the internal cerebral veins. The medial posterior choroidal arteries travel through the velum interpositum (tela choroidea), sending inconstant branches to the lateral ventricle through the choroidal fissure and foramen of Monro. The medial posterior choroidal artery supplies the choroid plexus in the roof of the third ventricle and sometimes the choroid plexus of the lateral ventricle [34, 36].

The distal pericallosal arteries that branch off of the anterior cerebral arteries (ACAs) are routinely encountered during transcallosal surgery. The ACAs arise from the internal carotid artery below the anterior perforated substance and course anteromedially above the optic nerve and chiasm to reach the interhemispheric fissure, where it ascends in front of the lamina terminalis to reach the area below the floor of the frontal horn [37]. It then passes below the rostrum and around the genu of the corpus callosum in close proximity to the floor, anterior wall, and roof of the frontal horn and the roof of the body of the lateral ventricle. Often the anterior cerebral artery on one side crosses the interhemispheric fissure to supply the medial part of the opposite hemisphere [38]. The distal part of the ACA may be exposed not only above but also below the corpus callosum because the terminal branch of the pericallosal artery may pass around the splenium and course forward in the roof of the third ventricle, reaching as far anterior as the foramen of Monro. The pericallosal branches that penetrate the corpus callosum reach the septum pellucidum and the fornix in the medial wall of the frontal horn and body [39].

The veins are useful as landmarks to direct the surgeon to the foramen of Monro, especially in cases in which hydrocephalus is present. In general, a line drawn from the bregma to the external auditory meatus should pass through the foramen of

Monro. When viewing the corpus callosum from above, the foramen of Monro is usually about 2.5 cm posterior to the rostrum.

There are many important veins composing the lateral and medial groups, but perhaps the best known for surgical and angiographic orientation is the thalamostriate vein. The thalamostriate vein courses from the lateral wall of the body of the ventricle through the sulcus between the caudate and thalamus toward the foramen of Monro. It then forms the venous angle with an acute posterior turn to empty into the internal cerebral veins. The veins, which drain the frontal horn and usually anterior lateral ventricle, drain into the internal cerebral vein as it travels in the roof of the third ventricle within the velum interpositum. When working within the lateral ventricle, a useful way to find the foramen of Monro is to trace the septal and thalamostriate veins. Their diameter increases as the approach the internal cerebral veins at the foramen. The veins in the temporal horn drain into the basal vein of Rosenthal as it passes through the ambient cistern. Veins from the atrium and occipital horn drain into the basal internal cerebral veins as well as the vein of Galen [6, 30, 36].

## 7.7    Technical Details

Instructions to the anesthesia team include prophylactic antibiotics (cefazolin every 8 h), dexamethasone, normal systolic blood pressure goal, wide MAP goal, end tidal $CO_2$ between 25 and 30 for brain relaxation. Mannitol is available if additional brain relaxation is required. Antiepileptics are generally not required unless there is cortical violation or concern for subarachnoid bleeding during the procedure.

Because the interhemispheric approach provides equal access to both lateral ventricles, the presence of midline draining cortical veins influences the side of the craniotomy; however, the nondominant hemisphere is the optimal choices if venous drainage is symmetrical. We will use the right-sided exposure in almost all cases and will describe the craniotomy from the right side here.

The patient is placed in the supine position with the brow up and elevated about 20 degrees (Fig. 7.3). An alternative position is to place the head parallel to the floor with the left side up and the right side down, to allow the right hemisphere to fall away during exposure. This enables the surgeon to use his or her hands next to each others and minimizes the need for retraction [40].

A coronal skin incision is the cosmetically acceptable and provides the most flexibility while demonstrating the surface landmarks for proper placement of the bone flap, though other scalp incisions e.g. (L-shaped, lazy S) can be used The incision extends most inferiorly on the right side to a point approximately 1 cm anterior to the external auditory meatus and approximately 2 cm above the zygoma. It is carried to the left far enough to allow reflection of the skin flap about 6 cm anterior to the coronal suture, which often requires an incision extending to a point approximately 5 cm above the left zygoma, depending on the age of the patient and the thickness of the scalp. The scalp flap is reflected anteriorly and secured with fish

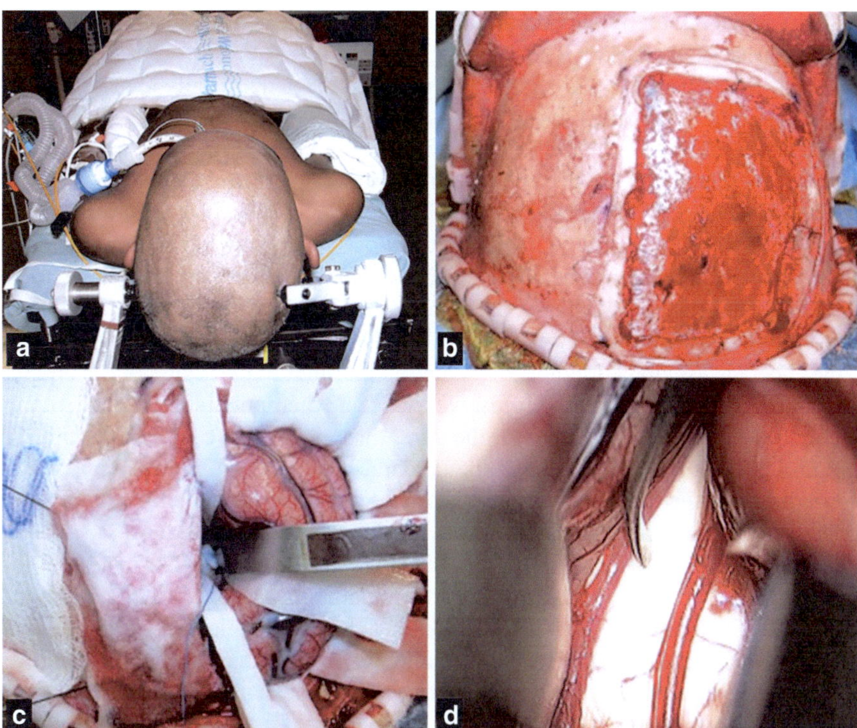

**Fig. 7.3** Anterior interhemispheric transcallosal exposure. (**a**) Supine positioning with brow up. (**b**) Quadrilateral bone flap with two burr holes over the sinus and two burr holes laterally, with the craniotomy 2/3 anterior and 1/3 posterior to the coronal suture. (**c**) Gentle retraction of the right hemisphere with the dural flap draped over the superior sagittal sinus. (**d**) Visualization of the pearly white corpus callosum with instrument pointing between bilateral pericallosal arteries

hooks. The coronal suture and the junction of the sagittal and coronal sutures at the bregma is identified on the skull surface [15].

A quadrilateral bone flap is fashioned to facilitate the midline interhemispheric approach. We place two lateral burr holes first, and then either two or three burr holes on the midline directly over the superior sagittal sinus (Fig. 7.3). Alternatively, the medial burr holes can be placed on either side of midline. The craniotomy usually extends 1 cm posterior to the bregma and 6 cm anterior to it. This allows for enough space to work around bridging veins from the cortex to the superior sagittal sinus. A triangular craniotomy can also be used. It is essential to remember that the approach to the corpus callosum is midline and necessitates reflecting the frontal lobe away from the falx while protecting the sagittal sinus.

The dura is stripped from the undersurface of the bone, with dissectors and a Gigli saw guide. Craniotome cuts from the anteromedial and posteromedial burr holes to the lateral burr holes are made directed away from the sinus. The midline cuts over the sagittal sinus are made last. The surgeon must always be prepared for injury to the sagittal sinus, which is why these cuts are made last, to allow the bone to be removed rapidly in the event of a sinus injury. Care is taken to avoid compression of the sagittal sinus.

The dura is opened in a U-shaped fashion and reflected medially toward the sagittal sinus. The bone overlying the sinus can be beveled with a drill to facilitate exposure of the midline. Care is taken to avoid kinking the sagittal sinus. At this point, if the ventricles are not enlarged, mannitol can be administered to decrease the need for hemisphere retraction. If there is hydrocephalus, no dehydrating agent is given because there will be marked relaxation of the brain when the ventricular system is opened. One or two cortical veins draining into the sinus may have to be divided to facilitate the exposure; the veins anterior to the coronal suture can generally be resected with impunity, but large draining veins should be preserved if possible. There is usually a draining vein entering the sinus at the region of the bregma or just behind it. We attempt to preserve this vein when possible. Traction sutures are placed to facilitate retraction of the dura, thus exposing the superior portion of the falx and the medial portion of the cerebral hemisphere. Only 3–4 cm of free space between the hemisphere and falx are required for adequate retraction. After the dura has been reflected, the operating microscope is introduced.

The right hemisphere is gently retracted (Fig. 7.3). As the inferior margin of the falx is reached, the corpus callosum is identified by its glistening white color and relative hypovascularity. The surgeon may mistake the cingulate gyrus for the corpus callosum, but with experience the distinction becomes more straightforward, as the cingulate gyrus looks like typical cortex with its gray color and pial vasculature. This misidentification can occur if the callosomarginal arteries overlying the cingulate gyrus are mistaken for the pericallosal arteries which are situated directly over the corpus callosum. The pericallosal arteries are separated and the corpus callosum is exposed for a few cm. Sometimes, the pericallosal arteries may be retracted to one side, depending on the anatomy (Fig. 7.3).

The right hemisphere is gently retracted away from the falx. A moist piece of Telfa is used to cover the cerebral hemisphere. An automatic retractor is placed on the hemisphere, or retraction can be achieved by using the suction catheter and bipolar forceps.

The corpus callosum is then divided for a length of about 2–3 cm in length, confined to the anterior third of the body. The exact length of the callosal sectioning is determined by the location and size of the tumor. As it is avascular, the corpus callosum can be divided using a blunt small dissector such as a Penfield 4, or using the bipolar forceps along with suction, and sharp dissection as needed. When the corpus callosum has been divided, CSF escapes from the ventricles. In the presence of hydrocephalus, the corpus callosum is usually quite thin. Entry into the ventricles is rapid, and the view of the intraventricular anatomy is excellent. With normal size ventricles, the corpus callosum is considerably thicker and the procedure takes more time, but the anatomical visualization is equally good. The self-retaining retractor along the right frontal lobe is deepened and may be placed over the cut edge of the corpus callosum.

Orientation is achieved by identifying the major landmarks within the right lateral ventricle: the choroid plexus, the thalamostriate vein, and the septal vein. The foramen of Monro is found by following the choroid plexus and thalamostriate vein anteriorly. It is useful to remember that there is no choroid plexus anterior to the foramen of Monro. The left rather than right lateral ventricle may be entered, but the anatomy makes this straightforward. Entry into a cavum septum pellucidum may be confusing until the surgeon realizes that no intraventricular structures are present. When increased magnification restricts the field of view through the operating microscope, it is frequently helpful to become reoriented to the normal anatomy to prevent wandering into the thalamus, hypothalamus, and fornix. Whenever possible, the plane between the tumor and ependymal surface should be maintained.

Lesions within the lateral ventricle or adjacent subependymal areas are generally seen as soon as the ventricle is entered, as the corpus callosum forms the roof of the lateral ventricle. If the foramen of Monro is patent, placement of a barrier will prevent blood from pooling into the third ventricle, minimizing the potential for ventricular obstruction. Third ventricular lesions in the anterior third ventricle are often seen through a dilated foramen of Monro (Fig. 7.4). Enlargement of the foramen may be necessary, in which case gentle pressure with a small blunt dissector in all directions except medially may be helpful. A wider view of the third ventricle can be obtained by opening the choroidal fissure, working between the tenia fornicis and the tenia thalami. Sometimes this widening can be created by the third ventricular tumor. The boundaries of the foramen are the column of the fornix anteriorly, the anterior commissure anteromedially, and the thalamus posteriorly. The fornix and commissure are difficult to visualize from the lateral ventricle, but their location must be kept in mind. An expanded foramen does not routinely need to be enlarged by sacrifice of a fornix, but if this is necessary, an incision is made anteriorly through one column of the fornix. When possible, and certainly when there is a lesion at a foramen of Monro, the septum pellucidum can be fenestrated to allow for biventricular communication. Or, if the callosal sectioning has led to the contralateral ventricle, the septum pellucidum can be opened to access the ipsilateral side. Should this occur, it is imperative to preserve the fornices at the base of the septum.

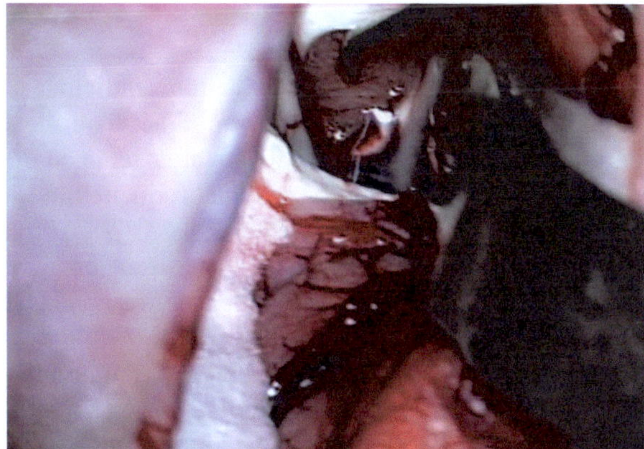

**Fig. 7.4** Germinoma of the third ventricle via transcallosal transforaminal approach

Alternatively, the third ventricle can be accessed through an interforniceal dissection. The anatomical definition of this space may be difficult to identify. The surgeon must work between the fornices and the internal cerebral veins. Bilateral forniceal injury can cause severe memory deficits and injury to the internal cerebral veins can be catastrophic. This approach is generally reserved for cases in which there is either a cavum septum pellucidum or significant mass effect that has anatomically separated the fornices.

Tumors arising in the choroid plexus such as papillomas and meningiomas receive their blood supply from the choroidal vessels. Early identification and transection of these vessels will reduce bleeding associated with piecemeal tumor resection. Lesions that arise from the ependymal surface and septum pellucidum (for example, gliomas and neurocytomas) receive blood supply from the small vessels of the ventricular walls. These small vessels create less intraoperative blood loss, but because they are frequently numerous and small, meticulous microscopic dissection is mandatory. Tumor resection is facilitated by maintaining the dissection plane between the ependyma and lesion.

When the tumor surgery is completed, meticulous hemostasis should be achieved. In some patients, an endoscope can provide a "last look" to ensure the absence of blood clot or residual tumor, and that interventricular communication is achieved. Extensive irrigation with Ringer's Lactate solution is used to evacuate blood that may have pooled in the lateral and third ventricles to aid in preventing delayed ventricular obstruction. The ventricles are filled with warmed Ringer's solution at the end of the surgery to remove air that may have become trapped. If, due to anatomy or residual tumor, there is concern that the patient may develop hydrocephalus, a ventricular catheter is left in either the ipsilateral or contralateral lateral ventricle postoperatively to monitor intracranial pressure and to demonstrate that the ventricular system is patent.

Postoperative imaging with MRI is performed to evaluate the extent of the tumor resection (Fig. 7.5).

## 7.8   Complications

Many of the complications seen with intraventricular surgery are related to the location and nature of the primary lesion rather than the approach [41]. For example, diabetes insipidus is seen in patients after removal of a sellar craniopharyngioma with extension into the third ventricle. Akinetic mutism can occur transiently with excessive retraction against both cingulate gyri. Aseptic meningitis is also seen in patients with tumors such as malignant astrocytomas which spill blood and necrotic tissue into the CSF spaces. This typically responds well to an extended course of corticosteroid therapy.

The major complications to avoid in the transcallosal approach, i.e., intraventricular hemorrhage or cerebral infarction, are related to compromise of venous drainage, either by occlusion of the superior sagittal sinus by retraction or by

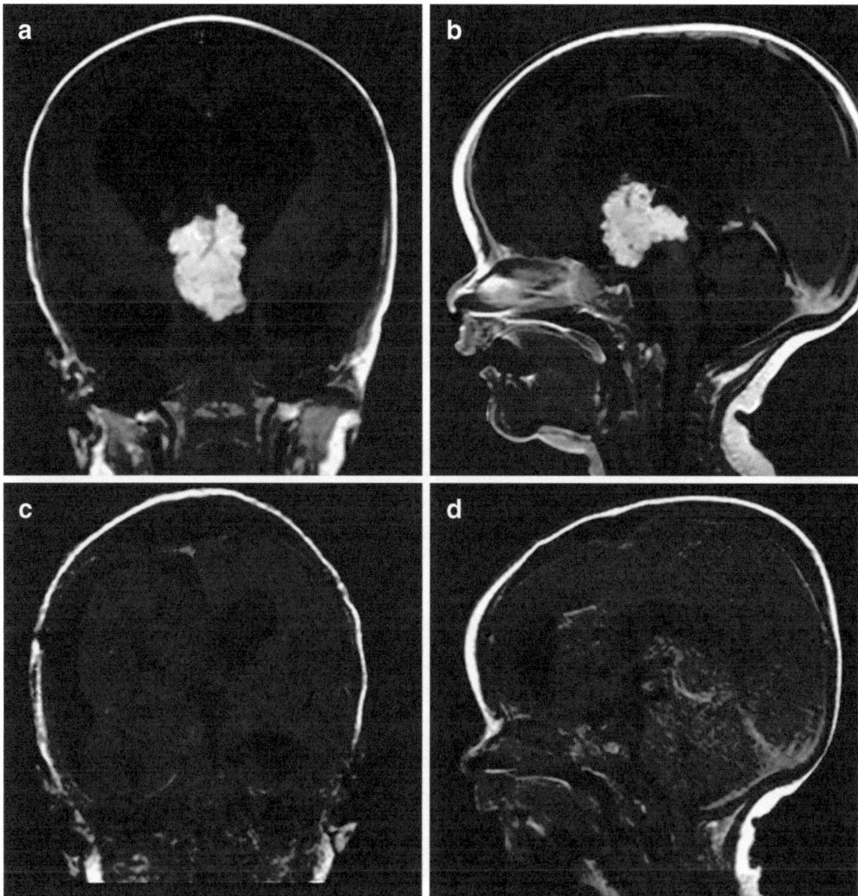

**Fig. 7.5** (**a**, **b**) Third ventricular choroid plexus papilloma in a two-month-old girl, MRI T1 with contrast, coronal and sagittal views. (**c**, **d**) Post-operative T1 with contrast, coronal and sagittal views of the same patient

division of very large draining veins, even if anterior to the coronal suture. These misadventures can be prevented with careful attention to retractor placement and to careful intraoperative decision making regarding draining veins [42]. We do not routinely see significant clinical deficits subsequent to division of the anterior third of the body of the corpus callosum. This includes acute disconnection syndromes, memory loss, affect difficulties, or other performance issues [43, 44]. However, excessive damage to the fornices can result in memory difficulties, and in severe cases, amnesia [45]. Postoperative neuropsychological assessment helps to identify subtle changes that may require additional therapy.

## 7.9 Conclusion

The interhemispheric transcallosal corridor can provide excellent access to lesions in the anterior ventricular system. It is a useful alternative to the transcortical approach and is effective even when the ventricles are not enlarged.

## References


1. Iyer RR, Shimony N, Jentoft ME, Jallo GI. Pathology of intraventricular tumors [internet]. Comprehensive overview of modern surgical approaches to intrinsic brain Tumors. Elsevier Inc.; 2019. p. 139–58. https://doi.org/10.1016/B978-0-12-811783-5.00007-0.
2. Agarwal A, Kanekar S. Intraventricular tumors. Semin Ultrasound CT MRI. [Internet]. 2016;37(2):150–8. https://doi.org/10.1053/j.sult.2015.12.003.
3. Dandy WE. Benign encapsulated tumors in the lateral ventricles of the brain: diagnosis and treatment. Ann Surg. 1933;98:841–5.
4. Ahmed SI, Javed G, Laghari AA, Bareeqa SB, Aziz K, Khan M, et al. Third ventricular tumors: a comprehensive literature review. Cureus. 2018;10:10.
5. Pendl G, Öztürk E, Haselsberger K. Surgery of tumours of the lateral ventricle. Acta Neurochir. 1992;116(2–4):128–36.
6. Ellenbogen RG. Transcortical surgery for lateral ventricular tumors. Neurosurg Focus. 2001;10:6.
7. Kasowski H, Piepmeier JM. Transcallosal approach for tumors of the lateral and third ventricles. Neurosurg Focus. 2001;10(6):6–10.
8. Delfini R, Pichierri A. Transcallosal approaches to intraventricular tumors. Cranial Craniofac Skull Base Surg. 2010:87–105.
9. Dandy WE. An operation for the removal of pineal tumors. Surg Gynec Obs. 1921;33(113)
10. Busch E. A new approach for the removal of tumors of the third ventricle. Acta Psychiatr Scand. [Internet]. 1944;19:57–60. https://doi.org/10.1111/j.1600-0447.1944.tb04560.x.
11. Kempe L, Blaylock R. Lateral-trigonal intraventricular tumors. A new operative approach. Acta Neurochir. 1976;35:233–42.
12. Hirsch J, Zouanaoui A, Renier D, Pierre-Kahn A. A new surgical approach to the third ventricle with interruption of the striothalamic vein. Acta Neurochir. 1979;47:135–47.
13. Ledoux JE, Risse GL, Springer SP, Wilson DH, Gazzaniga MS. Cognition and commissurotomy. Brain. 1977;100(1):87–104.
14. Milhorat TH, Baldwin M. A technique for surgical exposure of the cerebral midline: experimental transcallosal microdissection. J Neurosurg. 1966;24(3):687–91.
15. Shucart W, Stein B. Transcallosal Approach to the Anterior Ventricular System. Neurosurgery. 1978;3(3):0148-396X/78/0303-0339.
16. Ehni G. Interhemispheric and Percallosal (Transcallosal) Approach to the Cingulate Gyri, Intraventricular Shunt Tubes, and Certain Deeply Placed Brain Lesions. Neurosurgery. 1984;14(1):99–110.
17. Geffen G, Walsh A, Simpson D, Jeeves M. Comparison of the effects of transcortical and transcallosal removal of intraventricular tumours. Brain. 1980;103(4):773–88.
18. Yasargil M. Microneurosurgery of CNS tumors. Leipzig: Thieme; 1996.
19. Wen H, Rhoton AJ, de Oliveira E. Transchoroidal approach to the third ventricle: an anatomic study of the choroidal fissure and its clinical application. Neurosurgery. 1998;42:1205–17.
20. Rosenfeld JV, Harvey AS, Wrennall J, Zacharin M, Berkovic SF. Transcallosal resection of hypothalamic hamartomas, with control of seizures, in children with gelastic epilepsy. Neurosurgery. 2001;48(1):108–18.

21. Cikla U, Swanson KI, Tumturk A, Keser N, Uluc K, Cohen-Gadol A, et al. Microsurgical resection of tumors of the lateral and third ventricles: operative corridors for difficult-to-reach lesions. J Neuro-Oncol. 2016;130(2):331–40.
22. Stein B, Fraser R, Tenner M. Tumours of the third ventricle. Neurol India. 1977;25(3):166–9.
23. Sanford R, Laurent J. Intraventricular tumors of childhood. Cancer. 1985;56:1795–9.
24. John Silver A, Ramaiah Ganti S, Hilal SK. Computed tomography of tumors involving the atria of the lateral ventricles. Radiology. 1982;145:71–8.
25. Jelinek J, Smirniotopoulos JG, Parisi JE, Kanzer M. Lateral ventricular neoplasms of the brain: differential diagnosis based on clinical, CT, and MR findings. [published erratum appears in AJNR Am J Neuroradiol 1990 Jul-Aug;11(4):734]. AJNR Am J Neuroradiol. 1990;11(3):567–74.
26. Mani RL, Hedgcock MW, Mass SI, Gilmor RL, Enzmann DR, Eisenberg RL. Radiographic diagnosis of meningioma of the lateral ventricle. J Neurosurg. 1978;49(2):249–55.
27. Eichberg DG, Sedighim S, Buttrick S, Komotar RJ. Postoperative seizure rate after transcortical resection of subcortical brain tumors and colloid cysts: a single surgeon's experience. Cureus. 2018;10(1):1–8.
28. Milligan BD, Meyer FB. Morbidity of transcallosal and transcortical approaches to lesions in and around the lateral and third ventricles: a single-institution experience. Neurosurgery. 2010;67(6):1483–96.
29. Bellotti C, Pappadà G, Sani R, Oliveri G, Stangalino C. The transcallosal approach for lesions affecting the lateral and third ventricles—surgical considerations and results in a series of 42 cases. Acta Neurochir. 1991;111(3–4):103–7.
30. Türe U, Yaşargil MG, Al-Mefty O. The transcallosal—transforaminal approach to the third ventricle with regard to the venous variations in this region. J Neurosurg. 1997;87(5):706–15.
31. Nagasawa S, Miyake H, Ohta T. Transcallosal and transcortical approaches for tumors at the anterior part of the lateral ventricle: relations between visualized and ventricular size. No Shinkei Geka [Internet]. 1997;25(4):321–7. Available from: http://www.ncbi.nlm.nih.gov/pubmed/9125715
32. Joseph R. Reversal of cerebral dominance for language and emotion in a corpus callosotomy patient. J Neurol Neurosurg Psychiatry. 1986;49(6):628–34.
33. Lucas TH, Chowdhary M, Ellenbogen RG. Microsurgical approaches to the ventricular system. Principles Neurol Surg. 2018;21(1):666–681.e2.
34. Timurkaynak E, Rhoton A, Barry M. Microsurgical anatomy and operative approaches to the lateral ventricles. Neurosurgery. 1986;19(5):685–723.
35. Hofer S, Frahm J. Topography of the human corpus callosum revisited-comprehensive fiber tractography using diffusion tensor magnetic resonance imaging. NeuroImage. 2006;32(3):989–94.
36. Rhoton AJ, Fujii K, Fradd B. Microsurgical anatomy of the anterior choroidal artery. Surg Neurol. 1979;12:171–87.
37. Rosner SS, Rhoton ALJ, Ono M, Barry M. Microsurgical anatomy of the anterior perforating arteries. J Neurosurg. 1984;61:468–85.
38. Perlmutter D, Rhoton ALJ. Microsurgical anatomy of the distal anterior cerebral artery. J Neurosurg. 1978;49:204–28.
39. Perlmutter D, Rhoton AJ. Microsurgical anatomy of the anterior cerebral-anterior communicating-recurrent artery complex. J Neurosurg. 1976;45(3):259–72.
40. Chaddad-Neto F, Silva Da Costa MD, Bozkurt B, Doria-Netto HL, De Araujo PD, Da Silva Centeno R, et al. Contralateral anterior interhemispheric-transcallosal-transrostral approach to the subcallosal region: a novel surgical technique. J Neurosurg. 2018;129(2):508–14.
41. Jeeves MA, Simpson DA, Geffen G. Functional consequences of the transcallosal removal of intraventricular tumours. J Neurol Neurosurg Psychiatry. 1979;42(2):134–42.
42. Hassaneen W, Suki D, Salaskar AL, Levine NB, DeMonte F, Lang FF, et al. Immediate morbidity and mortality associated with transcallosal resection of tumors of the third ventricle. J Clin Neurosci [Internet]. 2010;17(7):830–6. https://doi.org/10.1016/j.jocn.2009.12.007.

43. Winkler PAMD, Ilmberger JPD, Krishnan KGMD, Reulen H-JMD. Transcallosal Interforniceal-transforaminal approach for removing lesions occupying the third ventricular space: clinical and neuropsychological results. Neurosurgery. 2000;46(4):879–90.
44. Oepen G, Schulz-Weiling R, Zimmermann P, Birg W, Straesser S, Gilsbach J. Neuropsychological assessment of the transcallosal approach. Eur Arch Psychiatry Neurol Sci. 1988;237(6):365–75.
45. McMackin D, Cockburn J, Anslow P, Gaffan D. Correlation of fornix damage with memory impairment in six cases of colloid cyst removal. Acta Neurochir. 1995;135(1–2):12–8.

# Chapter 8
# Treatment of Brain Arteriovenous Malformations

**Vladimír Beneš, Adéla Bubeníková, Petr Skalický, and Ondřej Bradáč**

## Contents




V. Beneš
Department of Neurosurgery and Neurooncology, Military University Hospital, First Faculty of Medicine, Charles University, Prague, Czech Republic
e-mail: vladimir.benes@uvn.cz

A. Bubeníková · P. Skalický · O. Bradáč (✉)
Department of Neurosurgery and Neurooncology, Military University Hospital, First Faculty of Medicine, Charles University, Prague, Czech Republic

Department of Neurosurgery, Motol University Hospital, Second Faculty of Medicine, Charles University, Prague, Czech Republic
e-mail: ondrej.bradac@uvn.cz



© The Author(s), under exclusive license to Springer Nature Switzerland AG 2024
C. Di Rocco (ed.), *Advances and Technical Standards in Neurosurgery*,
Advances and Technical Standards in Neurosurgery 49,
https://doi.org/10.1007/978-3-031-42398-7_8

## 8.1 Introduction

Arteriovenous malformations (AVMs) are abnormally developed fast-flow connections between venous and arterial circulation with the absence of a normal capillary bed, occurring in various organ systems in the body [1]. In the brain, AVMs' growth, pathophysiological patterns, and possible rupture cause a variety of serious problems that need to be taken into account before the decision to undergo active treatment is made [2].

Before the invention of angiography, computed tomography (CT), and magnetic resonance imaging (MRI), it was rather challenging to clearly elucidate the pathogenesis of the disease and even more difficult to provide efficient treatment. Nowadays, thanks to both technical and informational advances, there are four possible treatment modalities applied in clinical practice: active approaches that include (1) surgery, (2) radiosurgery, (3) endovascular embolization and passive one, and (4) observation, which is a justified therapy alternative in well-selected patients with intracerebral AVMs. Familiarity with the natural course of the disease is fundamental for any further decision-making in AVM treatment. The main aim of active treatment of AVMs is ensuring the prevention of haemorrhage, but the stabilization of seizures or neurological deficits are other possible indications for intervention.

This chapter overviews up-to-date findings of AVMs, from their pathogenesis, genetics, epidemiology, diagnostic methods, and treatment modalities, to final treatment outcome and prognosis. We present currently applied dogmas and introduce advances in each available treatment modality of AVM management.

## 8.2 Angioarchitecture and Classification

One of the most renowned classifications of cerebral vascular malformations by William F. McCormick was published in 1966 [1]. According to it, brain vascular malformations consist of four individual subcategories: (1) cavernous malformations, (2) venous malformations, (3) capillary telangiectasias, and finally (4) arteriovenous malformations. There are three most important morphological components of the AVM: (1) arterial feeders, (2) nidus (in Latin meaning the "nest"), and finally (3) draining veins. Arterial feeders can be both single or multiple and may originate from more than one main cerebral artery or its branches. The nidus is the racemose centre of the AVM composed of fragile and dysplastic vessels, mainly due to the significant deficiency of lamina muscularis. When there is intervening brain parenchyma between the vascular channels of the nidus, the nidus is called diffuse. If this is not true and no intervening brain tissue is present, the nidus is called compact, according to the classification of Valavanis and Yasargil [2]. There also might be more than one nidus within the AVM. Similarly to arterial feeders, also draining veins can be single or multiple and do not have to be in all cases exclusively devoted to the AVM itself. If a single draining vein divides into several vascular channels early in its course, it may sometimes resemble the drainage composed of multiple veins. The blood from superficial AVMs is typically drained through cortical veins towards the adjacent dural sinuses while the venous drainage of deep AVMs is primarily directed into the deep venous circulation.

Considering the high flow within the AVM and raised blood pressure towards the vascular wall, associated aneurysms may originate in some AVMs (the prevalence of brain AVMs with associated aneurysms varies, but it is reported to be between 3% and 58% [3, 4]). Associated aneurysms might be related or unrelated to the AVM nidus. Extranidal aneurysms typically originate on the walls of the feeding arteries or the draining veins [4]. Intranidal aneurysms are the most common type of AVM-associated aneurysms. They are typically most prone to rupture and correlate with symptomatic haemorrhage as they carry a higher risk of rupture when compared to AVMs without intranidal aneurysms. This fact is explained by their localization which is closer to the terminal arterial feeders and therefore is exposed to higher arterial pressure. The association between intranidal aneurysms and haemorrhage has been reported between 41% and 100% of patients with AVMs [4–6]. This might be even further illustrated in the results from Stapf et al. [7] where AVMs with associated aneurysms had a higher risk of haemorrhage at the initial presentation (odds ratio (OR) 2.27, 1.55–3.34; $p < 0.001$). Moreover, based on the performed analysis of multivariate Cox proportional hazards model on 622 untreated patients with cerebral AVM, besides variables such as age, previous history of haemorrhage, deep location, also associated aneurysms were shown to be predictors of haemorrhage (hazard ratio (HR) 1.62, 95% CI, 0.92–3.19). This is particularly important to bear in mind prior to the embolization of the AVM nidus since the pressure inside the arterial feeders increases following the embolization and associated aneurysms have therefore a higher tendency to rupture. This is why arterial feeders with flow-related aneurysms should be usually the first target to embolize [3]. In some cases, increased venous pressure analogously causes a pressure increase in the arterial side. As a result, the subsequent hypertension may increase the risk of aneurysms' rupture [8]. Other types of associated aneurysms may be flow-related and thus originate on proximal vessels due to the haemodynamic connection to the AVM nidus or may arise on distal small feeding arteries [4, 6]. Redekop et al. [6] in 1998 published a detailed classification of arterial AVM-associated intracranial aneurysms where the proximal wall aneurysms compose those found on the circle of Willis, the supraclinoid internal carotid artery, the middle cerebral artery, up to the primary bifurcation, the anterior cerebral artery, up to the anterior communicating artery, or the vertebrobasilar trunk. Distal aneurysms are those located distal to the abovementioned anatomical landmarks.

In children, the angioarchitecture of AVMs varies [9]. Paediatric AVMs tend to be smaller in size and have more frequent arteriovenous fistulas as well as deep venous drainage or mainly deep or central location of the AVM in the brain [7]. Some authors propose that adults are more likely to have AVM-associated aneurysms or venous ectasia compared to children, since these vascular features typically take time to originate completely [9]. Understanding the vascular component of the nidus, types of arterial feeders, modes of supply, and types of draining veins is necessary for adequate planning of AVM-related treatment.

## 8.3 Pathogenesis, Genetics, and Pathophysiology

Brain AVMs originate at the interface between arterial and venous endothelium where the capillary bed is under normal circumstances formed (Fig. 8.1) [10]. In earlier studies, it was believed that AVMs develop mainly congenitally during embryonic and early fetal development [2]. These hypotheses were argued, and the most recent findings have shown that the vast majority of AVMs develop sporadically during life, i.e. are typically not present at birth or neonatal period [11]. Nevertheless, there are some exceptions to inherited disorders, including Sturge-Weber syndrome, Louis-Barr syndrome, Wyburn-Mason syndrome, or Osler-Weber-Rendu syndrome. The last syndrome mentioned, also known as hereditary haemorrhagic telangiectasia (HHT), is a rare autosomal dominant disorder that might be classified into two groups: HHT1 and HHT2, based on the loss-of-function of two genes coding for activin-like kinase 1 (ALK1 gene) or activin A receptor, type II-like kinase 1 (ACVLR1 gene) and endoglin (ENG gene) that are fundamental for transforming growth factor-$\beta$ (TGF-$\beta$) signalling pathways [12]. This disease is characteristic of

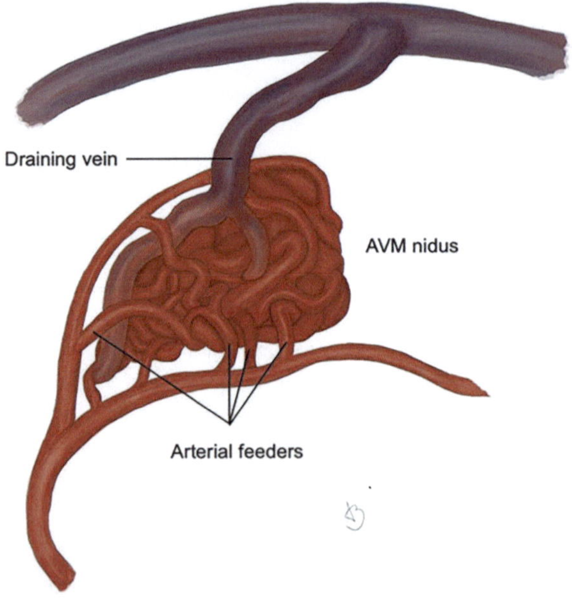


**Fig. 8.1** General anatomy of arteriovenous malformation, including three most important anatomical components relevant for subsequent decision-making of active treatment policy: (1) arterial feeders supplying the AVM, (2) AVM nidus, as a centre of the malformation itself, (3) draining vein (may be also multiple), directing the blood towards adjacent venous sinus

mucocutaneous fragility, disrupted vascular stabilization, and abnormally frequent AVMs. It is expected that the pathogenesis of AVMs in HHT (these cases account for approximately 3% of all brain AVMs [13]) may be closely linked to the pathological development of solitary AVMs [14]. The pathogenesis of AVMs is based on impaired signalling pathways and hyperexpression of angiogenic factors (such as VEGF, angiopoietin-2, MMP-9) along with inflammatory cytokines (most commonly TGF-β, TNF-α), and the members of the family of interleukins (mainly IL-1 and IL-6) [15]. Besides the fact that the abovementioned pathological factors are contributing members of inflammatory pathways involved in the abnormal development of the vasculature in the area of interest, they also have an inevitable impact on increasing the fragility of the vascular walls within the AVM and thus are associated with increased proneness of the AVM to rupture [16]. Histologically, it is suggested AVMs are lesions of dynamic and biologically active tissue, but still, very little is known about why some AVMs follow aggressive behaviour while others remain clinically silent during a patient's whole life [17]. Similarly to cavernous malformations, AVMs also follow Knudson's "two-hit" mechanism. This means that one inherited mutation in one copy of the studied gene responsible for the AVM development is accompanied by the second "hit" which is a somatic mutation, commonly of environmental origin [10]. Of note is that more than 900 genes were found to be involved in AVM development [11]. The concurrent interaction of many factors at once is the most likely explanation of the AVMs' pathogenesis, rather than only one, well-defined cause.

There is well-established evidence that AVMs smaller in size show a higher probability of rupture—it has been reported that the intraarterial pressure within feeding arteries tends to be significantly higher in smaller AVMs (those of <3 cm in size) [18–20]. It is also well known that the difference between mean intraarterial pressure and pressure within arterial feeder is typically significantly lower in ruptured compared to unruptured AVMs [20]. Besides the arterial side, disturbances on the venous side of the AVM have been shown to be involved in the disease development, in the formation of developmental venous anomalies or the risk of haemorrhage [21, 22]. Additionally, some authors have reported a decrease in venous intraluminal pressure following the resection of the AVM, which may consequently increase the risk of thrombus formation and potentially result in obliteration, which may not be a complication to the draining vein itself, but it may increase risk of thrombus formation and thus possible restrict the venous brain outflow [23]. However, clear consequences of decreased venous intraluminal pressure following the resection of the AVM have not been elucidated in the literature in more detail. Haemorrhagic complications may include stenoses of venous sinuses, retrograde venous thrombosis, or occlusion of smaller veins [24].

One of the widely discussed features of AVM pathophysiology is the so-called steal phenomenon, to some extent potentially responsible for clinical presentation in patients with neurological deficits. It has been demonstrated through single-photon emission computed CT that there is hypoperfusion in the adjacent brain to the AVM which may be the cause not only of mentioned neurological deficits but also seizures or cognitive disturbances [11]. The AVM "steals" the blood to its own feeding and supply, resulting in hypoperfusion in the surrounding brain parenchyma. However, a few reports have found no evidence supporting the vascular steal hypothesis or even a relationship between flow velocities or the pressure within arterial feeders and changes in cerebral blood flow or hypoperfusion. Nevertheless, the concept of both local and distant steal phenomenon has been supported by neuropsychological studies showing there is a deficit in cognitive tests mainly consisting of memory and verbal processing, regardless of whether the AVM is situated in a non-dominant or dominant cerebral hemisphere [25].

Another theory worth a short introduction is the *normal perfusion breakthrough*, described by Spetzler et al. in 1978 [26]. This theory describes the possibility of impaired reactivity of carbon dioxide along with vascular autoregulation in adjacent brain parenchyma to the AVM. Since the AVM is compared to a channel without any resistance, adjacent vessels tend to maintain their maximal dilatation in order to ensure the prevention of potential disturbances in cerebral perfusion—thus causing the loss of autoregulation. This phenomenon is particularly important to be aware of following the AVM resection when the increased pressure within the low-resistance vessels contributes to the formation of oedema and/or haemorrhage [27].

## 8.4 Epidemiology

The incidence of newly diagnosed AVMs is approximately 1–1.5 per 100,000 person-years. These numbers were derived from widely known population-based studies including NOMASS from 2002 (*Northern Manhattan Stroke Study* of 207 patients in this prospectively held database), *The New York Islands AVM Study* (performed on about 9.5 million New York's inhabitants between 2000 and 2002) from the same year or SIVMS (*Scottish Vascular Malformations Study*) which was published in 2003 [28–30]. It is expected that these values might increase prospectively, mainly due to better availability of non-invasive diagnostic methods and thus a more probable diagnosis of asymptomatic AVMs.

The majority of AVMs are diagnosed without previous history of rupture. This fact explains why the incidence of AVM haemorrhage compared to overall AVM incidence is significantly lower, approximately 0.5 per 100,000 person-years [28–30]. Overall, the AVM-related strokes account for around 2% of all intracerebral strokes, 3% of strokes in young adults, 9% of subarachnoid haemorrhages, and approximately 4% of all primary intracranial haemorrhages [31].

According to up-to-date reports, the prevalence of AVMs is likely to be a little higher in men than in women [30, 32, 33]. Reported ratios differ, but an illustrative example is the ratio of 1.22, derived from an international multicentre study of 1289 patients diagnosed at departments situated in Northern America, Europe, the Middle and South-East [30].

## 8.5 Clinical Presentation

The symptoms of intracranial AVM may originate at any age. The majority occur during the second or the third decade of life, but cases in children and adolescents are also reported [34]. On the contrary, the occurrence of AVM presentation for the first time in the elderly tends to be quite rare. Although some AVMs may remain clinically silent, other AVMs may cause a range of symptoms, mainly depending on the location, size, and haemodynamics of the malformation. The most common types of presentations are (1) consequences of bleeding, (2) seizures, or (3) focal neurological deficits. Approximately half of the patients with symptomatic AVMs have suffered from haemorrhage, most commonly caused by the rupture of fragile nidus or rupture of AVM-associated aneurysm(s) [35–37]. Only 10% of AVM-related haemorrhages are subarachnoid bleedings (those are mainly from cisternal AVMs), while the vast majority are intracerebral [3].

Between 20% and 40% of symptomatic AVMs present with epilepsy [29, 38, 39]. Seizures may be based on repeated micro-haemorrhages, which contribute to the deposition of hemosiderin in the adjacent brain parenchyma, activation of free radicals, and thus triggering the excitotoxic processes involving surrounding tissues [40]. Up-to-date reports have shown that the seizure presentation is specific to AVM localization (commonly in temporal lobes, insula, frontal lobes—generally superficial topography), size, feeding, venous outflow stenosis, and the presence of long pial course of the venous drainage [39].

Focal neurological deficits are present in approximately 10% of patients with intracranial AVM [41]. The pathophysiological mechanisms behind such presentation are likely to be similar to epilepsy, along with aforedescribed steal phenomenon, a higher number of draining veins, venous ectasias, and eloquent localization. It is worth noting that this presentation is quite rare, in the vast majority of cases predominantly present in females. According to the study of 302 consecutive AVM patients by Lv in 2013 [42], a non-haemorrhagic neurological deficit was present in 7.9% of analysed subjects. These authors verified previously mentioned factors, such as female gender, deep AVM location, more than three arterial feeders, as well as more than three draining veins or the presence of venous ectasias to be associated with such a clinical presentation.

## 8.6  Grading Schemes

Grading schemes regarding AVMs are based on used treatment so we differentiate surgical, radiosurgical, and endovascular embolization gradings.

### 8.6.1  Surgical Grading

Although there were historically several grading schemes, the most famous and most commonly used grading scheme was introduced by Spetzler and Martin (S-M grading) in 1986 [43]. This grading system is based on the evaluation of the diameter of the AVM nidus, the presence or absence of deep venous drainage, and finally the (non-)eloquence of adjacent brain tissue, which are those AVMs found in the brainstem, thalamus, hypothalamus, cerebellar peduncles, sensorimotor, language, or primary visual cortex (Table 8.1 and illustrative examples in Figs. 8.2, 8.3, and 8.4).

**Table 8.1** Spetzler-Martin grading scheme

| Parameter | Points |
|---|---|
| *Nidus diameter* | |
| <3 cm | 1 |
| 3–6 cm | 2 |
| >6 cm | 3 |
| *Deep venous drainage* | |
| No | 0 |
| Yes | 1 |
| *Eloquence of adjacent brain* | |
| No | 0 |
| Yes | 1 |

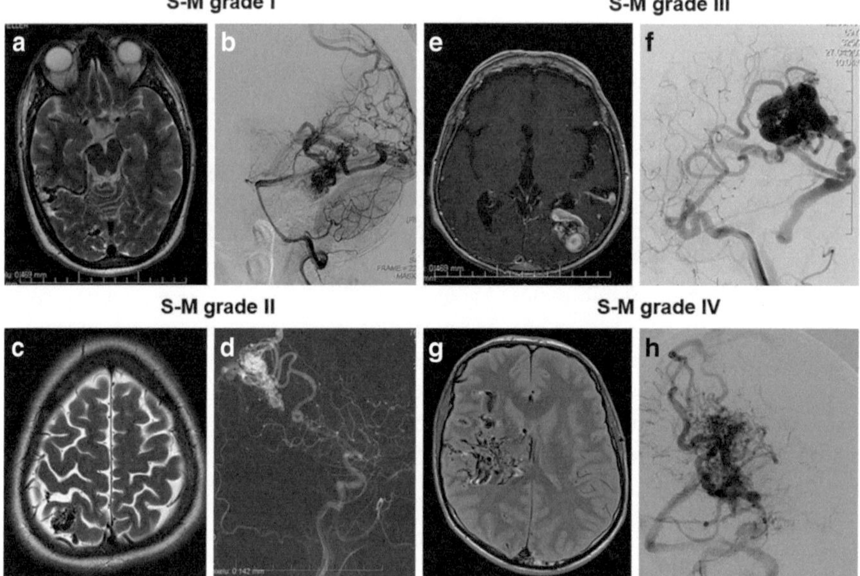


**Fig. 8.2** Illustrative examples of S-M grades I, II, III and IV. (**a**) Axial T2-weighted scan of right S-M grade I AVM. (**b**) DSA lateral view of the same AVM. (**c**) T2-weighted axial MRI scan of the right lobar AVM, S-M grade II, analogously shown (**d**) on magnetic resonance angiography from the lateral view. (**e**) T1-weighted axial MRI scan of left occipital AVM S-M grade III and (**f**) the same AVM on DSA. (**g**) S-M grade IV right hemispherical AVM in axial MRI with the involvement of deep eloquent areas and again depicted (**h**) on DSA

Less frequently, a supplementary grading system described by Lawton et al. is used in clinical practice, and it is called the Lawton-Young grading system. This scheme evaluates the age of patients, compactness of the AVM nidus, and history of haemorrhage (Table 8.2). The combination of Spetzler-Martin and Lawton-Young schemes (supplemented Spetzler-Martin grading system) was recently studied on a

## S-M grade V

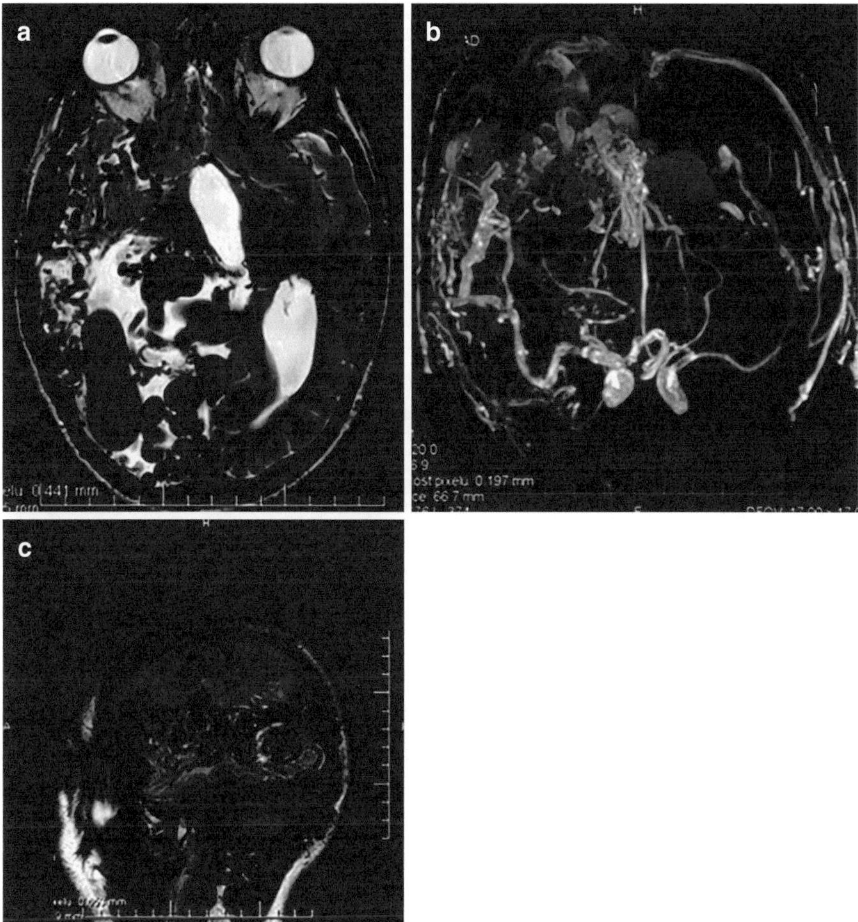

**Fig. 8.3** Illustrative example of large S-M grade V AVM. (**a**) T2 weighted axial scan of the AVM, involving eloquent areas. (**b**) Magnetic resonance angiography of the AVM with deep and superficial venous drainage. (**c**) Sagittal MRI view of the AVM

multicentre cohort of 1009 patients with a recommendation of its predictive accuracy which should be evaluated prior to the AVM resection [44]. This supplemented system is a sum of the two grading schemes we mentioned. Its clinical impact is primarily based on extended variables that are evaluated as well as the complementation of each other. Of note is also well-known Spezler-Ponce three-tier grading, classification AVMs into three groups according to their S-M grade: Class A is comprised of S-M grade I and II AVMs, Class B of S-M grade III, and Class C of S-M grade IV and V AVMs.

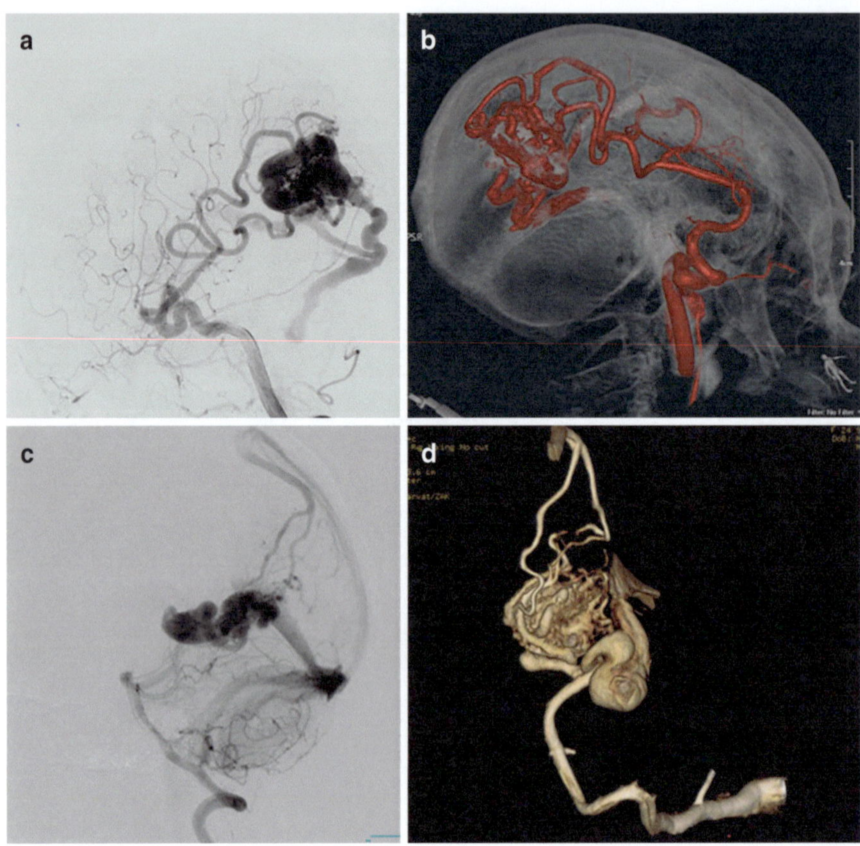

**Fig. 8.4** Two individual cases of temporo-occipital AVMs, upper (**a**, **b**) S-M grade III, lower (**c**, **d**) S-M grade II, both depicted on (**a**, **c**) DSA from the lateral view, and (**b**, **d**) different 3D projections

**Table 8.2** Lawton-Young grading scheme

| Parameter | Points |
| --- | --- |
| *Age* | |
| <20 | 1 |
| 20–40 | 2 |
| >40 | 3 |
| *Diffuse nidus* | |
| No | 0 |
| Yes | 1 |
| *Unruptured presentation* | |
| No | 0 |
| Yes | 1 |

## 8.6.2  Radiosurgical Grading

Radiosurgical gradings are commonly explained through two unique points of view. The first is represented by Karlsson's *K index* or by the *Obliteration Prediction Index* introduced by Schwartz [45, 46]. Both are using the ratio of radiation dose to the diameter of the AVM for the likelihood of AVM obliteration. The second point of view is based on Pollock's grading scheme (Pollock-Flickinger AVM score from 2002 and its modification from 2008 performed by the same authors), which is based on the correlation between age of patients, localization, the volume of the AVM, and the patients' outcome [47].

## 8.6.3  Endovascular Embolization Grading

Gradings regarding endovascular treatment have been developed recently and currently need prospective validation. There are two main grading schemes that should be mentioned: the Feliciano grading system (2014) and the Buffalo score (2015) [48]. The former evaluates the number of feeding vessels, (non-)eloquence of the lesion, and the presence/absence of arteriovenous fistula. On the other hand, the Buffalo score instead of the number of feeding vessels evaluates the number of arterial pedicles, and additionally arterial pedicle diameter along with the (non-)eloquence of the location.

## 8.7  Diagnostic Imaging

### 8.7.1  Digital Subtraction Angiography (DSA)

A gold standard for AVM investigation is digital subtraction angiography (DSA) since it allows detailed depiction of parameters based on AVM's angioarchitecture, including the nidus and its haemodynamic properties, anatomical characteristics, arterial feeders, and the pattern of venous drainage (deep or superficial). Moreover, associated aneurysms, signs of high-flow venous angiopathies such as venous ectasia or stenotic abnormalities, and other vasculopathies could be diagnosed through DSA. The time resolution of DSA is a crucial advantage mainly for the depiction of early draining veins. The availability of 3D model reconstruction may be helpful to study the anatomy of the angioarchitecture in more detail (Fig. 8.4). Superselective angiography is used for a more detailed depiction of AVM nidus's angioarchitecture along with the associated intranidal aneurysms as well as direct intranidal arteriovenous fistulas.

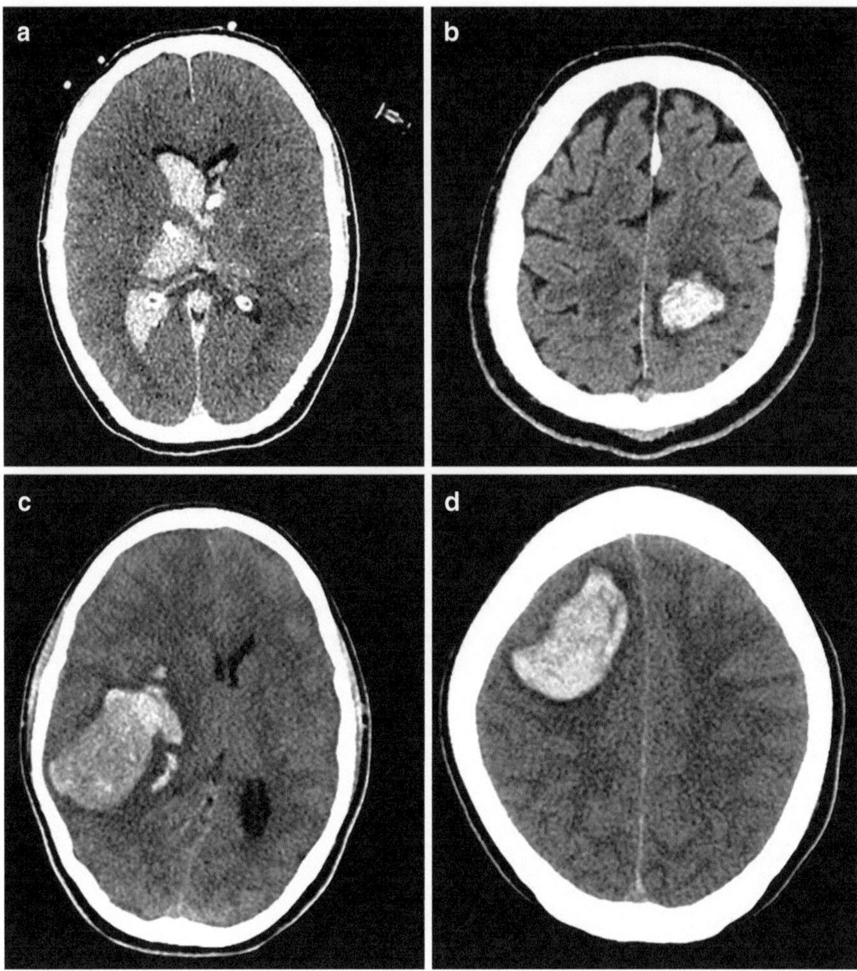

**Fig. 8.5** Various types of acute symptomatic haemorrhages from supratentorial AVMs depicted on the CT. (**a**) Right AVM S-M grade IV located in the basal ganglia with intraventricular haemorrhage. (**b**) Left parietal AVM, S-M grade I. (**c**) Fronto-parietal AVM S-M grade II. (**d**) Right frontal AVM, S-M grade II. S-M grades were subsequently defined based on DSA

## *8.7.2 Computed Tomography (CT) and CT Angiography (CTA)*

The CT is an inevitable diagnostic method in the acute phase in order to investigate the presence or absence of intracranial haemorrhage (Fig. 8.5). In combination with CT angiography (CTA), it is possible to evaluate the presence of the AVM during the acute phase, although the resolution of CTA is not as good as the DSA, and therefore CTA is not used as the decisive imaging for surgical planning [49]. Especially in atypical haematomas, CTA is an essential diagnostic method for

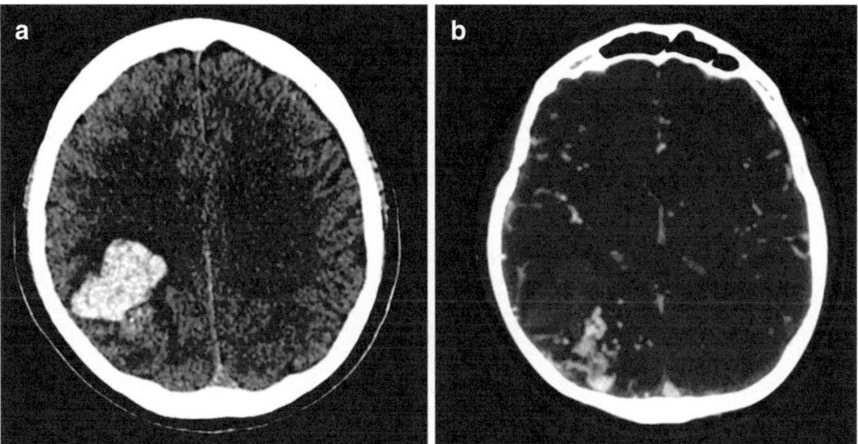

**Fig. 8.6** (**a**) Initial CT scan with an atypical lobar haematoma with a suspicion of ruptured AVM. (**b**) CTAg showing ruptured parieto-occipital AVM S-M grade II

further decision-making of active treatment policy. Its clinical relevance does not lay in the resolution and detailed evaluation of the AVM itself, but rather in the overall depiction of the draining veins, arterial feeding, etc., i.e. providing an easy-to-perform general diagnostic evaluation of the disease (Fig. 8.6). However, non-contrast enhanced CT in cases of unruptured AVMs would look normal or with curvilinear slightly hyperdense structures and thus suggest the diagnosis of AVM, potentially depicting the presence of calcifications. However, it is clear that only CT cannot be considered a decisive diagnostic method for AVMs.

### 8.7.3 Magnetic Resonance Imaging (MRI) and MR Angiography (MRA)

MRI is a fundamental tool for surgical planning in order to become familiar with the AVM's parts and their relations to the adjacent brain parenchyma. Compared to the CT, MRI is superior in terms of depicting subacute or chronic haemorrhage, while simultaneously evaluating further features such as oedema, mass effect, or perilesional gliosis [3]. Nowadays, if available, functional MRI (fMRI) along with diffusion tensor imaging (DTI) sequences for MR tractography are used and recommended to perform primarily in the decision-making of surgical intervention and surgical planning, especially in AVMs situated close to eloquent areas, including sensoric, motor, and speech centres (Fig. 8.7) [50]. Thromboses and signs of haemorrhage are well visualized on T2-weighted and gradient-echo (GRE) scans [51]. On susceptibility-weighted images (SWI), venous compartments show hypointense signals, thus it is possible to depict the unique difference between veins and arteries regardless of intravenous contrast or vessel

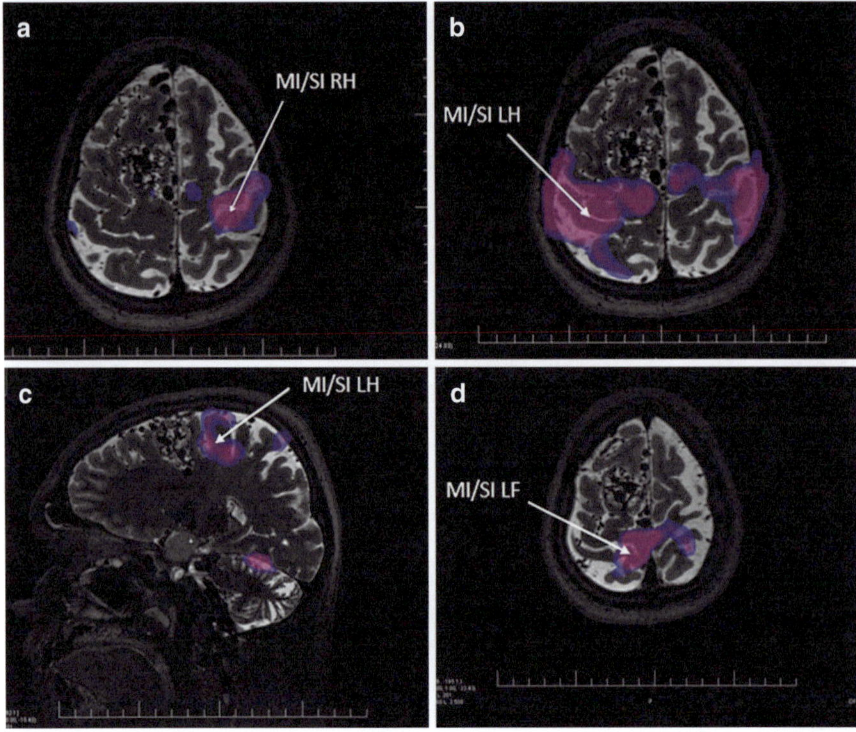


**Fig. 8.7** (**a–d**) Functional MRI in a patient with right frontal AVM S-M grade III depicting the activity of the primary motor (MI) and primary somatosensory (SI) cortex. Used abbreviations: *RH* right hand, *LH* left hand, *LF* left foot

calibre (Fig. 8.8) [52]. Hemosiderin is depicted as a hypointense area within the AVM itself or in its surroundings. Based on MR perfusion sequences, perfusion changes in the surrounding brain parenchyma can be evaluated—this option has been tested usually following the AVM resection or during the latency period after radiosurgery. Guo et al. evaluated the radiosurgical effect on brain perfusion in patients with cerebral AVMs [78]. They demonstrated changes in initial high transnidal flow and perinidal perfusion disturbances after radiosurgical intervention, but its clinical importance has not been well studied, and a clear benefit is unknown [53]. The MR angiography (MRA) is useful in providing 3D angiographic models of AVMs, dynamic contrast-enhanced MRA enables the depiction of the AVM in a time-resolved fashion (Fig. 8.8) [54, 55]. The combination of DSA, CT, and MRI is routinely performed for the completeness and most accurate diagnosis of AVM and thus cross-sectional imaging is crucial for decision-making about the final treatment plan and should therefore be well understood [53].

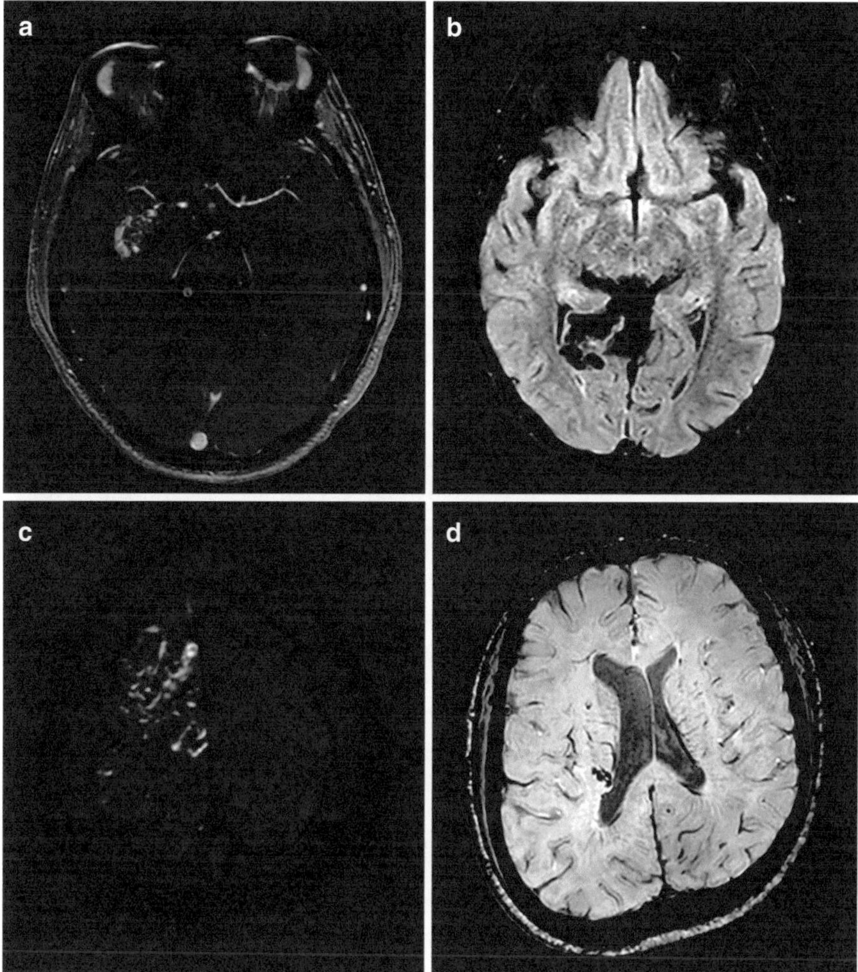

**Fig. 8.8** Summary of commonly used MRI sequences for the diagnosis of diverse brain AVMs. (**a**) GRE MRI scan of the AVM localized within the right Sylvian fissure. (**b**) Temporo-occipital AVM depicted in fluid attenuated inversion recovery (FLAIR) sequence. (**c**) Right frontal AVM depicted by susceptibility-weighted angiography (SWAN), 3D multi-echo gradient echo sequence, enabling delineation of small blood vessels, microbleedings, etc. (**d**) Right periventricular AVM in SWI MRI image

## 8.8   Natural History

As we have already mentioned in the previous paragraphs, besides modern technology, and approaches in terms of molecular and genetic aspects of AVMs, the natural history of this disease is yet not fully understood. The risk of unruptured AVM is approximately 2–4% per year, with an annual rehaemorrhage rate of 6–7% [18, 19].

The annual mortality rates vary but are typically between 0.7% and 2.9% [32, 56, 57]. Patients who suffer from AVM rupture are typically younger compared to patients who suffer other types of haemorrhage strokes, and the cause of the bleeding from AVM is not primarily based on factors causing typical spontaneous stroke, such as high cholesterol concentrations, hypertension, and smoking [58]. This further mirrors the fact that paediatric AVMs have a higher probability of bleeding, compared to adults [9, 59]. Of note is that almost 50% of all spontaneous intracranial haemorrhages in children younger than 18 years are caused by the rupture of the brain AVM [60].

The exact numbers dedicated to overall case fatality and permanent disability rates following the AVM rupture vary as well, typically ranging between 5% and 25% and from 10% to 40% [36, 41, 57, 61, 62]. Risk factors of haemorrhage based on AVM characteristics are smaller size, deep venous drainage, infratentorial and deep location, and high pressure inside the arterial feeders [7, 21, 22, 63–65]. However, we urge readers to understand that these predictions might be somewhat biased. For example, a lot of small AVMs may develop and subsequently present asymptomatically without any signs of haemorrhage (also considering lower intra-arterial and intranidal pressure, thus less associated aneurysms, etc.), whereas larger AVMs have significantly higher blood volumes within the feeding arteries and thus may result in much more severe haemorrhage if they rupture [3, 20].

The presence of AVMs and their anatomical features such as larger size, nidus, or deep feeding arteries suited in the cortical location, and the AVM found in temporal or parietal location has been reported to be associated with the development of seizures, the second most common presentation of AVMs [38, 66–69]. Tong et al. [33] investigated the effect of age, sex, and lesion location on AVM presentation, based on the data extracted from 3299 consecutive patients. They observed that younger age and female sex are associated with initial haemorrhage ($p < 0.05$). Of note is that ruptured AVMs were more common in eloquent locations, including the corpus callosum, brainstem, cerebellum, or the ventricles. Interestingly, the male gender was associated with initial epilepsy presentation ($p < 0.05$), as well as frontal, temporal, parietal, frontotemporal, and frontoparietal locations ($p < 0.05$). Temporal AVMs were, compared to frontal AVMs, more likely to present with haemorrhage and conversely less likely to present with seizure ($p < 0.05$).

## 8.9  Surgery

At the end of the nineteenth century, Giordano and later also Pean performed presumably the first surgeries of intracranial AVMs, followed by famous neurosurgeons including Cushing, Bailey, or Dandy [24]. Later on, in 1967, Yasargil was the first to use a microscope along with bipolar coagulation and automatic retractors [24]. The basic scheme of indications for "modern" surgical treatment of AVMs was introduced by Spetzler in 2011 [70] and remained rather stable over the years. Although there are some general indications for surgery of AVMs, each patient is unique, and each neurosurgeon should be well informed about each patient's clinical presentation. Detailed familiarity with the AVM itself is of no lesser importance, it is fundamental to study not only the lesion's anatomy but also its accessibility and angioarchitecture. Generally speaking, AVMs of S-M grade I or II are typically indicated for surgery, S-M grade III should be managed by multimodal cooperation with respect to the AVM anatomy, localization, and of course the patient's demographic characteristics [71]. Patients with AVMs of S-M grade IV and V are in the vast majority of cases not treated surgically since the risks of a surgical intervention exceed the risks of the natural course of the disease [72]. However, there are some cases where this classification cannot be straightforwardly applied. For example, in ruptured S-M grade IV or V AVMs with large intracranial haematoma, only the bleeding is very gently removed to decrease the intracranial pressure, but the AVM is usually treated afterwards.

Many paediatric patients with a history of symptomatic haemorrhage, uncontrollable seizures, or progressive neurological deficits undergo surgical intervention since the risk of deterioration is higher and the risk of AVM's rupture is known to increase prospectively [73]. Unruptured paediatric AVMs present a bigger challenge when it comes to the decision-making of active treatment policy. Simultaneously with the development of the brain, also AVMs tend to develop high-risk anatomical and pathophysiological features and therefore increase the risk of haemorrhage or the onset of symptomatic manifestation [9]. It is very important to evaluate not only the individual characteristics of the patient and its AVM but also objectively evaluate the physicians' and institutions' experience with this disease.

From the technical aspect of the surgery itself, we will discuss some important key steps and approaches that are useful to be well familiar with in every AVM surgery. The craniotomy should be larger than the AVM surface, beyond nidus margins. We routinely use neuronavigation to place the craniotomy and to enable an adequate surgical corridor. The dura needs to be opened carefully and the adhesions between the AVM surface and the dura should be sharply cut. Following the exposure of the nidus—when it is possible, we recommend having the long axis of the nidus in a vertical position. The neurosurgeon should subsequently inspect the brain surface to correlate ICG image and angiography with the surgical field. After the circumferential dissection of the arachnoid layer with respect to sulci, it is recommended to always start with the dissection from the arterial side. One should be very careful about en passage and transit vessels—until proven otherwise, all arteries should be considered as en passage ones (Figs. 8.9 and 8.10). The coagulation of vessels should be performed patiently and thoroughly, and we recommend the usage of miniclips to provide an effective alternative to normal coagulation mainly in deep feeding arteries (Figs. 8.11, 8.12, and 8.13). If necessary, non-stick, and high-power coagulation should be used exclusively for the brain tissue. Cutting of the coagulated vessels is done in a stepwise fashion. At the point of any

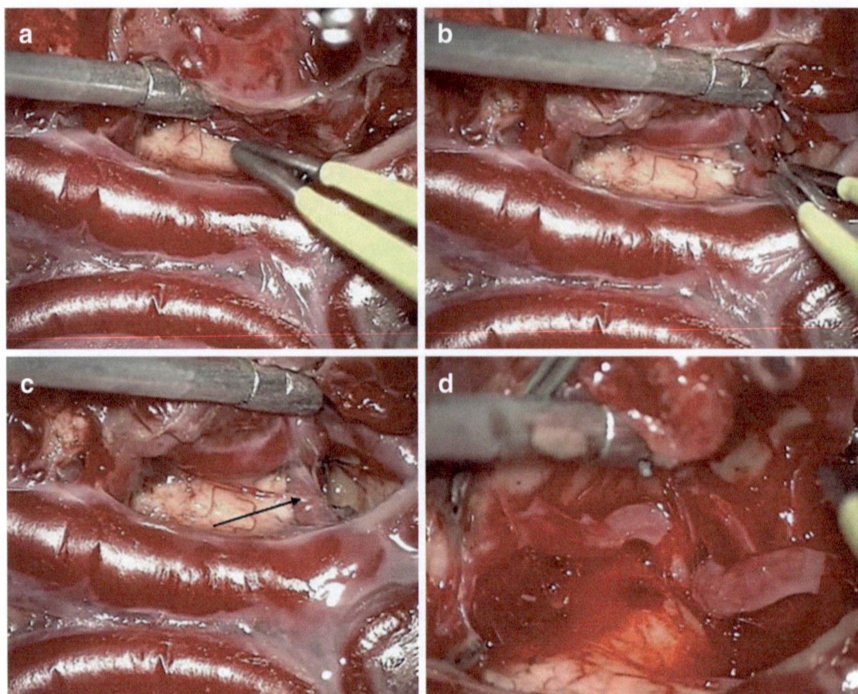

**Fig. 8.9** Intraoperative view of left temporal AVM. (**a**) The exposure of the nidus (above), feeding arteries and venous drainage. (**b**) Careful coagulation of the vessel that connects one of the vessels of the AVM nidus and the main draining vein. (**c**) The artery (arrow) might from this point of view misinterpreted as a feeding one, however, (**d**) after the complete dissection, it is obvious that the artery is the temporal branch of the middle cerebral artery. It has nothing to do with the AVM whatsoever and definitely must be preserved

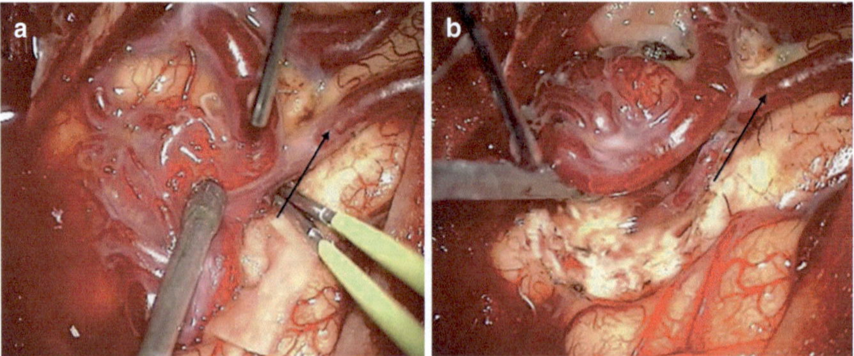

**Fig. 8.10** (**a**) Illustrative case of the transit artery which again erroneously resembles the AVM feeder (arrow). (**b**) Dissection, preserving the mentioned artery to make sure whether it is a feeder or not. (**c**) Coagulation of the vessels which are subsequently stepwise cut, the feeding artery is actually deeper below the transit artery. (**d**) As in the previous case, after the complete resection of the AVM, the first artery is a normal vessel supplying the adjacent brain and has nothing in common with the AVM

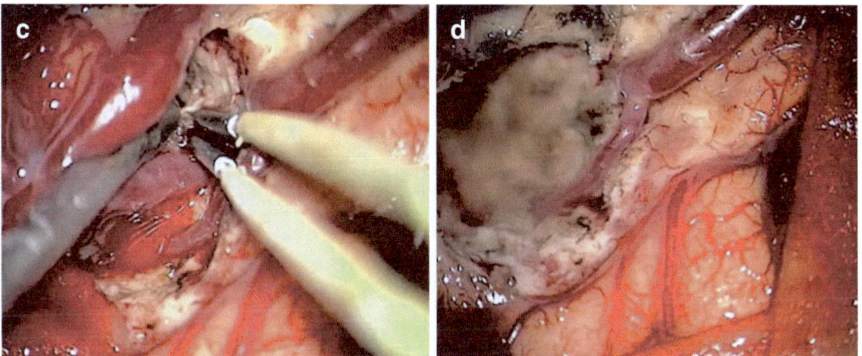

**Fig. 8.10** (continued)

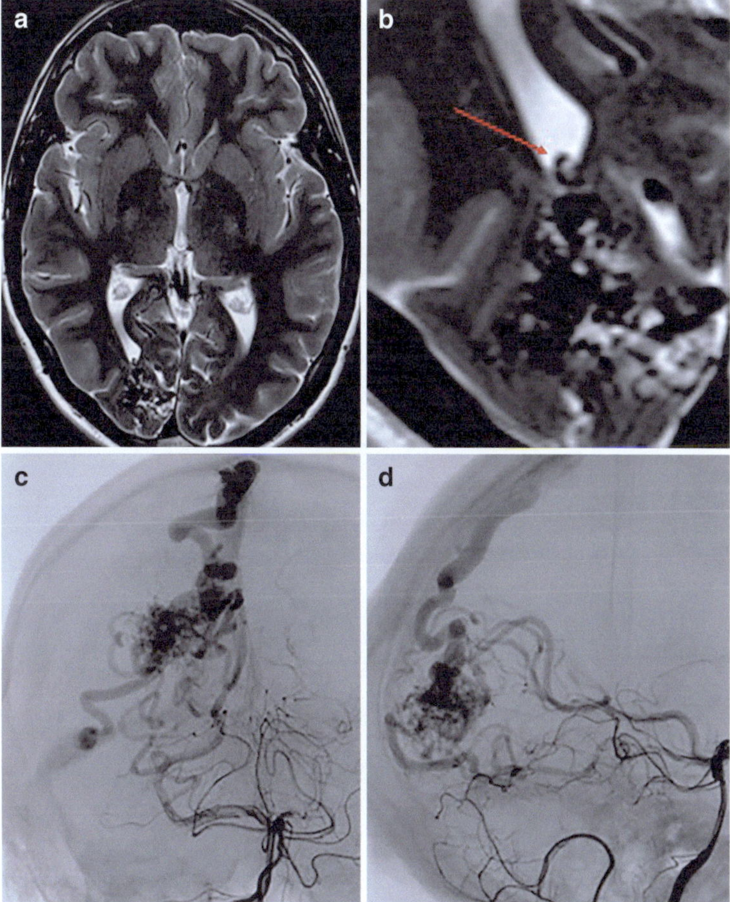

**Fig. 8.11** (**a**, **b**) Preoperative T2-weighted axial MRI scan with the occipital AVM. One of the feeding arteries is incorporated into the posterior horn of the lateral ventricle. (**c**, **d**) Angiography with apparent superficial venous drainage, (**c**) A-P and (**d**) lateral view

**Fig. 8.12** (**a**) Intraoperative identification of the feeding artery and (**b**) subsequent clip placement, providing safe occlusion of the feeder

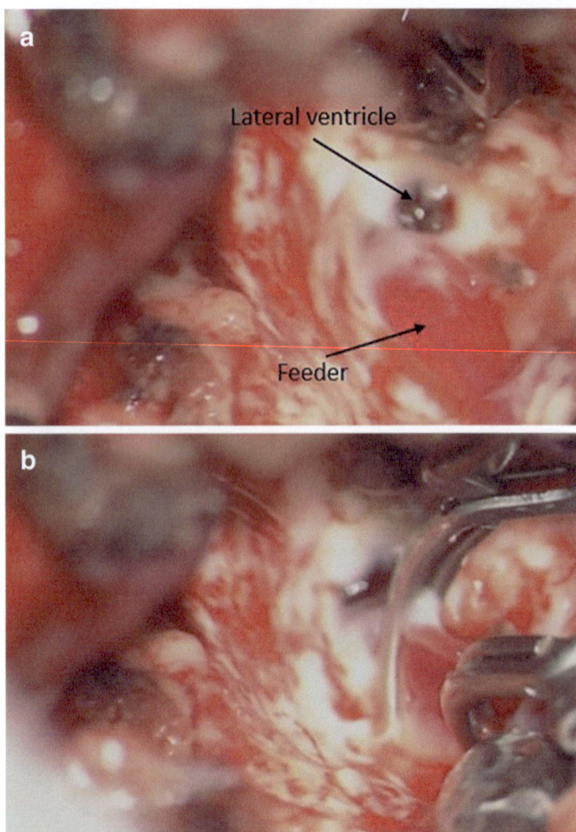



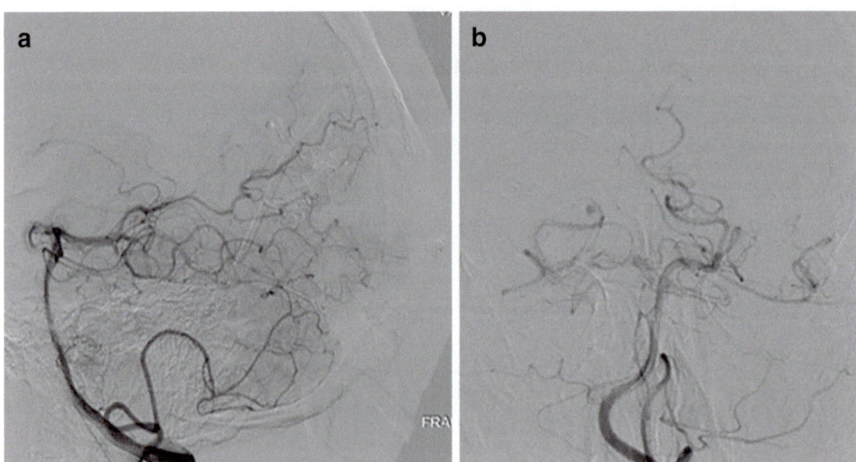



**Fig. 8.13** (**a**, **b**) Postoperative DSA of the previous case of the AVM with the intraventricular feeding artery, lateral and A-P view

**Table 8.3** Summary of key steps in AVM surgery. Most important in which extra attention should be paid are depicted in bold

| AVM surgery step by step |
| --- |
| 1. Plan thoroughly and patiently the surgery, understand well the anatomy |
| 2. Perform large enough craniotomy |
| 3. Position the patient to approach the AVM along the long axis, long axis should be vertical |
| **4. Open dura carefully, especially in AVMs situated on the surface** |
| 5. Correlate between angiography and surgical field |
| 6. Begin at the arterial side |
| 7. Dissect the arachnoid circumferentially, respect the sulci |
| **8. Identify and preserve en passage arteries** |
| 9. Coagulate patiently and thoroughly |
| 10. Cut the coagulated vessels stepwise |
| 11. Use miniclips |
| 12. Non-stick and high-power coagulation seldom |
| 13. Identify and deal with any bleeding before further resection |
| 14. Along the vein exceptionally |
| 15. Have important structures under control all the time |
| **16. Take extreme care with deep feeders** |
| 17. Choose the proper vein as last |
| 18. Use ICG |
| 19. Coagulate and cut the last draining vein |
| 20. Thorough haemostasis before closure |

bleeding, the first step is always to identify the source of the bleeding, subsequently to control the bleeding and not continue before these steps are properly performed. The work with deep feeding arteries should be always done with extreme care and awareness. The last step is to cut-off the draining vein—before it; however, ICG should be used to control the haemodynamics. After the resection, controlling ICG is always performed. Moreover, one must be aware of so-called perinidal vessels (also known as red veins). These are under influence of angiogenesis factors based on the drained blood from the AVM venous drainage. Routinely, the DSA and MRI are performed to confirm the completeness of the AVM resection. Summary of 20 most important steps in AVM surgery is presented in Table 8.3.

## 8.10  Endovascular Methods

The case of the first therapeutically embolized brain AVM was described in 1960 by Alfred J. Lessenhop and William T. Spence, using flow-directed spheres covered by methyl methacrylate injected through interval carotid artery [74]. In 1969, Newton and Cronqvist published a classification of intracranial AVMs according to the involvement of dural blood supply. Some of the brain AVMs receive blood "feeding" from meningeal branches of external and internal carotid arteries, or possibly branches of vertebral arteries [75]. The first group includes pure dural AVMs, i.e. those receiving blood supply from meningeal arteries. On the other hand, pure pial AVMs are those supplied by cerebral or cerebellar arteries. The last group comprises mixed dural-pial AVMs that are supplied by both cerebral/cerebellar arteries along with meningeal arterial contribution [75]. These AVMs tend to vary in their angioarchitecture characteristics and natural course. This fact is important to bear in mind in therapy decision-making, in this case especially in targeting the embolization and/or further interventions [76].

A few years later, Serbinenko used a detachable balloon connected to a flexible flow-directed catheter in 1974 [77], and in 1976, Kerber described a technique of using a microcatheter with a calibrated-leak balloon with isobutyl-2-cyanoacrylate, a liquid embolic agent [78]. Kerber's technique had one major advantage over the first two mentioned—when using diagnostic catheters, the manipulation and regulation of the agent infusion were rather difficult, carrying a higher risk of unwanted occlusion of proximal feeding arteries without the obliteration of the AVM nidus itself or possible embolization of normal cerebral arteries unrelated to the AVM. The advances in the developing embolic agents and techniques have enabled both better precision of endovascular methods and benefits of embolization in multidisciplinary AVM therapy.

Taken from a current technical perspective, endovascular therapy as a primary treatment is usually performed in very specific cases, mainly including patients with smaller AVMs with a few feeding arteries which are carrying a higher surgical risk based on their location. More commonly, endovascular embolization is typically used as (1) adjuvant therapy prior to surgical or radiosurgical intervention or as (2) a palliative treatment modality for embolization of flow-related aneurysms or in order to ease the symptoms related to mechanical or vascular compression (Fig. 8.14) [5, 79]. Embolic agents used in clinical practice can be divided into liquid (more commonly used) and solid ones. The former group consists of cyanoacrylate monomers and polymeric precipitates in solutions including the modern embolic agent ethylene-vinyl alcohol copolymer, known by its trade name Onyx. The mechanism of how cyanoacrylates work is based on their ability to polymerize to a solid state when they are exposed to an ionic environment, for example blood. This process, which typically takes approximately only 1 s, further causes vessel occlusion by forming a thrombosis. On the other hand, the functioning of Onyx relies on sedimentary deposits of the embolic agent itself, which is held in a solution by a solvent, in this case dimethyl sulfoxide [79].

The method of partial embolization may be also beneficial for patients suffering from drug-refractory epilepsy or from progressive neurological deficits which might be also partially attributable to venous hypertension, or the steal phenomenon

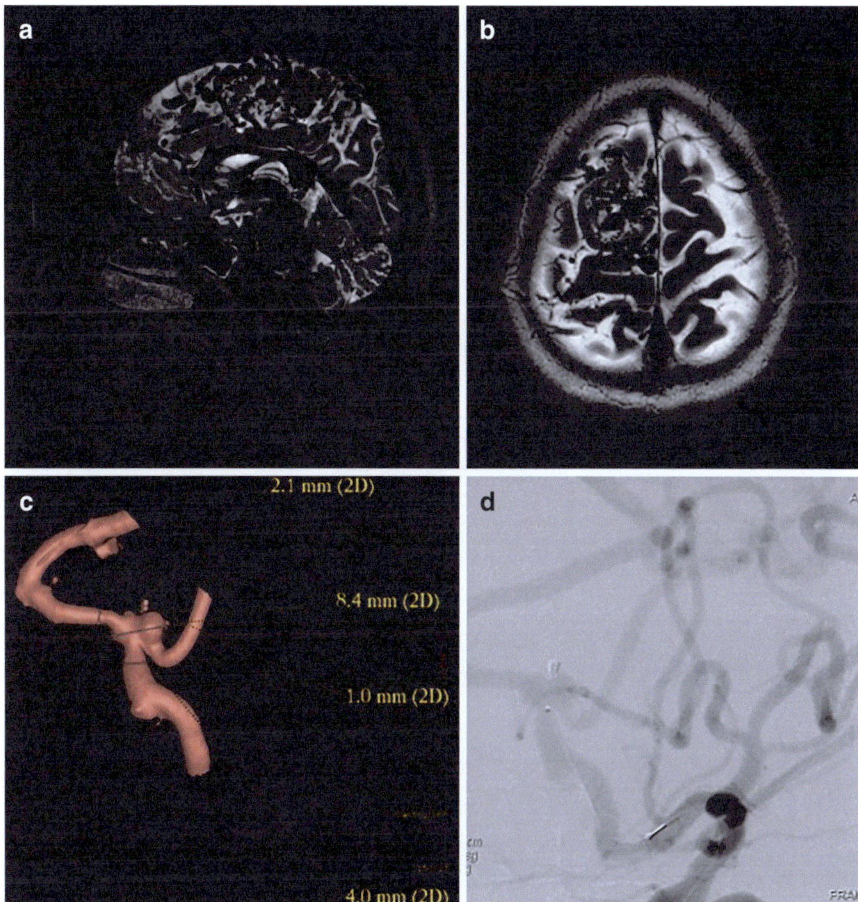



**Fig. 8.14** (**a, b**) Example of asymptomatic AVM S-M grade III with (**c**) flow-related aneurysm. (**d**) The flow-related aneurysm was subsequently coiled due to a relatively high risk of rupture; the AVM is under observation

described earlier. However, the question of whether palliative embolization should be also applied for hardly surgically accessible and large AVMs remains controversial. There is no significant evidence stating that the benefits of partial embolization in these causes exceed the benefits of the natural course of the disease [5, 79–81]. The surgery of well-embolized AVMs may be easier in terms of the nidus dissection from the adjacent brain parenchyma and the fact that main feeders are occluded at the time of surgery (Fig. 8.15). Nevertheless, in some cases, even embolized arteries may extensively bleed and the coagulation is as a consequence exceedingly challenging [3].

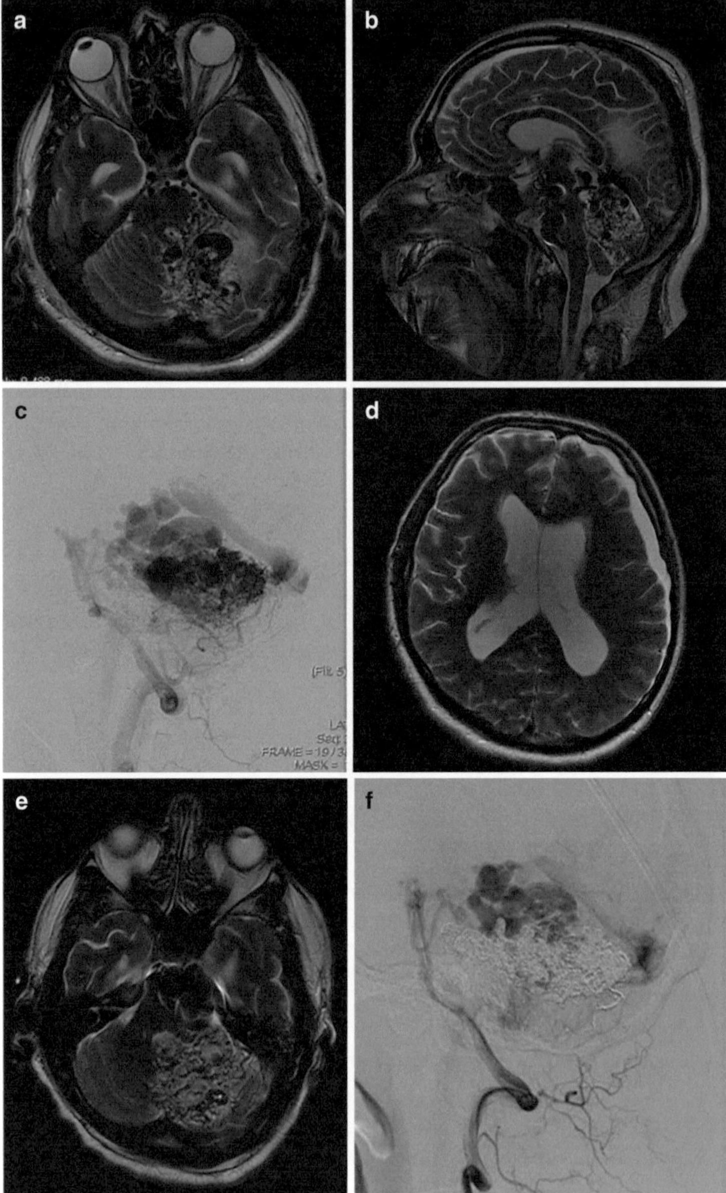

**Fig. 8.15** Case of partial embolization of AVM S-M grade IV, subsequently microsurgically resected. (**a**, **b**) Left cerebellar AVM depicted on T2-weighted MRI, (**c**) DSA of the AVM with deep venous drainage. (**d**) Associated obstructive hydrocephalus. The AVM was primarily partially embolized with Onyx. (**e**) T2-weighted MRI, depicting partially embolized AVM, as also proved on (**f**) the DSA. Due to unchanged clinical status and unceasing bulbar syndrome and oculomotor deficit, the patient agreed to undergo surgical resection of the AVM. (**g**) Intraoperative view of partially embolized part of the AVM, surgery was performed 7 days after the primary embolization. (**h**) Postoperative T2-weighted MRI and (**i**) DSA, depicting successful complete resection. The patient afterwards underwent ventriculoperitoneal shunt implantation, due to the (**d**) hydrocephalus depicted earlier

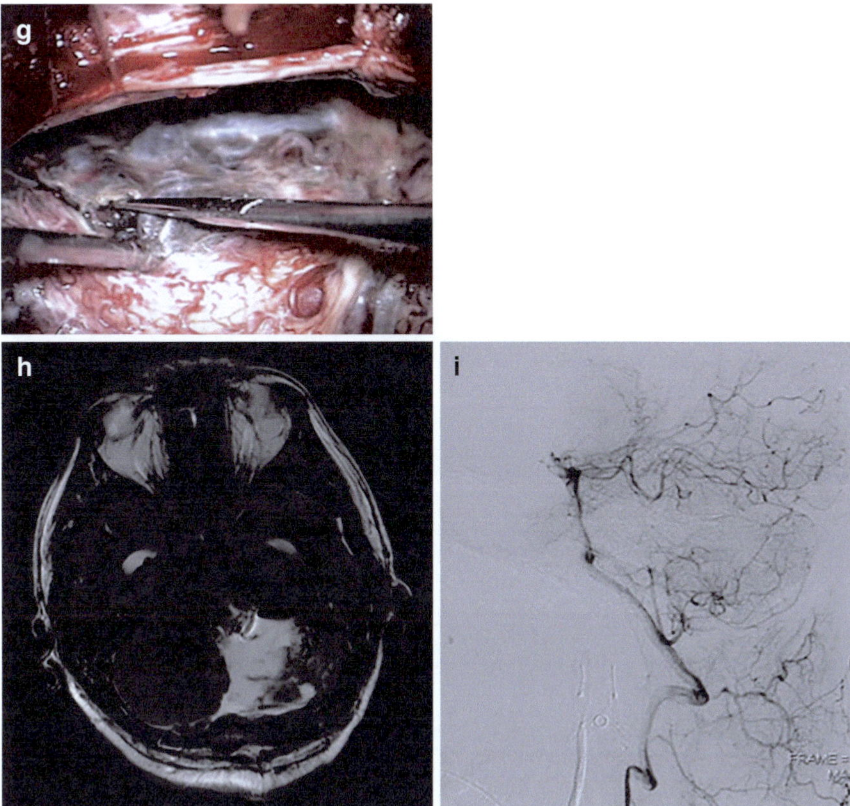

**Fig. 8.15** (continued)

## 8.11 Radiosurgery

The last treatment alternative applied in clinical practice for AVM management is radiosurgery—a diverse therapy modality including a variety of techniques and used radiosurgical instruments (Gamma Knife most commonly, Cyberknife, Linear Accelerator, etc.). The first case report of treated AVM by radiosurgery is dated to 1972, published by Steiner et al. [82]. Since then, radiosurgery has become a well-established treatment modality for cerebral AVMs. The main advantage of radiosurgical intervention is its minimally invasive nature, which may be particularly beneficial for patients having eloquently-seated AVMs where surgical risks would exceed the benefits of conservative management, but still harbour not negligible risk of bleeding (Figs. 8.16 and 8.17) [83]. Moreover, older patients and/or patients with various comorbidities that would increase the risk of surgical intervention may be radiosurgical candidates as well.

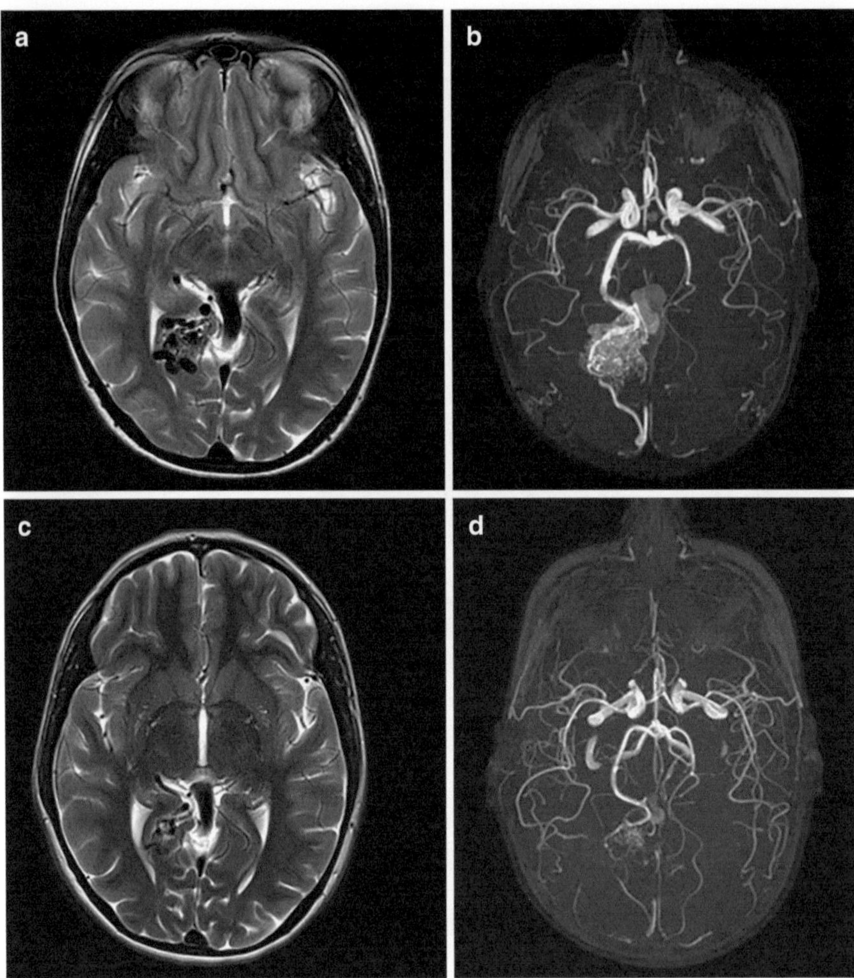

**Fig. 8.16** Case of a 25-year-old lady with asymptomatic temporo-occipital AVM depicted in (**a**) T2-weighted MRI and (**b**) MRA, subsequently managed by Gamma Knife. During the 2-year follow-up, (**c, d**) there is an evident shrinkage of the AVM

In 2012, Kano et al. comprehensively analysed radiosurgically treated AVMs from a Pittsburgh database in order to unite and evaluate both adequate indications and final treatment outcomes [83, 84]. The obliteration rate of low S-M grade has been reported to be approximately 90% with minimal mortality and morbidity rates. However, along with increasing S-M grade, the efficacy of radiosurgical treatment tended to decrease, with simultaneously increasing complication rates [85]. On the other hand, very high efficacy of radiosurgery in the management of AVM large in size was reported after single or multiple irradiation, supported by conclusions by Karlsson et al. [86] who calculated efficacy of 62% for AVM exceeding 9 cm$^3$, and

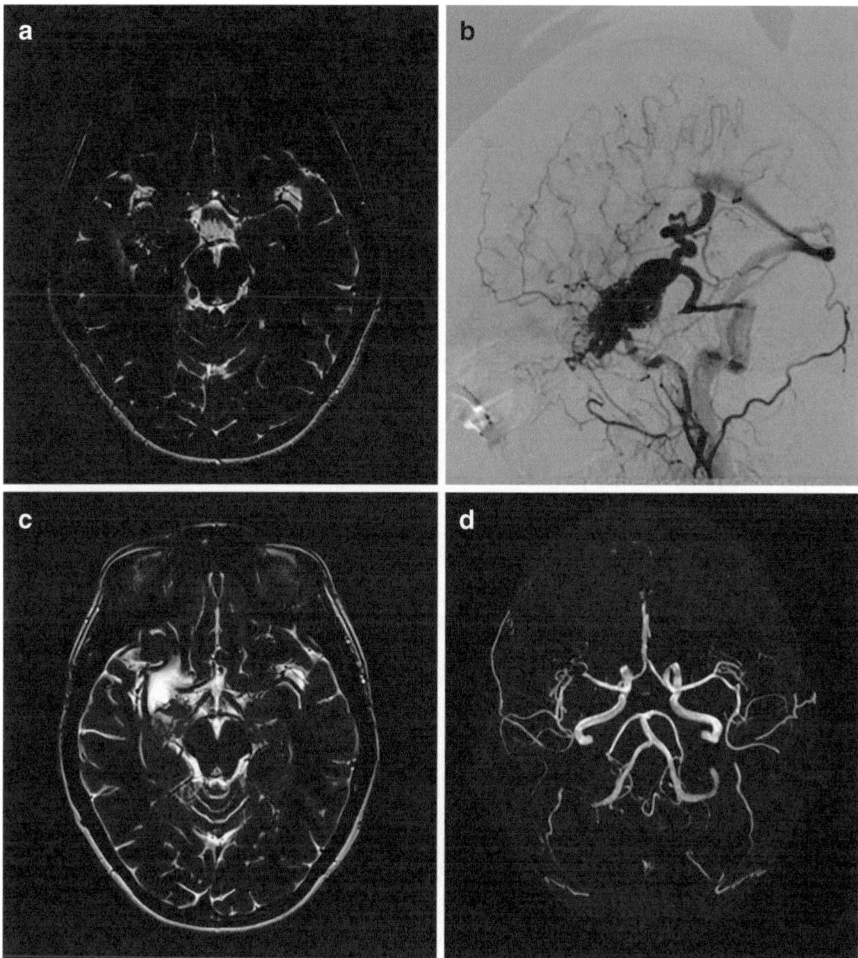

**Fig. 8.17** Second case of a 23-year-old patient with the AVM localized within the right Sylvian fissure, also managed by Gamma Knife. (**a, b**) T2-weighted scan and DSA of the AVM before irradiation, (**c, d**) T2-weighted MRI and MRA scan at the last follow-up

a study by Sirin et al. [87] which observed efficacy of 50% for AVMs larger 15 cm$^3$ in size.

Morphological studies of postradiated AVMs differentiated histological examinations of incompletely and completely obliterated AVMs, considering various stages of pathological mechanisms within targeted tissues. The specimens are characteristic of various stages of endothelial destruction, formulations of granulation tissue which are followed by hyaline degeneration [88]. The proliferation of modified myofibroblasts present in the subendothelial layer is most likely involved in vessel occlusion following the radiation [88].

Of note is an interesting study by Simon et al. [89] focused on developing a deep learning approach to automatically segment cerebrovascular-anatomical maps from multiple high-resolution MRI/MRA sequences in patients with brain AVM. This idea was built upon known variability in the appearance of the AVM nidus among different imaging methods, which may be a challenge for adequate radiosurgical mapping. The authors used a hybrid semi-automated and manual approach to label MRI/MRA with cerebrospinal fluid, vasculature, brain tissue, and also embolized vessels, since 66% of patients underwent partial embolization prior to radiosurgery. Based on the data from high-resolution MRI and using a convolutional neural network, they developed a single 3D synthetic image volume that represents the AVM image which may be useful in radiosurgery planning. This image can help to outline the target tissue (in this case the AVM nidus, arteries, vessels) from tissue that should be preserved (brain parenchyma). As a result, this method enables a high-resolution anatomical map of the whole intracranial volume. The algorithm showed satisfactory discriminatory performance across an anatomically highly diverse set of validation images, which is an interesting conclusion worth further investigation [89]. Currently used stereotactic techniques may potentially benefit from such an approach, especially due to improved resolution enabling more accurate and improved targeting of radiosurgical treatment.

## 8.12   Outcome and Prognosis

The aim of an active treatment policy in AVM management is to ensure the prevention of haemorrhage. This may be successfully performed by various approaches, but without complete resection or obliteration of the AVM, there is still a risk of haemorrhage that may have a detrimental effect on the patient's performance. Surgery is generally considered the principal treatment method since it provides early obliteration of the AVM along with the decompression of surrounding structures. However, radiosurgery has been discussed as an effective and safe alternative to surgery or embolization for the management of small AVMs or those in which surgical risks would be unacceptably high [90]. The question regarding the best treatment modality is almost impossible to answer in general, since it is highly dependent on the individual patient and its AVM. There is still a lack of randomized control trials that would be suitable for evaluating this question more in detail. One of the most famous randomized control trials is A Randomized Trial of Unruptured Brain Arteriovenous Malformations (ARUBA), published in 2013 [91]. It was performed within 39 centres in nine countries on 223 patients with a mean follow-up time of 33 months. The main aim of the ARUBA study was to compare the best medical treatment with active therapy, i.e. surgery, radiosurgery, and endovascular treatment as a single modality or in combination. Although it was initially supposed to randomize a total of 800 patients for at least 5 years, it was stopped prematurely because of the evident superiority of medical treatment over the interventional approach in the sixth year. According to its results, the authors concluded that medical treatment alone is superior to medical management with interventional therapy, in terms of the prevention of stroke or death in patients having unruptured AVMs since the hazard ratio of stroke or death was 0.27 (95% CI, 0.14–0.54) for patients randomized to medical management when compared to patients randomized to interventional therapy. Since then, there has been a significant body of criticism about ARUBA, and possible biases that likely importantly affected final conclusions, including lax criteria in terms of site selection, relatively short follow-up, or low proportion of enrolled patients. Moreover, contradictory, and inconclusive findings led to studies with a new approach towards randomized trials, including the Beyond ARUBA—Randomized Low-grade Brain AVM Study: Observation versus Surgery (BARBADOS) [92], aiming to compare surgical management and the natural course of the disease in S-M grade I and II AVMs or Treatment of Brain AVMs (TOBAS) [93], which is currently ongoing. These two trials may help to deliver the required tailored management approaches suitable for individual patients with specific AVM.

Complication rates of surgical management for brain AVMs are similar across various studies. Major morbidity and mortality in S-M grade I AVMs are typically ranging between 0% and 1%, in S-M grade II it is approximately 4%, in S-M grade IV 7% and around 12% in S-M grade V AVMs [94]. A meta-analysis of 2668 patients evaluating seizure outcome after active treatment for brain AVMs showed that surgical resection was associated with a higher probability of seizure freedom and overall seizure improvement, when compared to radiosurgical, endovascular or multimodal treatment [95]. In other study [96], complete seizure-free rates in patients with AVM-associated or haemorrhage-related seizures were 82.6% (95% CI, 80.0–85.3%) after surgery, 46.4% (95% CI, 43.6–49.2%) after radiosurgery, and 44.6% (95% CI, 32.5–56.7%) after embolization.

Brosnan et al. [97] performed a systematic review and meta-analysis of randomized trials and cohort studies that investigated the role of preoperative embolization as an adjunct to surgery. Embolization-related complications were observed in 29.4% of patients (95% CI, 16.9–40.2%). Generally, lower complications rates are observed in these cases, i.e. patients who subsequently undergo surgery and therefore complete obliteration is not the primary aim of presurgical embolization. The main aim of presurgical embolization is typically to obliterate deeper feeding arteries that are less accessible by surgery itself. Conversely, higher complication rates are more commonly reported in intended curative endovascular embolization [3, 98]. Although some authors published significantly higher proportions of successfully managed patients via presurgical embolization followed by microsurgical resection [99], there is a lack of evidence to more clearly evaluate the benefits of preoperative embolization and larger prospective studies are needed [97].

The combined treatment of embolization/surgery prior to radiosurgery may be primarily useful in reducing the risk of haemorrhage within the latency period, however, there is a potential risk of various complications [84]. Conversely, radiosurgery may be performed prior to surgery, although this approach has not been widely studied yet and therefore there is a significant lack of relevant clinical evidence based on a wider amount of primary patient data. In 2009, authors Sanchez-Mejia compared 21 radiosurgically treated to surgically resected AVMs [100]. Radiosurgery had achieved decreasing mean AVM volume (in 78% of patients; $p < 0.01$) and decreasing S-M grade (in 52% of patients; $p < 0.001$). It has been also demonstrated that radiosurgery prior to surgical resection of the AVM facilitates surgical outcomes and decreases operative morbidity. Although there is no well-established classification that would differentiate AVMs that should or should not be treated through such management, surgery should be generally recommended for radiated AVMs that show no signs of complete obliteration after the latency period of at least 3 years, those increasing in size or causing significant clinical deterioration. Radiosurgically treated patients with AVMs are exposed to a higher risk of haemorrhage during the latency period, while the risk of AVM rupture may be as high as 8% within the first year following the radiosurgical intervention [101]. The question of whether surgery should be promptly offered after radiosurgical intervention needs to be studied prospectively more in detail, especially in the mentioned specific cases showing high risk of clinical deterioration, high risk of rupture or significant increase in size [100].

Recently published population-based study of 1515 patients diagnosed with brain AVM between 1997 and 2003 reported that the post-treatment bleeding risk of ruptured AVMs was significantly lower in patients who underwent radiosurgical intervention than in those who did not (adjusted HR 0.34, 95% CI, 0.19–0.62) [102]. Overall bleeding risk from both ruptured and unruptured AVMs was in a similar manner lower in the group of patients who were treated radiosurgically (adjusted HR 0.61, 95% CI, 0.40–0.92). Interestingly, the bleeding risk from unruptured AVMs was higher in the radiosurgical group, compared to the natural history of the disease (adjusted HR 1.95, 95% CI, 1.04–3.65). Additionally, the incidence of haemorrhage within the unruptured AVMs was significantly higher in patients over 40 years of age who underwent radiosurgical intervention (adjusted HR 3.21, 95% CI, 1.12–9.14) [102]. In terms of complication rate, Herbert et al. [103] found that 17% of radiosurgically treated patients with AVM volume smaller than 28 cm and an exact half of their cohort post-radiosurgically suffered from some degree of radiation injury. Similar results were obtained from younger reports. Complications related to irradiation, such as the onset of intractable seizures, delayed neural degeneration or radiosurgery-induced intracranial tumour are not impossible to occur, but they are rather rare entities [104–106].

Similar results were observed in paediatric patients with AVMs, although children AVMs are known to be more malignant in terms of the risk of haemorrhage [59]. In 2017, Starke et al. [107] performed international multicentre cohort study of 357 children with brain AVMs to evaluate post-radiosurgery outcomes of unruptured versus ruptured paediatric AVMs, along with the aim to define predictive factors of favourable clinical outcome. AVM obliteration was achieved in 63%. During a cumulative latency period of 2748 years, the annual haemorrhage rate after radiosurgery was 1.4%, and the majority of patients (59%) reached a favourable clinical outcome. Symptomatic and permanent radiation-induced changes occurred in 8% and 3%, respectively. Interestingly, children who did not undergo prior embolization and those treated with a higher margin dose were more likely to reach a favourable outcome ($p = 0.001$ and $p < 0.001$, respectively). The annual bleeding rates following the irradiation were 0.8% for unruptured and 1.6% for ruptured AVMs. Börcek et al. [108] evaluated the obliteration rate, post-radiosurgical de novo haemorrhage rate, neurological deficit rate and new mortality rate in paediatric AVMs in a recent meta-analysis. Single session radiosurgical intervention delivered complete obliteration of the AVM in 65.9% of cases (95% CI, 60.5–71.1%). Overall complication rate (including de novo bleeding, neurological deficit, and mortality) was 8.0% (95% CI, 5.1–11.5%). De novo neurological deficit rate after radiosurgery was 3.1% (95% CI, 1.3–5.4%), and new haemorrhage rate was 4.2% (95% CI, 2.5–6.3%). The authors did not find any statistically significant difference between studies when divided according to used radiosurgical modality (Gamma Knife versus other modalities), treatment year (before the year 2000 versus after the year 2000), reported median volume of the AVM ($\geq$3 cm$^3$ versus <3 cm$^3$), median dose reported ($\geq$20 Gray versus <20 Gray), or follow-up period ($\geq$36 months versus <36 months) [115].

The possibility to use embolization prior radiosurgery is mainly performed in mid- and large-sized AVMs where it is useful in reducing the AVM size or in occluding the arterial or intranidal aneurysms. Moreover, it may be used to occlude arteriovenous fistulas which are known to be less sensitive to radiosurgical intervention [109–112]. The general idea of pre-radiosurgical embolization is primarily to shrink the AVM, thus making the radiosurgical planning easier and simultaneously reducing the risks of radiosurgical intervention [5]. However, these statements were questioned by Kano et al. [84] and Andrade-Souza [113], who showed a decrease in the obliteration, but they did not observe any benefit in terms of haemorrhage risk during the latency period. Interestingly, embolization prior radiosurgical intervention was even associated with an increased risk of complications, compared to radiosurgery itself [114]. There were also controversies about whether embolization with Onyx should be applied prior to radiation therapy, mainly speaking of possible reduction of the radiation dose and inaccuracies in imaging and thus possible inadequate radiosurgical planning [115–117]. Therefore, these uncertainties were evaluated by Chen et al. in 2021 in a multicentric retrospective study [115]. Their results are suggestive of no or not significant effect of using Onyx before radiosurgery on final treatment outcome. The efficacy and safety of combined endovascular embolization and radiosurgery for the management of intracranial AVMs were evaluated in a recent meta-analysis of 19 studies including 3454 patients [118]. Interestingly, embolization as adjuvant therapy of radiosurgery was associated with a lower obliteration rate, compared to single treatment management by radiosurgical intervention ($p < 0.001$). These results mirror earlier findings, for example meta-analysis by Zhu et al. [119] in an alike manner showed that the obliteration rate is significantly lower in patients with prior embolization followed by irradiation, again compared to patients who underwent only radiosurgery (49.5% versus 70.4%; OR 2.29, 95% CI, 1.55–3.38; $p < 0.001$). Aforedescribed results, verified also by other authors, are suggestive of the trend when endovascular embolization adjuvant to radiosurgery decreases the obliteration rate, along with no effect on reduction of haemorrhage or persistent neurological deficits [115, 118, 119]. This trend was verified in radiosurgically treated paediatric AVMs in a similar fashion [107].

## 8.13  Experience at Our Institution

Our own surgical experience with brain AVMs during the past 22 years has shown 97.3% efficacy in the completeness of AVM's radical resection with an overall 2.6% mortality/mortality rate. Of a total of 188 surgically treated patients, 3 patients died and 2 developed de novo major neurological deficit, both groups comprising only AVM of S-M grade III and IV. Three surgically partially resected AVMs were subsequently sent to Gamma Knife and two cases were postsurgically embolized. The surgical efficacy in solving S-M grade I and II AVMs has been 100% with zero mortality morbidity rates, thus clearly reflecting statements of previously cited study [94]. In cases of S-M grade III and S-M grade IV/V, the efficacy has been 95.5% (mortality/morbidity rate of 6.3%) and 71.4% (mortality/morbidity rate of 27.0%), respectively.

In the endovascular group of 64 patients, the efficacy of successful AVM obliteration was 35.9% per patient and 21.3% per session. Total number of sessions performed was 108. Twelve patients developed major deficit and/or were clinically evaluated according to the Glasgow Come Scale by less than eight points upon admission. There were 6 major complications reflecting the endovascular mortality and morbidity rate of 9.4% per patient and 5.5% per session. Three patients died (4.7%), three patients experienced bleeding following the partial embolization and four patients developed deficit after 1 year as a result of the initial bleeding. Thirteen patients were after partial embolization sent to Gamma Knife, the rest were observed or surgically resected based on their clinical status, bleedings, etc. An example of partially embolized cerebellar AVM, subsequently surgically resected, was presented in Fig. 8.15.

Last but not least, the radiosurgery group consisted of 69 patients, of who 53 were sent directly to Gamma Knife, 13 were irradiated after partial embolization and 3 patients were sent to radiosurgery after partial surgical resection. Only one serious complication (blindness) occurred after radiosurgery. Two patients died because of bleeding during the latency period, therefore, the overall mortality and morbidity rate of the radiosurgical group was 4.3%. Complete obliteration was proven in 58% of cases. Four patients experienced bleeding after radiosurgical intervention (6%).

## 8.14  Future Directions

Although it was not the principal core of our chapter, future investigations dedicated to the pathogenesis and pathophysiology may help to elucidate the disease dynamics more clearly. There is still a lack of information about genetic aspects of the disease, whether and possibly how they may affect the very unique tendency of growth or rupture in specific AVMs. More specific molecular findings could help us to answer why some AVMs show aggressive dynamic behaviour and some remain clinically silent over decades. There are interesting imaging novelties that may be particularly useful in the decision-making and planning of the most effective treatment approach for individual patients with intracranial AVM. However, these are to date not applied in ongoing clinical practice. Finally, due to the rarity of the disease, high-quality population-based prospective databases with larger population samples are of great importance to more clearly describe the disease manifestation as well as to more efficiently tailor known treatment modalities to individual patients.

## 8.15   Conclusion

There are well-established treatment algorithms that play an important role in the decision-making of active treatment policy in AVM management. Although the natural course of the disease is far away from being fully understood, the pathogenesis is likely to be invoked by various factors at once, rather than by one, well-defined cause. Notably, mainly due to the advances in imaging modalities and treatment approaches, overall mortality and morbidity rates have decreased over time. This progress happens regardless of the used modality, which reflects an evident improvement and better experience with the disease itself. Surgery is often called "superior" over the other treatment modalities. Although providing the highest probability of prevention of haemorrhage, each patient should be managed individually, and the risks of an active treatment policy should not exceed the benefits of the natural course of the disease. The radiosurgical intervention plays a fundamental role, especially as the primary treatment for eloquent AVMs which carry unacceptably high surgical risks. Endovascular embolization is rarely performed as a primary treatment, and if so, then mainly in patients with smaller AVMs carrying a higher surgical risk based on their location. It is more frequently used as adjuvant therapy prior to surgical or radiosurgical intervention or as a palliative treatment modality. All treatment modalities are therefore justified but need to be meticulously applied in well-selected individuals with accurate indications regarding the clinical and radiological findings specific to each patient.

**Compliance with Ethical Standards**   The authors declare no conflict of interest, no funding sources and confirm that any experiments which would involve humans or animals were conducted by respecting the corresponding ethical guidelines and that all figures (intraoperative or radiological) were fully anonymized.

## References


1. McCormick WF. The pathology of vascular ("arteriovenous") malformations. J Neurosurg. 1966;24(4):807–16.
2. Valavanis A, Yaşargil MG. The endovascular treatment of brain arteriovenous malformations. Adv Tech Stand Neurosurg. 1998;24:131–214. https://doi.org/10.1007/978-3-7091-6504-1_4.

3. Beneš V, Bradáč O. Brain arteriovenous malformations: pathogenesis, epidemiology, diagnosis, treatment and outcome. Berlin: Springer; 2017.

4. Rammos SK, Gardenghi B, Bortolotti C, Cloft HJ, Lanzino G. Aneurysms associated with brain arteriovenous malformations. Am J Neuroradiol. 2016;37(11):1966–71. https://doi.org/10.3174/ajnr.A4869.

5. Ogilvy CS, Stieg PE, Awad I, Brown RD Jr, Kondziolka D, Rosenwasser R, et al. AHA scientific statement: recommendations for the management of intracranial arteriovenous malformations: a statement for healthcare professionals from a special writing group of the Stroke Council, American Stroke Association. Stroke. 2001;32(6):1458–71. https://doi.org/10.1161/01.str.32.6.1458.

6. Redekop G, TerBrugge K, Montanera W, Willinsky R. Arterial aneurysms associated with cerebral arteriovenous malformations: classification, incidence, and risk of hemorrhage. J Neurosurg. 1998;89(4):539–46. https://doi.org/10.3171/jns.1998.89.4.0539.

7. Stapf C, Mast H, Sciacca RR, Choi JH, Khaw AV, Connolly ES, et al. Predictors of hemorrhage in patients with untreated brain arteriovenous malformation. Neurology. 2006;66(9):1350–5. https://doi.org/10.1212/01.wnl.0000210524.68507.87.

8. Piotin M, Ross IB, Weill A, Kothimbakam R, Moret J. Intracranial arterial aneurysms associated with arteriovenous malformations: endovascular treatment. Radiology. 2001;220(2):506–13. https://doi.org/10.1148/radiology.220.2.r01au09506.

9. Hetts SW, Cooke DL, Nelson J, Gupta N, Fullerton H, Amans MR, et al. Influence of patient age on angioarchitecture of brain arteriovenous malformations. Am J Neuroradiol. 2014;35(7):1376–80. https://doi.org/10.3174/ajnr.a3886.

10. Leblanc GG, Golanov E, Awad IA, Young WL. Biology of vascular malformations of the brain. Stroke. 2009;40(12):e694–702. https://doi.org/10.1161/strokeaha.109.563692.

11. Moftakhar P, Hauptman JS, Malkasian D, Martin NA. Cerebral arteriovenous malformations. Part 1: cellular and molecular biology. Neurosurg Focus. 2009;26(5):E10. https://doi.org/10.3171/2009.2.Focus09316.

12. Marchuk DA, Srinivasan S, Squire TL, Zawistowski JS. Vascular morphogenesis: tales of two syndromes. Hum Mol Genet. 2003;12 Spec No 1:R97–112. https://doi.org/10.1093/hmg/ddg103.

13. Bharatha A, Faughnan ME, Kim H, Pourmohamad T, Krings T, Bayrak-Toydemir P, et al. Brain arteriovenous malformation multiplicity predicts the diagnosis of hereditary hemorrhagic telangiectasia: quantitative assessment. Stroke. 2012;43(1):72–8. https://doi.org/10.1161/strokeaha.111.629865.

14. Komiyama M. Pathogenesis of brain arteriovenous malformations. Neurol Med Chir (Tokyo). 2016;56(6):317–25. https://doi.org/10.2176/nmc.ra.2016-0051.

15. Achrol AS, Kim H, Pawlikowska L, Trudy Poon KY, McCulloch CE, Ko NU, et al. Association of tumor necrosis factor-alpha-238G>A and apolipoprotein E2 polymorphisms with intracranial hemorrhage after brain arteriovenous malformation treatment. Neurosurgery. 2007;61(4):731–9. https://doi.org/10.1227/01.Neu.0000298901.61849.A4; discussion 40.

16. Mouchtouris N, Jabbour PM, Starke RM, Hasan DM, Zanaty M, Theofanis T, et al. Biology of cerebral arteriovenous malformations with a focus on inflammation. J Cereb Blood Flow Metab. 2015;35(2):167–75. https://doi.org/10.1038/jcbfm.2014.179.

17. Rothbart D, Awad IA, Lee J, Kim J, Harbaugh R, Criscuolo GR. Expression of angiogenic factors and structural proteins in central nervous system vascular malformations. Neurosurgery. 1996;38(5):915–24. https://doi.org/10.1097/00006123-199605000-00011; discussion 24–5.

18. Crawford PM, West CR, Chadwick DW, Shaw MD. Arteriovenous malformations of the brain: natural history in unoperated patients. J Neurol Neurosurg Psychiatry. 1986;49(1):1–10. https://doi.org/10.1136/jnnp.49.1.1.

19. Itoyama Y, Uemura S, Ushio Y, Kuratsu J, Nonaka N, Wada H, et al. Natural course of unoperated intracranial arteriovenous malformations: study of 50 cases. J Neurosurg. 1989;71(6):805–9. https://doi.org/10.3171/jns.1989.71.6.0805.

20. Spetzler RF, Hargraves RW, McCormick PW, Zabramski JM, Flom RA, Zimmerman RS. Relationship of perfusion pressure and size to risk of hemorrhage from arteriovenous malformations. J Neurosurg. 1992;76(6):918–23. https://doi.org/10.3171/jns.1992.76.6.0918.
21. Langer DJ, Lasner TM, Hurst RW, Flamm ES, Zager EL, King JT Jr. Hypertension, small size, and deep venous drainage are associated with risk of hemorrhagic presentation of cerebral arteriovenous malformations. Neurosurgery. 1998;42(3):481–6. https://doi.org/10.1097/00006123-199803000-00008; discussion 7–9.
22. Stefani MA, Porter PJ, terBrugge KG, Montanera W, Willinsky RA, Wallace MC. Angioarchitectural factors present in brain arteriovenous malformations associated with hemorrhagic presentation. Stroke. 2002;33(4):920–4. https://doi.org/10.1161/01.str.0000014582.03429.f7.
23. al-Rodhan NR, Sundt TM Jr, Piepgras DG, Nichols DA, Rüfenacht D, Stevens LN. Occlusive hyperemia: a theory for the hemodynamic complications following resection of intracerebral arteriovenous malformations. J Neurosurg. 1993;78(2):167–75. https://doi.org/10.3171/jns.1993.78.2.0167.
24. Yaşargil M. Microneurosurgery: AVM of the brain: clinical considerations, general and special operative techniques, surgical results, nonoperated cases, cavernous and venous angiomas, neuroanesthesia. Stuttgart: Thieme; 1988.
25. Mahalick DM, Ruff RM, Heary RF, U HS. Preoperative versus postoperative neuropsychological sequelae of arteriovenous malformations. Neurosurgery. 1993;33(4):563–70. https://doi.org/10.1227/00006123-199310000-00003; discussion 70–1.
26. Spetzler RF, Wilson CB, Weinstein P, Mehdorn M, Townsend J, Telles D. Normal perfusion pressure breakthrough theory. Clin Neurosurg. 1978;25:651–72. https://doi.org/10.1093/neurosurgery/25.cn_suppl_1.651.
27. Moftakhar P, Hauptman JS, Malkasian D, Martin NA. Cerebral arteriovenous malformations. Part 2: physiology. Neurosurg Focus. 2009;26(5):E11. https://doi.org/10.3171/2009.2.Focus09317.
28. Stapf C, Labovitz DL, Sciacca RR, Mast H, Mohr JP, Sacco RL. Incidence of adult brain arteriovenous malformation hemorrhage in a prospective population-based stroke survey. Cerebrovasc Dis. 2002;13(1):43–6. https://doi.org/10.1159/000047745.
29. Stapf C, Mast H, Sciacca RR, Berenstein A, Nelson PK, Gobin YP, et al. The New York Islands AVM study: design, study progress, and initial results. Stroke. 2003;34(5):e29–33. https://doi.org/10.1161/01.Str.0000068784.36838.19.
30. Al-Shahi R, Bhattacharya JJ, Currie DG, Papanastassiou V, Ritchie V, Roberts RC, et al. Prospective, population-based detection of intracranial vascular malformations in adults: the Scottish Intracranial Vascular Malformation Study (SIVMS). Stroke. 2003;34(5):1163–9. https://doi.org/10.1161/01.Str.0000069018.90456.C9.
31. Al-Shahi R. A systematic review of the frequency and prognosis of arteriovenous malformations of the brain in adults. Brain. 2001;124(10):1900–26. https://doi.org/10.1093/brain/124.10.1900.
32. ApSimon HT, Reef H, Phadke RV, Popovic EA. A population-based study of brain arteriovenous malformation: long-term treatment outcomes. Stroke. 2002;33(12):2794–800. https://doi.org/10.1161/01.str.0000043674.99741.9b.
33. Tong X, Wu J, Lin F, Cao Y, Zhao Y, Ning B, et al. The effect of age, sex, and lesion location on initial presentation in patients with brain arteriovenous malformations. World Neurosurg. 2016;87:598–606. https://doi.org/10.1016/j.wneu.2015.10.060.
34. Petridis AK, Fischer I, Cornelius JF, Kamp MA, Ringel F, Tortora A, et al. Demographic distribution of hospital admissions for brain arteriovenous malformations in Germany—estimation of the natural course with the big-data approach. Acta Neurochir. 2016;158(4):791–6. https://doi.org/10.1007/s00701-016-2727-2.
35. Abecassis IJ, Xu DS, Batjer HH, Bendok BR. Natural history of brain arteriovenous malformations: a systematic review. Neurosurg Focus. 2014;37(3):E7. https://doi.org/10.3171/2014.6.Focus14250.

36. Brown RD Jr, Wiebers DO, Torner JC, O'Fallon WM. Frequency of intracranial hemorrhage as a presenting symptom and subtype analysis: a population-based study of intracranial vascular malformations in Olmsted Country, Minnesota. J Neurosurg. 1996;85(1):29–32. https://doi.org/10.3171/jns.1996.85.1.0029.

37. Hillman J. Population-based analysis of arteriovenous malformation treatment. J Neurosurg. 2001;95(4):633–7. https://doi.org/10.3171/jns.2001.95.4.0633.

38. Hoh BL, Chapman PH, Loeffler JS, Carter BS, Ogilvy CS. Results of multimodality treatment for 141 patients with brain arteriovenous malformations and seizures: factors associated with seizure incidence and seizure outcomes. Neurosurgery. 2002;51(2):303–9; discussion 9–11.

39. Garcin B, Houdart E, Porcher R, Manchon E, Saint-Maurice JP, Bresson D, et al. Epileptic seizures at initial presentation in patients with brain arteriovenous malformation. Neurology. 2012;78(9):626–31. https://doi.org/10.1212/WNL.0b013e3182494d40.

40. Ruan D, Yu XB, Shrestha S, Wang L, Chen G. The role of hemosiderin excision in seizure outcome in cerebral cavernous malformation surgery: a systematic review and meta-analysis. PLoS One. 2015;10(8):e0136619. https://doi.org/10.1371/journal.pone.0136619.

41. Choi JH, Mast H, Hartmann A, Marshall RS, Pile-Spellman J, Mohr JP, et al. Clinical and morphological determinants of focal neurological deficits in patients with unruptured brain arteriovenous malformation. J Neurol Sci. 2009;287(1–2):126–30. https://doi.org/10.1016/j.jns.2009.08.011.

42. Lv X, Li Y, Yang X, Jiang C, Wu Z. Characteristics of brain arteriovenous malformations in patients presenting with nonhemorrhagic neurologic deficits. World Neurosurg. 2013;79(3–4):484–8. https://doi.org/10.1016/j.wneu.2012.04.006.

43. Spetzler RF, Martin NA. A proposed grading system for arteriovenous malformations. J Neurosurg. 1986;65(4):476–83. https://doi.org/10.3171/jns.1986.65.4.0476.

44. Kim H, Abla AA, Nelson J, McCulloch CE, Bervini D, Morgan MK, et al. Validation of the supplemented Spetzler-Martin grading system for brain arteriovenous malformations in a multicenter cohort of 1009 surgical patients. Neurosurgery. 2015;76(1):25–31. https://doi.org/10.1227/neu.0000000000000556; discussion 2; quiz 2–3.

45. Karlsson B, Lindquist C, Steiner L. Prediction of obliteration after gamma knife surgery for cerebral arteriovenous malformations. Neurosurgery. 1997;40(3):425–30. https://doi.org/10.1097/00006123-199703000-00001; discussion 30–1.

46. Schwartz M, Sixel K, Young C, Kemeny A, Forster D, Walton L, et al. Prediction of obliteration of arteriovenous malformations after radiosurgery: the obliteration prediction index. Can J Neurol Sci. 1997;24(2):106–9. https://doi.org/10.1017/S0317167100021417.

47. Pollock BE, Flickinger JC. Modification of the radiosurgery-based arteriovenous malformation grading system. Neurosurgery. 2008;63(2):239–43. https://doi.org/10.1227/01.Neu.0000315861.24920.92; discussion 43.

48. Dumont TM, Kan P, Snyder KV, Hopkins LN, Siddiqui AH, Levy EI. A proposed grading system for endovascular treatment of cerebral arteriovenous malformations: Buffalo score. Surg Neurol Int. 2015;6:3. https://doi.org/10.4103/2152-7806.148847.

49. Mossa-Basha M, Chen J, Gandhi D. Imaging of cerebral arteriovenous malformations and dural arteriovenous fistulas. Neurosurg Clin N Am. 2012;23(1):27–42. https://doi.org/10.1016/j.nec.2011.09.007.

50. Bérubé J, McLaughlin N, Bourgouin P, Beaudoin G, Bojanowski MW. Diffusion tensor imaging analysis of long association bundles in the presence of an arteriovenous malformation. J Neurosurg. 2007;107(3):509–14. https://doi.org/10.3171/JNS-07/09/0509.

51. Atlas SW, Mark AS, Fram EK, Grossman RI. Vascular intracranial lesions: applications of gradient-echo MR imaging. Radiology. 1988;169(2):455–61. https://doi.org/10.1148/radiology.169.2.3174993.

52. Jagadeesan BD, Delgado Almandoz JE, Moran CJ, Benzinger TLS. Accuracy of susceptibility-weighted imaging for the detection of arteriovenous shunting in vascular malformations of the brain. Stroke. 2011;42(1):87–92. https://doi.org/10.1161/strokeaha.110.584862.

53. Guo WY, Wu YT, Wu HM, Chung WY, Kao YH, Yeh TC, et al. Toward normal perfusion after radiosurgery: perfusion MR imaging with independent component analysis of brain arteriovenous malformations. Am J Neuroradiol. 2004;25(10):1636–44.
54. Machet A, Portefaix C, Kadziolka K, Robin G, Lanoix O, Pierot L. Brain arteriovenous malformation diagnosis: value of time-resolved contrast-enhanced MR angiography at 3.0T compared to DSA. Neuroradiology. 2012;54(10):1099–108. https://doi.org/10.1007/s00234-012-1024-x.
55. Togao O, Obara M, Helle M, Yamashita K, Kikuchi K, Momosaka D, et al. Vessel-selective 4D-MR angiography using super-selective pseudo-continuous arterial spin labeling may be a useful tool for assessing brain AVM hemodynamics. Eur Radiol. 2020;30(12):6452–63. https://doi.org/10.1007/s00330-020-07057-4.
56. Forster DM, Steiner L, Håkanson S. Arteriovenous malformations of the brain. A long-term clinical study. J Neurosurg. 1972;37(5):562–70. https://doi.org/10.3171/jns.1972.37.5.0562.
57. Ondra SL, Troupp H, George ED, Schwab K. The natural history of symptomatic arteriovenous malformations of the brain: a 24-year follow-up assessment. J Neurosurg. 1990;73(3):387–91. https://doi.org/10.3171/jns.1990.73.3.0387.
58. Ko NU, Johnston SC, Young WL, Singh V, Klatsky AL. Distinguishing intracerebral hemorrhages caused by arteriovenous malformations. Cerebrovasc Dis. 2003;15(3):206–9. https://doi.org/10.1159/000068829.
59. Fullerton HJ, Achrol AS, Johnston SC, McCulloch CE, Higashida RT, Lawton MT, et al. Long-term hemorrhage risk in children versus adults with brain arteriovenous malformations. Stroke. 2005;36(10):2099–104. https://doi.org/10.1161/01.STR.0000181746.77149.2b.
60. Meyer-Heim AD, Boltshauser E. Spontaneous intracranial haemorrhage in children: aetiology, presentation and outcome. Brain Dev. 2003;25(6):416–21. https://doi.org/10.1016/s0387-7604(03)00029-9.
61. van Beijnum J, Lovelock CE, Cordonnier C, Rothwell PM, Klijn CJ, Al-Shahi Salman R. Outcome after spontaneous and arteriovenous malformation-related intracerebral haemorrhage: population-based studies. Brain. 2009;132(Pt 2):537–43. https://doi.org/10.1093/brain/awn318.
62. Da Costa L, Wallace MC, Ter Brugge KG, O'Kelly C, Willinsky RA, Tymianski M. The natural history and predictive features of hemorrhage from brain arteriovenous malformations. Stroke. 2009;40(1):100–5. https://doi.org/10.1161/strokeaha.108.524678.
63. Kader A, Young WL, Pile-Spellman J, Mast H, Sciacca RR, Mohr JP, et al. The influence of hemodynamic and anatomic factors on hemorrhage from cerebral arteriovenous malformations. Neurosurgery. 1994;34(5):801–7. https://doi.org/10.1227/00006123-199405000-00003; discussion 7–8.
64. Duong DH, Young WL, Vang MC, Sciacca RR, Mast H, Koennecke H-C, et al. Feeding artery pressure and venous drainage pattern are primary determinants of hemorrhage from cerebral arteriovenous malformations. Stroke. 1998;29(6):1167–76. https://doi.org/10.1161/01.str.29.6.1167.
65. Stefani MA, Porter PJ, Terbrugge KG, Montanera W, Willinsky RA, Wallace MC. Large and deep brain arteriovenous malformations are associated with risk of future hemorrhage. Stroke. 2002;33(5):1220–4. https://doi.org/10.1161/01.str.0000013738.53113.33.
66. Ding D, Starke RM, Quigg M, Yen CP, Przybylowski CJ, Dodson BK, et al. Cerebral arteriovenous malformations and epilepsy, part 1: predictors of seizure presentation. World Neurosurg. 2015;84(3):645–52. https://doi.org/10.1016/j.wneu.2015.02.039.
67. Englot DJ, Young WL, Han SJ, McCulloch CE, Chang EF, Lawton MT. Seizure predictors and control after microsurgical resection of supratentorial arteriovenous malformations in 440 patients. Neurosurgery. 2012;71(3):572–80. https://doi.org/10.1227/neu.0b013e31825ea3ba.
68. Turjman F, Massoud TF, Sayre JW, Viñuela F, Guglielmi G, Duckwiler G. Epilepsy associated with cerebral arteriovenous malformations: a multivariate analysis of angioarchitectural characteristics. Am J Neuroradiol. 1995;16(2):345–50.

69. Crawford PM, West CR, Shaw MD, Chadwick DW. Cerebral arteriovenous malformations and epilepsy: factors in the development of epilepsy. Epilepsia. 1986;27(3):270–5. https://doi.org/10.1111/j.1528-1157.1986.tb03539.x.

70. Spetzler RF, Ponce FA. A 3-tier classification of cerebral arteriovenous malformations. Clinical article. J Neurosurg. 2011;114(3):842–9. https://doi.org/10.3171/2010.8.Jns10663.

71. Schramm J, Schaller K, Esche J, Boström A. Microsurgery for cerebral arteriovenous malformations: subgroup outcomes in a consecutive series of 288 cases. J Neurosurg. 2017;126(4):1056–63. https://doi.org/10.3171/2016.4.jns153017.

72. Han PP, Ponce FA, Spetzler RF. Intention-to-treat analysis of Spetzler-Martin grades IV and V arteriovenous malformations: natural history and treatment paradigm. J Neurosurg. 2003;98(1):3–7. https://doi.org/10.3171/jns.2003.98.1.0003.

73. Ding D, Starke RM, Kano H, Mathieu D, Huang PP, Feliciano C, et al. International multicenter cohort study of pediatric brain arteriovenous malformations. Part 1: predictors of hemorrhagic presentation. J Neurosurg Pediatr. 2017;19(2):127–35. https://doi.org/10.3171/2016.9.peds16283.

74. Luessenhop AJ, Spence WT. Artificial embolization of cerebral arteries. Report of use in a case of arteriovenous malformation. J Am Med Assoc. 1960;172:1153–5. https://doi.org/10.1001/jama.1960.63020110001009.

75. Newton TH, Cronqvist S. Involvement of dural arteries in intracranial arteriovenous malformations. Radiology. 1969;93(5):1071–8. https://doi.org/10.1148/93.5.1071.

76. Jin H, Qiu H, Chen C, Ge H, Li Y, He H. Embolization of feeding arteries and symptom alleviation of mixed dural-pial arteriovenous malformations. Chin Neurosurg J. 2018;4:5. https://doi.org/10.1186/s41016-018-0111-1.

77. Serbinenko FA. Balloon catheterization and occlusion of major cerebral vessels. J Neurosurg. 1974;41(2):125–45. https://doi.org/10.3171/jns.1974.41.2.0125.

78. Kerber C. Balloon catheter with a calibrated leak. A new system for superselective angiography and occlusive catheter therapy. Radiology. 1976;120(3):547–50. https://doi.org/10.1148/120.3.547.

79. Bruno CA, Meyers PM. Endovascular management of arteriovenous malformations of the brain. Interv Neurol. 2012;1(3–4):109–23. https://doi.org/10.1159/000346927.

80. Miyamoto S, Hashimoto N, Nagata I, Nozaki K, Morimoto M, Taki W, et al. Posttreatment sequelae of palliatively treated cerebral arteriovenous malformations. Neurosurgery. 2000;46(3):589–94. https://doi.org/10.1097/00006123-200003000-00013; discussion 94–5.

81. Lv X, Wu Z, Li Y, Yang X, Jiang C. Hemorrhage risk after partial endovascular NBCA and ONYX embolization for brain arteriovenous malformation. Neurol Res. 2012;34(6):552–6. https://doi.org/10.1179/1743132812y.0000000044.

82. Steiner L, Leksell L, Greitz T, Forster DM, Backlund EO. Stereotaxic radiosurgery for cerebral arteriovenous malformations. Report of a case. Acta Chir Scand. 1972;138(5):459–64.

83. Kano H, Kondziolka D, Flickinger JC, Yang HC, Flannery TJ, Niranjan A, et al. Stereotactic radiosurgery for arteriovenous malformations, part 4: management of basal ganglia and thalamus arteriovenous malformations. J Neurosurg. 2012;116(1):33–43. https://doi.org/10.3171/2011.9.Jns11175.

84. Kano H, Lunsford LD, Flickinger JC, Yang HC, Flannery TJ, Awan NR, et al. Stereotactic radiosurgery for arteriovenous malformations, part 1: management of Spetzler-Martin Grade I and II arteriovenous malformations. J Neurosurg. 2012;116(1):11–20. https://doi.org/10.3171/2011.9.Jns101740.

85. Koltz MT, Polifka AJ, Saltos A, Slawson RG, Kwok Y, Aldrich EF, et al. Long-term outcome of gamma knife stereotactic radiosurgery for arteriovenous malformations graded by the Spetzler-Martin classification. J Neurosurg. 2013;118(1):74–83. https://doi.org/10.3171/2012.9.Jns112329.

86. Karlsson B, Jokura H, Yamamoto M, Söderman M, Lax I. Is repeated radiosurgery an alternative to staged radiosurgery for very large brain arteriovenous malformations? J Neurosurg. 2007;107(4):740–4. https://doi.org/10.3171/jns-07/10/0740.

87. Sirin S, Kondziolka D, Niranjan A, Flickinger JC, Maitz AH, Lunsford LD. Prospective staged volume radiosurgery for large arteriovenous malformations: indications and outcomes in otherwise untreatable patients. Neurosurgery. 2008;62(Suppl 2):744–54. https://doi.org/10.1227/01.neu.0000316278.14748.87.

88. Szeifert GT, Levivier M, Lorenzoni J, Nyáry I, Major O, Kemeny AA. Morphological observations in brain arteriovenous malformations after gamma knife radiosurgery. Prog Neurol Surg. 2013;27:119–29. https://doi.org/10.1159/000341772.

89. Simon AB, Hurt B, Karunamuni R, Kim GY, Moiseenko V, Olson S, et al. Automated segmentation of multiparametric magnetic resonance images for cerebral AVM radiosurgery planning: a deep learning approach. Sci Rep. 2022;12(1):786. https://doi.org/10.1038/s41598-021-04466-3.

90. Starke RM, Yen CP, Ding D, Sheehan JP. A practical grading scale for predicting outcome after radiosurgery for arteriovenous malformations: analysis of 1012 treated patients. J Neurosurg. 2013;119(4):981–7. https://doi.org/10.3171/2013.5.Jns1311.

91. Mohr JP, Parides MK, Stapf C, Moquete E, Moy CS, Overbey JR, et al. Medical management with or without interventional therapy for unruptured brain arteriovenous malformations (ARUBA): a multicentre, non-blinded, randomised trial. Lancet. 2014;383(9917):614–21. https://doi.org/10.1016/s0140-6736(13)62302-8.

92. Teo M, St George J, Lawton MT. Time for BARBADOS after ARUBA trial. Br J Neurosurg. 2015;29(5):635–6. https://doi.org/10.3109/02688697.2015.1096909.

93. Darsaut TE, Magro E, Gentric JC, Batista AL, Chaalala C, Roberge D, et al. Treatment of brain AVMs (TOBAS): study protocol for a pragmatic randomized controlled trial. Trials. 2015;16:497. https://doi.org/10.1186/s13063-015-1019-0.

94. Davidson AS, Morgan MK. How safe is arteriovenous malformation surgery? A prospective, observational study of surgery as first-line treatment for brain arteriovenous malformations. Neurosurgery. 2010;66(3):498–504. https://doi.org/10.1227/01.Neu.0000365518.47684.98; discussion 5.

95. Lak AM, Cerecedo-Lopez CD, Cha J, Aziz-Sultan MA, Frerichs KU, Gormley WB, et al. Seizure outcomes after interventional treatment in cerebral arteriovenous malformation-associated epilepsy: a systematic review and meta-analysis. World Neurosurg. 2022;160:e9–22. https://doi.org/10.1016/j.wneu.2021.09.063.

96. Mamaril-Davis JC, Aguilar-Salinas P, Avila MJ, Nakaji P, Bina RW. Complete seizure-free rates following interventional treatment of intracranial arteriovenous malformations: a systematic review and meta-analysis. Neurosurg Rev. 2022;45(2):1313–26. https://doi.org/10.1007/s10143-021-01724-w.

97. Brosnan C, Amoo M, Javadpour M. Preoperative embolisation of brain arteriovenous malformations: a systematic review and meta-analysis. Neurosurg Rev. 2022;45(3):2051–63. https://doi.org/10.1007/s10143-022-01766-8.

98. Taylor CL, Dutton K, Rappard G, Pride GL, Replogle R, Purdy PD, et al. Complications of preoperative embolization of cerebral arteriovenous malformations. J Neurosurg. 2004;100(5):810–2. https://doi.org/10.3171/jns.2004.100.5.0810.

99. Saatci I, Geyik S, Yavuz K, Cekirge HS. Endovascular treatment of brain arteriovenous malformations with prolonged intranidal Onyx injection technique: long-term results in 350 consecutive patients with completed endovascular treatment course. J Neurosurg. 2011;115(1):78–88. https://doi.org/10.3171/2011.2.Jns09830.

100. Sanchez-Mejia RO, McDermott MW, Tan J, Kim H, Young WL, Lawton MT. Radiosurgery facilitates resection of brain arteriovenous malformations and reduces surgical morbidity. Neurosurgery. 2009;64(2):231–8. https://doi.org/10.1227/01.Neu.0000338068.44060.Ea; discussion 8–40.

101. Zabel-du Bois A, Milker-Zabel S, Huber P, Schlegel W, Debus J. Risk of hemorrhage and obliteration rates of LINAC-based radiosurgery for cerebral arteriovenous malformations treated after prior partial embolization. Int J Radiat Oncol Biol Phys. 2007;68(4):999–1003. https://doi.org/10.1016/j.ijrobp.2007.01.027.

102. Chye C-L, Wang K-W, Chen H-J, Yeh S-A, Tang JT, Liang C-L. Haemorrhage rates of ruptured and unruptured brain arteriovenous malformation after radiosurgery: a nationwide population-based cohort study. BMJ Open. 2020;10(10):e036606. https://doi.org/10.1136/bmjopen-2019-036606.
103. Herbert C, Moiseenko V, McKenzie M, Redekop G, Hsu F, Gete E, et al. Factors predictive of symptomatic radiation injury after linear accelerator-based stereotactic radiosurgery for intracerebral arteriovenous malformations. Int J Radiat Oncol Biol Phys. 2012;83(3):872–7. https://doi.org/10.1016/j.ijrobp.2011.08.019.
104. Kaido T, Hoshida T, Uranishi R, Akita N, Kotani A, Nishi N, et al. Radiosurgery-induced brain tumor. Case report. J Neurosurg. 2001;95(4):710–3. https://doi.org/10.3171/jns.2001.95.4.0710.
105. Husain AM, Mendez M, Friedman AH. Intractable epilepsy following radiosurgery for arteriovenous malformation. J Neurosurg. 2001;95(5):888–92. https://doi.org/10.3171/jns.2001.95.5.0888.
106. Yeo SS, Jang SH. Delayed neural degeneration following gamma knife radiosurgery in a patient with an arteriovenous malformation: a diffusion tensor imaging study. NeuroRehabilitation. 2012;31(2):131–5. https://doi.org/10.3233/nre-2012-0780.
107. Starke RM, Ding D, Kano H, Mathieu D, Huang PP, Feliciano C, et al. International multicenter cohort study of pediatric brain arteriovenous malformations. Part 2: outcomes after stereotactic radiosurgery. J Neurosurg Pediatr. 2017;19(2):136–48. https://doi.org/10.3171/2016.9.peds16284.
108. Börcek A, Çeltikçi E, Aksoğan Y, Rousseau MJ. Clinical outcomes of stereotactic radiosurgery for cerebral arteriovenous malformations in pediatric patients: systematic review and meta-analysis. Neurosurgery. 2019;85(4):E629–40. https://doi.org/10.1093/neuros/nyz146.
109. Deruty R, Pelissou-Guyotat I, Amat D, Mottolese C, Bascoulergue Y, Turjman F, et al. Complications after multidisciplinary treatment of cerebral arteriovenous malformations. Acta Neurochir. 1996;138(2):119–31. https://doi.org/10.1007/bf01411350.
110. Pollock BE, Flickinger JC, Lunsford LD, Maitz A, Kondziolka D. Factors associated with successful arteriovenous malformation radiosurgery. Neurosurgery. 1998;42(6):1239–44. https://doi.org/10.1097/00006123-199806000-00020; discussion 44–7.
111. Gobin YP, Laurent A, Merienne L, Schlienger M, Aymard A, Houdart E, et al. Treatment of brain arteriovenous malformations by embolization and radiosurgery. J Neurosurg. 1996;85(1):19–28. https://doi.org/10.3171/jns.1996.85.1.0019.
112. Friedman WA, Bova FJ. Radiosurgery for arteriovenous malformations. Neurol Res. 2011;33(8):803–19. https://doi.org/10.1179/1743132811y.0000000043.
113. Andrade-Souza YM, Ramani M, Scora D, Tsao MN, terBrugge K, Schwartz ML. Embolization before radiosurgery reduces the obliteration rate of arteriovenous malformations. Neurosurgery. 2007;60(3):443–51. https://doi.org/10.1227/01.Neu.0000255347.25959.D0; discussion 51–2.
114. Van Beijnum J, Van Der Worp HB, Buis DR, Salman RA-S, Kappelle LJ, Rinkel GJE, et al. Treatment of brain arteriovenous malformations. JAMA. 2011;306(18):2011. https://doi.org/10.1001/jama.2011.1632.
115. Chen CJ, Ding D, Lee CC, Kearns KN, Pomeraniec IJ, Cifarelli CP, et al. Embolization of brain arteriovenous malformations with versus without Onyx before stereotactic radiosurgery. Neurosurgery. 2021;88(2):366–74. https://doi.org/10.1093/neuros/nyaa370.
116. Akakin A, Ozkan A, Akgun E, Koc DY, Konya D, Pamir MN, et al. Endovascular treatment increases but gamma knife radiosurgery decreases angiogenic activity of arteriovenous malformations: an in vivo experimental study using a rat cornea model. Neurosurgery. 2010;66(1):121–9. https://doi.org/10.1227/01.Neu.0000363154.88768.34; discussion 9–30.
117. Pollock BE, Kondziolka D, Lunsford LD, Bissonette D, Flickinger JC. Repeat stereotactic radiosurgery of arteriovenous malformations: factors associated with incomplete obliteration. Neurosurgery. 1996;38(2):318–24. https://doi.org/10.1097/00006123-199602000-00016.

118. Jiang Z, Zhang X, Wan X, Wei M, Liu Y, Ding C, et al. Efficacy and safety of combined endovascular embolization and stereotactic radiosurgery for patients with intracranial arteriovenous malformations: a systematic review and meta-analysis. Biomed Res Int. 2021;2021:6686167. https://doi.org/10.1155/2021/6686167.
119. Zhu D, Li Z, Zhang Y, Fang Y, Li Q, Zhao R, et al. Gamma knife surgery with and without embolization for cerebral arteriovenous malformations: a systematic review and meta-analysis. J Clin Neurosci. 2018;56:67–73. https://doi.org/10.1016/j.jocn.2018.07.008.

# Chapter 9
# The Father of Wisdom: "The Influence of Surgical Experience on Overall Survival in Patients with Malignant Gliomas"


Ioan Stefan Florian, Lehel Beni, Zorinela Andrasoni, Cristina Aldea, and Ioan Alexandru Florian


## Contents




I. S. Florian · I. A. Florian (✉)
Department of Neurosurgery, "Iuliu Hatieganu" University of Medicine and Pharmacy Cluj-Napoca, Cluj-Napoca, Romania

Department of Neurosurgery, Cluj County Clinical Emergency Hospital Cluj-Napoca, Cluj-Napoca, Romania

I. Beni · Z. Andrasoni
Department of Neurosurgery, Cluj County Clinical Emergency Hospital Cluj-Napoca, Cluj-Napoca, Romania

C. Aldea
Department of Neurosurgery, "Iuliu Hatieganu" University of Medicine and Pharmacy Cluj-Napoca, Cluj-Napoca, Romania



© The Author(s), under exclusive license to Springer Nature Switzerland AG 2024
C. Di Rocco (ed.), *Advances and Technical Standards in Neurosurgery*, Advances and Technical Standards in Neurosurgery 49, https://doi.org/10.1007/978-3-031-42398-7_9

## 9.1 Introduction

In spite of the insurmountable effort behind the research, number of studies both published or otherwise, breakthroughs regarding intraoperative adjuvants, and innovations in delivery of chemotherapeutic agents and radiotherapy, the prognostic of high-grade gliomas (HGG) has remained generally unaltered in the last few decades. The attempts at individualizing therapy according to molecular and genetic features of these tumors have yet to yield the long-awaited improvement in overall survival (OS) and progression-free survival (PFS). Currently, multimodal treatment of HGG consists of surgery, radiotherapy, and chemotherapy, a triad that, in principle, has remained unchanged for over half a century. If the trial led by Stupp et al. in 2005 led to a transient decrease in the role of surgery [1], a growing body of more recent research has favorably reappraised its importance in prolonging survival, as well as quality of life [2–4]. The implementation of surgical adjuvants such as 5-aminolevulinic acid (5-ALA) [5, 6], intraoperative MRI (iMRI) [7], intraoperative ultrasonography [8] and more recently contrast-enhanced ultrasonography [9], employment of live fluorescence imaging in association with iMRI [10], and neuronavigation superimposed on diffusion tensor imaging (DTI) tractography [11] have aided in the enhancement of surgical resection and also offered sufficient data to support the advantages of gross total removal (GTR) over subtotal removal (STR) or biopsy of HGG concerning patient survival. Concurrently, awake surgery and cortical and subcortical mapping have led to an improvement in functional results of surgical treatment, especially for lesions located in highly functional areas [12, 13]. Contrariwise, the last few decades have experienced a tendency toward a markedly defensive medical practice, tumors with a higher risk of postoperative neurological deficit benefitting from a more conservative approach favoring biopsy to large cytoreduction [14]. Although frequently mentioned, surgical experience has only rarely been the subject of more comprehensive studies in the specialized literature [14–16]. Within this article, our aim is to demonstrate the role of an expansive surgical experience in the prolonging of OS using objective statistical methods.

## 9.2 Material and Methods

### 9.2.1 Study Model and Hypothesis

The hypothesis behind this study stems from the idea that, along with increased surgical experience, by improving the technique, intraoperative decision-making, and an enhanced familiarity regarding the difference between clearly pathological and apparently normal brain tissue, the degree of tumor resection is improved and, implicitly, the OS of the patient. In order to test this premise, it is necessary to compare two distinct and sufficiently extensive time intervals encompassing a significant and comparable number of cases so that the OS evaluation remains eloquent, while surgical interventions are performed by the same surgeon under similar technical circumstances. In order to avoid the possible bias brought on by intraoperative adjuvants, in the country in which this study was performed there is no iMRI available in the public healthcare system, whereas the use of 5-ALA is costly and has not been regulated and was therefore not possible.

This study model has been made possible by the experience of over two decades of the main author (ISF) who, between the years of 2000 and 2020, has treated a number of 1591 of new cases of gliomas out of a total of 1878 surgical interventions from the 6281 surgeries encompassing all brain tumors within the same timeframe. To demonstrate the difference that the experience of a single surgeon can provide for the OS of HGG patients, we selected two distinct intervals: between 2000 and 2009 and between 2012 and 2020, respectively. Only cases which had undergone current standard treatment incorporating surgery and adjuvant radio-chemotherapy were included in this study. We also mention that prior to the publication of the trial by Stupp et al. [1], some of the cases operated underwent radiotherapy and concomitant temozolomide (TMZ), whereas others followed an earlier protocol of radiotherapy associated with lomustine (CCNU). After the results of the aforementioned trial were made public, the standard adjuvant therapy in our center was replaced by radiotherapy and TMZ.

### 9.2.2  Extent of Resection and Surgical Technique

Concerning the extent of resection, our main goal was GTR whenever possible. For deep-seated tumors, STR was the principal aim, preserving preoperative neurological functions as much as possible. We are in favor of lesionectomy, lobectomy being reserved only for cases wherein the tumor involves the entire affected lobe.

It is not the purpose of this article to discuss in detail the surgical technique, although it must be stated that it has not changed significantly in the last few years. Cortical tumors that possess a gyral limitation can be easily isolated along the sulci, yet the extreme fragility of neoplastic vessels imposes the meticulous use of the bipolar coagulator. Once the tumor is isolated, the resection continues deeper, along the hypervascularized surface of the lesion, proceeding within the lowermost portion of the gyrus where normal arteries offer numerous neoplastic feeders. Identifying, isolating, and coagulating these feeders while preserving normal cortical arteries guarantees a critical reduction of intraoperative blood loss on the one hand, and on the other ensures a satisfactory neurological function (Fig. 9.1). Of significant importance are also the subpial dissection and preservation of large drainage veins (Fig. 9.2) in order to prevent postoperative hemorrhagic infarctions, as well as an extensive peritumoral edema. Intratumoral debulking with the ultrasonic aspirator or the normal aspirator combined with bipolar coagulation allow for a more facile progressive circumferential isolation of the tumor from the normal parenchyma and are, in the opinion of the main author, the most useful strategies in the resection of HGG.

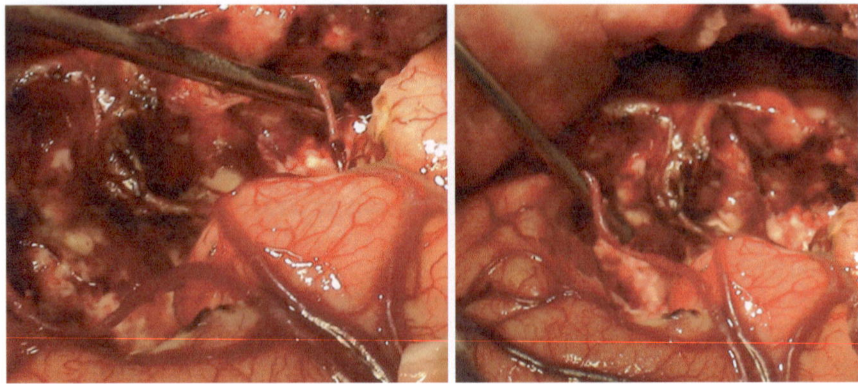

**Fig. 9.1** Surgical removal of a cortical HHG. As seen, the major cortical vessels are carefully preserved as the surgeon aspirates around them while avoiding excessive traction

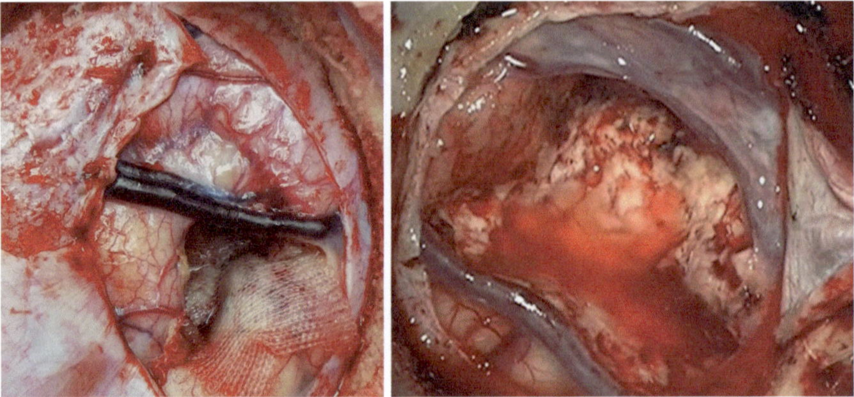

**Fig. 9.2** Surgical removal of a subcortical HHG alongside the affected cortical area. As seen, the major draining vein is preserved so as to prevent postoperative edema and hemorrhagic infarction

As for deep-seated lesions, we are in favor of using the natural pathways that direct us closest to the tumor, thus the transsulcal approach is our solution for a large number of HGG. The identification of a target sulcus is facilitated by intraoperative ultrasonography, this device being also helpful in detecting any potential tumor residue. According to our observations, the majority of deep-seated HGG come into contact with or even invade the lateral ventricle, with a contiguity existing between the innermost aspect of the tumor and the ipsilateral choroid plexus. Some of the neoplastic vessels originate from the very choroid plexus, making resection of this structure at least partially a crucial step of surgery in achieving GTR and adequate hemostasis. Generally, after opening the lateral ventricle, we insert an external ventricular drainage (EVD) and maintain it for up to 4 days after surgery.

The only intraoperative adjuvant available within the latter interval (2012–2019) was intraoperative ultrasonography, introduced in our department in 2012, having proven its usefulness in localizing deep-seated lesions and of eventual significant tumor residue, yet with limitations in detecting smaller tumor remnants due to exogeneity artefacts. Contrast-enhanced ultrasonography has also been used for a short period of time, yet in our opinion it was not superior to classic ultrasonography regarding EOR. Neuronavigation (Brainlab Curve™ Image-Guided Surgery and Buzz™ Digital OR) was introduced only in the third trimester of 2019, too recently to influence the results of this study.

### 9.2.3   Patient Population and Statistical Tools

The population included in this retrospective study was selected from the cohort of patients harboring tumors of glial origin and operated at the Neurosurgery Department of the Cluj County Clinical Emergency Hospital, Romania, between the years 2000 and 2020 by the main author (FIS). In order to gather patient data, we reviewed all written patient records and operative protocols corresponding to the studied intervals, as well as the electronic patient files which were available from 2012 onwards. This arduous process was made more difficult by the inevitable deterioration of some of the older written records that in some cases yielded incomplete information and made it obligatory to exclude some of the patients from this study. Inclusion criteria for our patients were: having been diagnosed and operated for HGG resection within the interval of January 2000 to December 2020, the main author was the principal surgeon for all interventions (including recurrences and immediate complications such as postoperative hematomas), the patient data was complete, and patients had also undergone adjuvant radio-chemotherapy. Patients with tumors other than HGG or those who had only undergone biopsy instead of resection, were operated at a time different from the specified interval or by a surgeon different from the main author, cases with incomplete data or those who had no evidence of adjuvant therapies were excluded from this study.

Regarding descriptive statistical methods for our group, we used the distribution values (mean ± standard deviation), confidence interval, min/max values, contingency tables, and frequencies. For analytical statistics, we employed the survival analysis and the disease-free interval depending on age, pathological diagnostic, surgical procedure/resection type through Kaplan–Meier method, and the evaluation of differences concerning survival.

## 9.3 Results

### *9.3.1 Patient Cohort*

The total number of patients with pathologically confirmed tumors of glial origin operated in the aforementioned interval was 1591. Out of these, 682 (42.8%) were 'de novo' low-grade glioma (LGG) cases, and the remaining 909 (57.1%) were HGG patients. Within the HGG cohort, 495 (54.5%) were male and 414 (45.5%) were female. The mean age in this cohort was 51.9 years (SD ±15.8). While examining the age distribution, an incidence peak between the ages of 50–59 years could be observed, followed by a sharp decline after the age of 70. When comparing LGG and HGG population in respects to age distribution, it is apparent that LGG in our practice presented two peaks respective of the pediatric age and between the fourth decade of life, in contrast to the HGG group (Fig. 9.3).

For the 909 HGG patients a total of 1103 surgical interventions were performed. The number of surgeries showed a steady yearly increase with an average of 15 additional interventions, adding up to the highest number of 90 cases in 2017, followed by a slight decrease to 86 operations for HGG in 2019 by the main author. The mean number of operations for HGG per year between 2000 and 2009 was 34.3 ± 11.47, mounting to 71.555 ± 15.61 surgeries between 2012 and 2020. Contextually, the mean number of operations per year for brain tumors in in the former time period was 199.9 (SD ±76.74) and in the latter 401 (SD ±27.1), thus effectively doubling the average number of surgeries per year from one interval to the other.

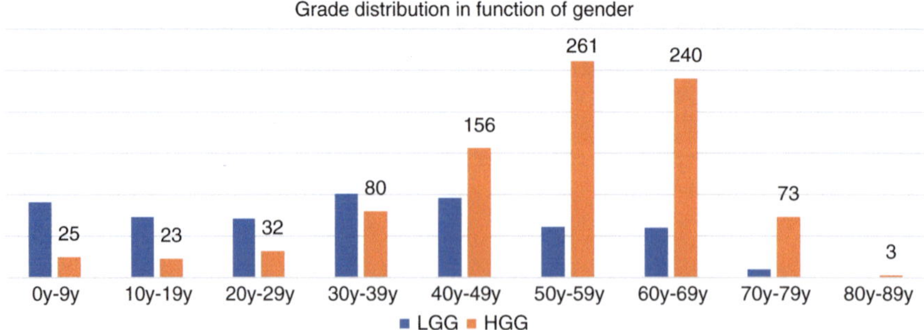


**Fig. 9.3** Distribution of low-grade gliomas (LGG) and high-grade gliomas (HGG) according to age group

## 9.3.2   Histological Features

Out of the total number of HGG patients, 254 (27.9%) had WHO grade III and 655 (72.1%) harbored WHO grade IV tumors. The most common HGG subtype according to our findings were glioblastomas (GBM) with a total number 620 cases (68.2%) from the total of HGG, and also the single most common glial tumor of any kind (33.01%). A total of 763 operations was performed for these 620 patients, 143 (23.0%) of these cases undergoing two or more surgeries for tumor recurrences. The next most common type of tumor encountered in our experience was the anaplastic astrocytoma with 185 (20.4%) cases, representing 11.6% of all patients with gliomas. Combined, these two histological entities amounted to 88.5% out of all HGG.

## 9.3.3   Localization

In our casuistry, we found that the most common site was the frontal lobe 142 (34.5%), followed by temporal lobes 120 (29.2%), parietal lobes 91(22.1%), and occipital lobes 54 (13.1%). Fourteen of these cases had tumors exclusively in the basal ganglia, ten diencephalic, ten corpus callosum, nine brain stem, seven cerebellar, and four pineal region cases of HGG.

## 9.3.4   Survival Analysis

The analysis of patient OS at 12 months, 18 months, and 24 months, respectively, confers an accurate outlook of the progression of HGG. In order to assess our study hypothesis, we compared the Kaplan–Maier curves and the OS of patients between the patients treated within the specified intervals.

The OS of HGG patients at 12 months is similar in both time periods with 48.6% for the former and 47.00% for the latter period (Table 9.1). At 18 months, the OS was 26.3% in the first timeframe, versus 38.4% in the second, showing a 12.1%

**Table 9.1**  Comparison of the OS between the two intervals from 2000 to 2012 and 2012 to 2020

| | 2000–2009 | | | |
|---|---|---|---|---|
| | Total $N$ | $N$ of events | Censored $N$ | Percent (%) |
| 24 months | 266 | 108 | | 16.70 |
| 18 months | 228 | 123 | | 26.30 |
| 12 months | 228 | 164 | | 47 |
| | 2012–2020 | | | |
| 24 months | 490 | 321 | 169 | 34.50 |
| 18 months | 490 | 302 | 188 | 38.40 |
| 12 months | 490 | 252 | 238 | 48.60 |

difference in the number of patients having survived at the 18-month mark between the two intervals. Furthermore, at 2 years, the OS in the first time period reached 16.7%, whereas in the second period, it amounted to 34.5%, thus demonstrating a difference of 17.8% (Fig. 9.4).

In our experience, out of the 172 patients surgically treated between 2012 and 2015, only 4 remain alive at the writing of this manuscript; therefore, the 5-year survival of HGG only reached 2.40%, with a mean survival time of 13.141 months (SD ±1.169 month) (Fig. 9.5).

The mean OS time in HGG patients in the first period was 11.000 months, compared to 13.441 months in the second (CI, 12.642–14.24), thus patients treated between 2012 and 2020 benefitted from an additional survival time of 2.441 months in average.

Dividing the HGG cohort into two age groups, namely patients below 65 years of age and those 65 or older, it can be noticed that 36.9% of the younger patients were alive at 24 months, as opposed to 22.6% of the elderly patients. The average OS below 65 years was 14.081 months (CI, 13.211–14.951) and 10.345 months (CI, 12.642–14.240) in the older patient group.

Additionally, GBM patients at 24 months show a 30.9% survival rate, whereas anaplastic ependymomas reach 25.0%, anaplastic oligoastrocytomas 38.50%, and anaplastic astrocytoma 48.20%.

Finally, the indicator that most accurately expresses the experience of a surgeon can be observed in the OS according to EOR. Patients who had benefited from STR show a 18.6% survival rate at 24 months after the intervention with a mean OS of 9.512 months (CI, 6.952–12.071), as opposed to cases with GTR that show a 36.0% survival rate at 24 months, with a mean survival of 13.819 months.

## 9.4 Discussions

After the first few attempts at removing these tumors (the first glioma was operated on 25th November 1884 by Rickman John Golee [17]) and a reserved optimism regarding these procedures, the decades that ensued experienced a more defensive and defeatist ambience. As Maxwell once stated, interventions for GBM are generally met as definitive failures, since a large number of these tumors spread into the contralateral hemisphere via the corpus callosum and eventually recur [18]. It has also been argued that although brain gliomas challenge the proficiency and ingenuity of neurosurgeons, there has been little to no progress made in the surgical management of these tumors [19]. Even if some of the surgical series are astonishing in volume, such as the series of Olivecrona, which encompassed 2008 verified gliomas [20], HHG have long represented, and in some centers still do, a training ground for young neurosurgeons. This was also the result of the dogma that neurosurgeons in training should acquire their experience on glial tumors, wherein no surgeon, regardless of talent, would accomplish anything significant [21].

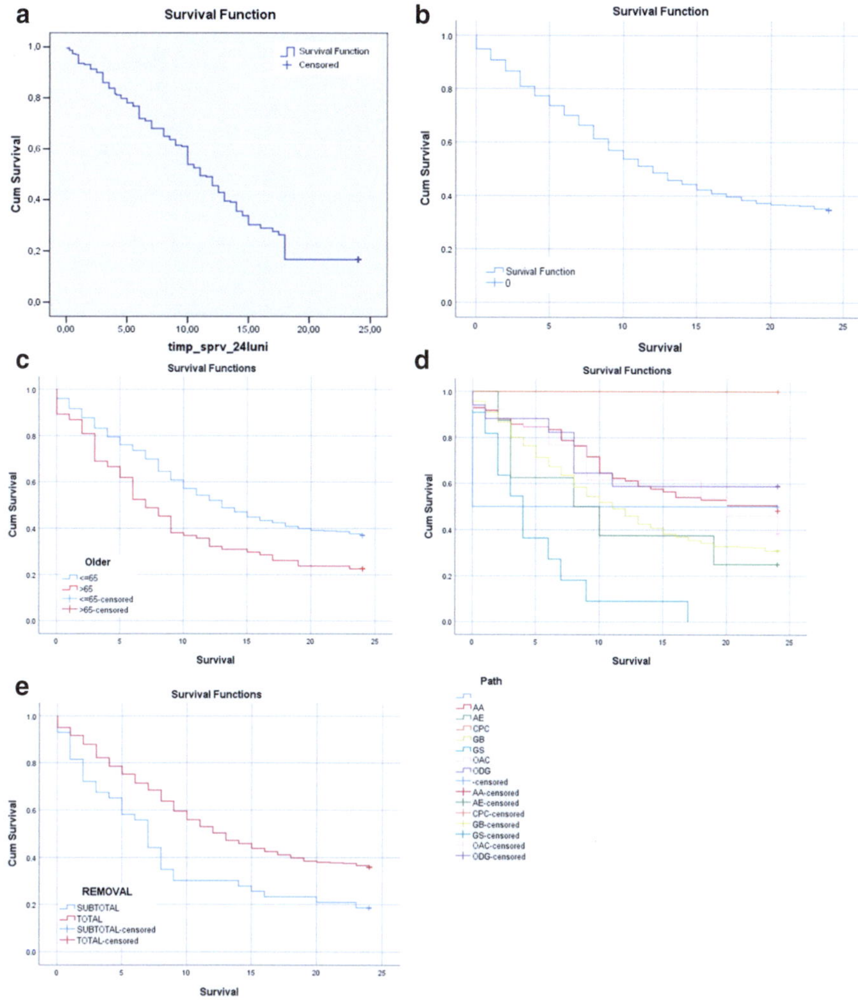

**Fig. 9.4** (**a**) The survival function of all high-grade gliomas in the time period from 2000 to 2009 the overall survival being and 16.7% patients being alive at 24 months. (**b**) The survival function of all high-grade gliomas in the time period from 2012 to 2020 the overall survival is 13.41 months and 34.5% of the patients being alive at 24 months. (**c**) The survival of patients with ages below 65 and above 65. Patients below 65 years showing 14.08 months of median survival with 36.9% of the patients being alive at 24 months, compared to patients above 65 years with 10.23 months of median survival and 22.6% being alive at 24 months. (**d**) The comparison of overall patient survival in function of histopathological findings. The worst prognosis being associated with gliosarcomas (GS), anaplastic ependymomas (AE), and glioblastomas (GB) at 24 months. (**e**) The comparison in survival with patient undergoing subtotal removal versus total removal. Patients with subtotal removal showing a median survival of 9.5 months and 18.6% being alive at 24 months, compared to patients with total removal showing a 13.8-month survival with 36.0% of the patients being alive at 24 months

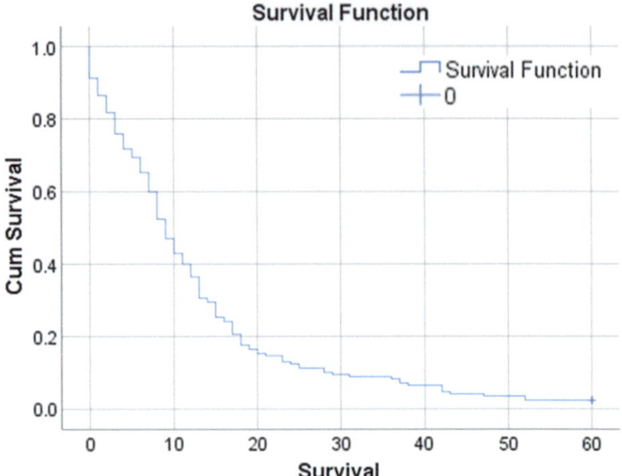



**Fig. 9.5** The OS of HGG at 5 years shows a 2.4% survival rate (4 patients), with a mean survival of 13.141 months

It was Yasargil who shifted the paradigm from both a neuroanatomical understanding of the brain itself, and of the localization and distribution of malignant gliomas, their progression and implicitly their surgical treatment [22]. His concept that gliomas implicate certain segments or sectors of the encephalon such as the neopallial or paleopallial gyri, specific regions of the white matter, basal ganglia, diencephalon, clear aspects of the brainstem or vermis, and even the ventricles denotes a vast microsurgical experience and a profound understanding of the cerebral anatomy. Our own experience supports these observations and we adhere to the belief that malignant gliomas in these aforementioned areas generally display a sharp, occasionally even linear, boundary to the adjacent compartments. We also agree that the pattern of gliomas is virtually identical on MRI studies for lesions involving the same compartments. For example, as Yasargil mentioned, the majority of neopallial lesions possess a pyramidal shape on coronal MRI sections, the tip pointing toward the ventricle, similarly to brain AVMs. Furthermore, we too confirm that each of these compartments possesses a particular vascularization concerning arterial feeders and draining veins alike. Although contrary to Yasargil's opinion that glioma growth is predominantly expansive and in a retrograde manner towards the ventricles, our impression is that migration occurs in the opposite direction, from the periventricular region towards the cortex, closely following the embryological vascular print of that compartment. As we have proven in previous studies, the role of glial stem cells in the development of malignant gliomas cannot be neglected. The invasive expansion of these neoplastic cells resembles the migration of glial and neuronal cells and their precursors during brain embryogenesis, with surmounting proof advocating that GBM most likely arise from neural stem cells rather than dedifferentiated mature astrocytes [23]. It is no mere coincidence that the neural stem cell compartment is situated principally in the subventricular zone of the lateral ventricles and adjacent to the ependyma of the dentate gyrus of the temporal horn [24–26], regions described by Yaşargil as glioma-specific. On the other hand, according to our own observations, the choroid plexuses demonstrate modifications in both aspect and dimensions in patients suffering from GBM, denoting a potential activity alteration during oncogenesis [27]. The role and placement of the choroid plexus in the development of HHG, as well as AVMs, the intercellular communication and information transfer as well as tumor progression represent our research target, in the hopes of developing personalized and specific multimodal therapies [28, 29]. Concerning surgical treatment in itself, we adhere to the principles expounded by Yasargil even as early as 1996 [30], our own experience confirming GTR can be achieved in the majority of HHG patients, offering a real benefit in regard to quality of life and OS.

In the case of superficial lesions, the gyral delineation facilitates a sulcal dissection of the tumor along almost the entirety of its circumference. Even in areas where cortical modifications are not as obvious (a slightly pale cortical surface), the existence of intensely reddish and enlarged pial vessels with a more sinusoidal trajectory represents a macroscopic clue for a subcortical lesion. By following the plane of the selected sulcus until its innermost aspects, one can progressively identify the feeder arteries of the tumor, which generally emerge from a normal-appearing artery. Thusly, these pathological feeders can be sequentially coagulated at 1–2 mm from their origin while sparing the main artery. Large cortical veins should also be preserved through pial dissection and careful mobilization off the tumoral plane. Tumor draining veins, which bring an outflow of arterialized blood from the lesion, are coagulated and ligated at a distance from the main vein so as to avoid its retraction. Internal debulking then allows for an easier progressive circumferential dissection of the tumor. Nevertheless, after crossing the level of the sulcus within the white matter, the lesion borders are much more difficult to identify for an inexperienced eye. In this step of the surgery, intraoperative adjuvants such as 5-ALA and iMRI usually come into play [6, 7]. However, the existence of a microvascular plane formed by neoplastic vessels, the behavior of the brain tissue when in contact with the bipolar forceps, the ease of aspiration of coagulated regions, and the layer-by-layer removal of the tumor allow for GTR in the majority of cases in the hands of a skilled and experienced surgeon. Similar to Yasargil, we are in favor of lesionectomy, lobar resection being reserved only for tumors involving an entire lobe [30].

Concerning subcortical and deep-seated HHG, our observation is that these tumors are always connected to the nearest ventricle in some degree. The transsulcal approach via the most direct sulcus in the least eloquent area and facilitated by intraoperative ultrasonography favors the identification of the tumor plane. Once the lesion is recognized and tissue samples are obtained, we initiate intratumoral debulking. We avoid excessive corticotomies as much as possible, being adepts of dynamic progressive retractions. As the tumor volume is reduced via aspiration (either ultrasonic or simple in combination with bipolar coagulator), the tumor–brain interface is easily identifiable, allowing for progressive cauterization of superficial vessels. In our surgical experience, we found that there is always a contiguity between the neoplastic vessels and the adjacent choroid plexus within the nearest ventricle. In many cases, the choroid plexus itself has a modified appearance due to significant vacuolization, thromboses, and even areas of tumoral infiltration. Considering these aspects, we believe it necessary to coagulate and remove the modified portion of the choroid plexus to achieve GTR, which of course implies opening the ventricle. As we have previously stated, we are convinced that the choroid plexus plays an important yet insufficiently studied role in tumorigenesis, being a veritable field of research in the near future. Furthermore, the choroid plexus may also be the target of adjuvant therapies, utilizing nanotechnologies as a supraselective transportation vector for various chemotherapeutic agents [31–33].

The aforesaid microsurgical principles have dominated the strategy of the main author for the last 20 years of practice, all of which benefitted from a series of refinements and improvements while gaining experience. Although a part of the utilized equipment has been replaced along the years, such as the intraoperative microscopes, ultrasonic aspirators, bipolar coagulators, and nonstick forceps, they had little to no impact on the degree of resection of HHG in itself. While 5-ALA and iMRI have apparently increased the rates of GTR attainment [10, 34], these were not available in our department due to prohibitive costs. Fluorescein angiography, a cheaper alternative to 5-ALA, proven as useful in vascular neurosurgery [35], and advocated for HHG resection [36, 37], did not demonstrate its effectiveness in improving the degree of tumor resection in the few cases we employed it for. Furthermore, because of the lack of specificity it did increase the risk of morbidity by also highlighting the normal cerebral tissue surrounding the tumor. Other authors also came to this conclusion [38]. As a result, we have completely abandoned intraoperative fluorescein visualization for tumors in our department. However, it is not just according to our own opinion that intraoperative ultrasonography is an extremely useful adjuvant, enabling real time cerebral imaging that is both repeatable and accurate, all the while being incomparably cheaper than the iMRI [9]. We address a special mention to microsurgical techniques with 6× magnification loupes possessing an individual light source and 420 mm focal distance (Heine Optotechnik GmbH & Co KG, Germany). For superficial tumors, these offer similar magnification and lightening to an operative microscope with the added bonus of not hindering the head mobility of the wearer, who can also see beneath the corner and avoid unnecessary brain traction and large cortical incisions. Speaking from experience, these too require training, yet just like the microscope and endoscope, after the steep learning curve follow an obvious series of advantages, especially in shortening surgical time. Nonetheless, it is preferable to use the microscope whenever a larger magnification is needed.

Our goal is GTR whenever possible and when this does not involve risks related to the deep location of these tumors (brainstem or thalamo-mesencephalic region). Otherwise, maximal safe cytoreduction with the preservation of neurological functions becomes our aim. Regarding gliomas highly functional areas, most patients already have a neurological deficit when undergoing surgery, therefore any additional postoperative deficit is usually recovered in a matter of weeks or up to 3 months after the intervention [39, 40]. It is believed that brain reorganization begins even before the surgical removal of the tumor. Nevertheless, recovery is more apparent in patients with LGG than in those with HGG. Moreover, surgery itself seems to contribute little to the pattern of functional brain remodeling [41]. As such, the decision to operate in these scenarios depends on several factors aside from the neurological status, tumor features, as well as prognostic. Psychological and emotional factors pertaining to both the patient and their family, pressure and persistence to 'do anything and everything possible,' the assumption of risks tied to the possible postoperative consequences, and even just the postponement of the inevitable to allow accommodation with this dreaded diagnostic reflect a certain cultural, religious and last but not least educational background that is different in our country to that of Western Europe or North America. While certain operative risks are considered inadmissible in Western European countries, they may be taken for granted and more freely accepted by the patients and their families in Eastern Europe. Under these circumstances, maximal safe cytoreduction in our practice is offered more frequently than diagnostic biopsy, even for tumors possessing a high chance of neurological deficit.

The role of GTR in prolonging OS for HHG has been underscored in numerous retrospective personal or institutional studies. Conversely, the trial led by Stupp et al. that resulted in the current standard therapy for HHG [1] paradoxically led to the widespread belief that importance of surgery should be undermined in the multimodal treatment of these lesions, especially of GBM. The passing reference and lack of a consistent analysis regarding the role of surgery, as well as the insistent emphasis on the association with TMZ resulted in the impression that neurosurgical treatment is not as significant as once thought. This is further evidenced by the data provided in the Supplementary Appendix of the same article, showing a significant difference in median survival time between patients subjected to biopsy (5 months shorter survival than the radiotherapy only group, and 6.4 months shorter than the radiotherapy + TMZ group), compared to cases with decompressive surgery [1]. Despite being a well-structured randomized trial, it was centered on the benefits of adjuvant therapy while forgoing the advantages corresponding to the extent of resection (GTR 40% in the radiotherapy group, and 39% in the Radiotherapy + TMZ group, compared to cu STR in 45% and 44% of these two groups, respectively). This only accentuated the controversy, since a prospective study published in 2001 demonstrated that only GTR (defined as removing 98% or more of the tumor volume) had a positive impact on the patients with GBM [42]. Because of research ethics and professional reasons, there were no prospective randomized trials regarding EOR for HHG, the only data in this aspect arising from a study analyzing the influence of 5-ALA on the grade of resection [6]. The authors discovered a 4.9-month survival benefit (16.7 months for GTR compared to 11.8 months for STR), yet the value of STR could not be evaluated further. A more recent retrospective study based on preoperative and postoperative volumetric analysis of tumors demonstrated that a 78% degree of resection was the threshold that could positively influence OS, becoming the minimal target in cases where GTR is not achievable [43]. Our own research published in 2011 revealed that age and type of surgery behaved as prognostic factors influencing OS at 12, 18, and 24 months in a series of 266 patients. We discovered a difference of mean survival at 12, 18, and 24 months at postoperative monitoring equal to 2.8 months, 4.4 months and 5.1 months, respectively, in favor of patients subjected to GTR [44]. Several other studies, the majority of which being retrospective, have demonstrated the benefit of GTR versus STR or biopsy in both young and elderly individuals [45] and that heightening the EOR was linked to improved OS independent of increasing extent of resection was associated with improved survival independent of age, degree of disability, WHO grade, of the tumor, or succeeding treatment methods employed [46, 47].

In the absence of intraoperative adjuvants, there is the issue of quantifying surgical experience and its influence on increasing EOR and, implicitly, patient OS. Surgical experience is often mentioned, yet seldom analyzed, despite it being one of the decisive factors in improving interventional outcome. Moreover, there seems to be little difference concerning PFS and OS between HGG patients undergoing awake surgery and those under general anesthesia [48]. It may be argued that a neurosurgical intervention in itself is comparable to a severe traumatic head injury (TBI) in terms of impact upon the contents of the cranium. Although this may seem a brutal statement, subtle gestures on the brain may affect the vegetative system in a manner similar to actual trauma. Therefore, in the opinion of the main author, surgical experience may be compared to reducing the traumatic effect of a neurosurgical intervention from a severe to a mild TBI via improving gestures and reducing hand tremor, recognizing and anticipating potential risks, as well as the ability to mend more of the damage caused. As Howell so knowledgeably explained, a neophyte first travels through stages of 'unconscious incompetence,' followed by 'conscious incompetence' and finally 'unconscious competence' [49]. Surgical expertise is intimately associated with the relative experience of that surgeon, in turn posing the issue concerning the correlation between the number of interventions and operative outcome. Consistency in the outcomes of a specific surgical intervention or a certain procedure is linked to the number of times that surgeon executed it, even after eliminating related variables, such as total hospital volume [50]. Thus, an increased frequency of performing a specific procedure may yield a superior outcome [51]. In the field of surgery, an expert may be characterized as a practitioner who has amassed experience and achieves consistently better outcomes while also displaying a superior performance in various surgical skills in contrast to nonexperts [52]. An association between reasoning and fine motor skills is crucial, especially since these two facets of surgery are interconnected, an association that is earned through learning, practice, and constant feedback [53].

Several studies performed in the last two decades have proven that surgical experience, in the neurosurgical field or otherwise, as quantified by the volume of procedures performed is independently correlated with an improvement in outcome for both adult [54, 55] and pediatric patients alike [15]. Concerning neurosurgery and its multitude of subspecialties and procedures, better outcomes are attained by high-volume surgeons practicing at high-volume centers, results being measured by surgery-related mortality, rate of complications, and length of stay (LOS) [14, 56].

To our knowledge, a single study in the recent literature makes an analysis on personal neurosurgical experience, investigating four distinct intervals on a period of 17 years of patients operated for brain tumors by the same surgeon. The researched factor referred to the accuracy with which the surgeon evaluates the EOR in comparison to postoperative volumetric MRI studies, demonstrating a linear increase in accuracy over the studied period (gross perception of 70.0–85.7% and quantitative perception 66.7–100.0%), indicating the learning curve. The neurosurgeon in question had a high-volume tumor practice, with an average 176 tumor surgeries/year and more than 3000 interventions for tumors in this period, including both asleep and awake patients. As the authors of this study concluded, there is a learning curve accompanying the personal estimation of EOR, and it might take more than 10 years and thousands of surgeries to become "actually" skilled [16]. Yet our study follows the effect of experience on lengthening OS for HHG, as proficiency does not solely signify a more precise EOR estimation, but also an improvement in the act of surgery itself and preventing intraoperative and postoperative complications, as well as reducing surgery-related morbidity and mortality. Experience also means being more capable in decision-making in regard to surgical indication, timing, approach, identification, and avoidance of potential risks, as well as the ability to differentiate between the intraoperative behavior of normal and pathological brain tissues. Similar to the abovementioned study, the main author of this manuscript has a vast experience of 6281 surgeries for brain tumors in the last 20 years, equating to an average of 314.05 interventions/year, with a total number of glioma surgeries of 1878, or 93.9 interventions/year in this timeframe. The starting point of this study does not correspond to the beginning of the main author's career, which had started approximately a decade prior. We can confirm the existence of the learning curve corroborated with a gradual increase of surgical volume. For example, for the 909 new cases of HGG in the studied period, a total of 1103 interventions were performed. From 23 HGG operated cases out of a total of 93 surgeries for cerebral tumors in the year 2000, the number of interventions for brain tumors increased by an average of 15 each year, adding up to 80 surgeries for HGG out of 395 operated brain tumors in 2020. The mean number of operations for brain tumors per year within the first studied interval was 199.9 (SD: ±76.74), whereas for the second interval (2012–2020), the mean more than doubled for a total of 404.6 (SD: ±27.02). The same was also applicable for HGG, as the mean number was initially 34.3 (SD: ±11.47) between 2000 and 2009 and 71.666 (SD: ±15.61) cases between 2012 and 2020.

We reiterate that as no significant intraoperative adjuvants were used apart from ultrasonography; therefore, surgical experience may be incriminated for OS improvement. In order to establish the influence of experience and surgical volume increase influenced OS, we compared the two patient lots in terms of survival at 12, 18, and 24 months using the Kaplan–Maier curves. Afterward, we analyzed and compared data according to EOR, patient age, and last but not least pathological subtype for the most frequent HHG operated in our department. The OS of HGG patients at 12 months was almost equivalent for both time periods (48.6% for the former and 47.00% for the latter). The marked difference that surgical experience yields begins to be visible at later intervals. At 18 months, the OS of patients was 26.3% for the first period versus 38.4% in the second, hence a 12.1% difference in the number of surviving patients at 18 months after initial surgery. At 2 years, the average OS for the first time period was 16.7%, compared to the second time period wherein it reached 34.5%, thus showing a difference of 17.8%. The mean OS time at 24 months in 2000–2009 period was 11.000 months, compared to 2012–2020 when it equaled 13.441 months (CI, 12.642–14.24), thus patients operated in the latter period possessed an average OS longer by 2.441 months. In other words, we can safely assume that surgical experience as an independent factor offers an average benefit of two additional months in terms of OS for HHG, equivalent to adjuvant TMZ therapy.

The indicator that expresses EOR and thus the experience of a surgeon can be observed on OS. Patients that had benefited from a STR showed a 18.6% survival rate with a mean OS of 9.512 months (CI, 6.7952–12.071) at 24 months after surgery, whereas patients with GTR demonstrated a 36.0% OS with a mean survival of 13.819 months at the two-year mark. This is again clear evidence that GTR is more beneficial to STR in terms of prolonging life expectancy for these patients and that experienced neurosurgeons should strive for total resection whenever feasible.

Regarding pathological subtypes, patients harboring anaplastic astrocytomas lived on average an additional 3 months in the latter period (15.261 months) compared to those from the former (11.946), whereas those with GBM had an added 1.6 month of survival time when comparing the same intervals (12.816 months vs. 11.205 months). This fact brings the median OS strikingly close to that obtained in a resembling high-volume center (12.2 months) that has modern technical facilities at its disposal (*Department of Neurological Surgery, University of California, San Francisco, California)* [43]. This finding may be an argument in favor of surgical experience compensating (at least partially) for the lack of recent neurosurgical intraoperative adjuvants.

The current study has a series of limitations, such as it being retrospective in nature, and that incomplete case data led to the exclusion of several patients. Moreover, the lack of electronic data before 2012 made data retrieval extremely arduous. Some of the individuals treated between 2000 and 2005 received CCNU instead of the current standard adjuvant therapy (TMZ), whereas radiotherapy was still in its infant stages of standardization at that time. These facts might have influenced the outcome of approximately 40 patients in the earlier study interval. Additionally, being an expansive study on 20 years of practice within a neurosurgical resident training department, operating teams have changed over time, resulting in a slight increase of postoperative complications such as CSF fistulas and hematomas with the succession of each generation. This too might have vaguely affected postinterventional morbidity and mortality. We also acknowledge that the lack of intraoperative adjuvants may not represent a reason to gloat; however, this is due to the public healthcare administration on a national level and does not reflect the desires and intentions of our own department and its surgeons.

The strong point of this study is that all patients included were operated by the same neurosurgeon (ISF), alongside the same neuroanesthesiologist (AZ) for the grand majority of cases. The follow-up on such a large scale (20 years) of patients treated in similar conditions represents an almost singular opportunity to demonstrate the influence surgical experience may bring in the highly disputed field of malignant gliomas.

## 9.5  Conclusions

Surgical treatment represents a crucial first step in the multimodal treatment of HHG. Surgical experience is a factor that influences not only survival time in a manner equivalent to chemotherapy but also the quality of life. Therefore, a special competence in neurooncology should be required to offer these patients a second chance at life. The main author of this manuscript is a member of a European initiative group that promotes the competence in Neurooncological surgery, and the present study is a strong argument in supporting this project.

## References


1. Stupp R, Mason WP, van den Bent MJ, et al. Radiotherapy plus concomitant and adjuvant temozolomide for glioblastoma. N Engl J Med. 2005;352(10):987–96. https://doi.org/10.1056/NEJMoa043330.
2. Silva da Costa MD, Camargo NC, Dastoli PA, Nicácio JM, Benevides Silva FA, Sucharski Figueiredo ML, Chen MJ, Cappellano AM, Saba da Silva N, Cavalheiro S. High-grade gliomas in children and adolescents: is there a role for reoperation? J Neurosurg Pediatr. 2020;11:1–10. https://doi.org/10.3171/2020.7.PEDS20389. PMID: 33307529.
3. Hervey-Jumper SL, Berger MS. Maximizing safe resection of low- and high-grade glioma. J Neuro Oncol. 2016;130(2):269–82. https://doi.org/10.1007/s11060-016-2110-4. Epub 2016 May 12. PMID: 27174197.
4. Hardesty DA, Sanai N. The value of glioma extent of resection in the modern neurosurgical era. Front Neurol. 2012;18(3):140. https://doi.org/10.3389/fneur.2012.00140. PMID: 23087667; PMCID: PMC3474933.
5. Stummer W, Pichlmeier U, Meinel T, et al. Fluorescence-guided surgery with 5-aminolevulinic acid for resection of malignant glioma: a randomised controlled multicentre phase III trial. Lancet Oncol. 2006;7(5):392–401. https://doi.org/10.1016/S1470-2045(06)70665-9.
6. Gandhi S, Tayebi Meybodi A, Belykh E, Cavallo C, Zhao X, Syed MP, Borba Moreira L, Lawton MT, Nakaji P, Preul MC. Survival outcomes among patients with high-grade glioma treated with 5-aminolevulinic acid-guided surgery: a systematic review and meta-analysis. Front Oncol. 2019;9:620. https://doi.org/10.3389/fonc.2019.00620. PMID: 31380272; PMCID: PMC6652805.
7. Kelly PJ. Image-directed tumor resection. Neurosurg Clin N Am. 1990;1(1):81–95.
8. Chadduck WM. Perioperative sonography. J Child Neurol. 1989;4(Suppl):S91–S100. https://doi.org/10.1177/0883073889004001s14.
9. Mahboob S, McPhillips R, Qiu Z, et al. Intraoperative ultrasound-guided resection of gliomas: a meta-analysis and review of the literature. World Neurosurg. 2016;92:255–63. https://doi.org/10.1016/j.wneu.2016.05.007.
10. Gessler F, Forster MT, Duetzmann S, et al. Combination of intraoperative magnetic resonance imaging and intraoperative fluorescence to enhance the resection of contrast enhancing gliomas. Neurosurgery. 2015;77(1):16–22. https://doi.org/10.1227/NEU.0000000000000729.
11. Barone DG, Lawrie TA, Hart MG. Image guided surgery for the resection of brain tumours. Cochrane Database Syst Rev. 2014;2014(1):CD009685. Published 2014 Jan 28. https://doi.org/10.1002/14651858.CD009685.pub2.
12. Surbeck W, Hildebrandt G, Duffau H. The evolution of brain surgery on awake patients. Acta Neurochir. 2015;157(1):77–84. https://doi.org/10.1007/s00701-014-2249-8.

13. Sanai N, Berger MS. Mapping the horizon: techniques to optimize tumor resection before and during surgery. Clin Neurosurg. 2008;55:14–9.
14. Trinh VT, Davies JM, Berger MS. Surgery for primary supratentorial brain tumors in the United States, 2000-2009: effect of provider and hospital caseload on complication rates. J Neurosurg. 2015;122(2):280–96. https://doi.org/10.3171/2014.9.JNS131648.
15. McAteer JP, LaRiviere CA, Drugas GT, Abdullah F, Oldham KT, Goldin AB. Influence of surgeon experience, hospital volume, and specialty designation on outcomes in pediatric surgery: a systematic review. JAMA Pediatr. 2013;167(5):468–75. https://doi.org/10.1001/jamapediatrics.2013.25.
16. Lau D, Hervey-Jumper SL, Han SJ, Berger MS. Intraoperative perception and estimates on extent of resection during awake glioma surgery: overcoming the learning curve. J Neurosurg. 2018;128(5):1410–8. https://doi.org/10.3171/2017.1.JNS161811.
17. Oliver K, Strangman S. The first documented modern-day brain tumor surgery for a glioma. London: International Brain Tumor Alliance; 2009.
18. Maxwell HP. The incidence of interhemispheric extension of glioblastoma multiforme through the corpus callosum. J Neurosurg. 1946;3(1):54–7.
19. Ley A, Lay A Jr, Guitard JM, Oliveras C. Surgical management of intracranial gliomas. J Neurosurg. 1962;19(5):365–74.
20. Olivecrona H. The cerebellar angioreticulomas. J Neurosurg. 1952;9(4):317–30. https://doi.org/10.3171/jns.1952.9.4.0317.
21. Grant FC. A study of the results of surgical treatment in 2326 consecutive patients with brain tumor. In: The seventh annual max M: Peet lecture, November 18, 1955. Ann Arbor: University Hospital.
22. Yaşargil MG, Kadri PA, Yasargil DC. Microsurgery for malignant gliomas. J Neuro Oncol. 2004;69(1–3):67–81.
23. Tomuleasa C, Soritau O, Rus-Ciuca D, et al. Functional and molecular characterization of glioblastoma multiforme-derived cancer stem cells. J BUON. 2010;15(3):583–91.
24. Sanai N, Alvarez-Buylla A, Berger MS. Neural stem cells and the origin of gliomas. N Engl J Med. 2005;353(8):811–22. https://doi.org/10.1056/NEJMra043666. PMID: 16120861.
25. Alvarez-Buylla A, Kohwi M, Nguyen TM, Merkle FT. The heterogeneity of adult neural stem cells and the emerging complexity of their niche. Cold Spring Harb Symp Quant Biol. 2008;73:357–65. https://doi.org/10.1101/sqb.2008.73.019. Epub 2008 Nov 6. PMID: 19022766.
26. Doetsch F, Petreanu L, Caille I, Garcia-Verdugo JM, Alvarez-Buylla A. EGF converts transit-amplifying neurogenic precursors in the adult brain into multipotent stem cells. Neuron. 2002;36(6):1021–34. https://doi.org/10.1016/s0896-6273(02)01133-9. PMID: 12495619.
27. Şuşman S, Leucuţa DC, Kacso G, Florian ŞI. High dose vs low dose irradiation of the subventricular zone in patients with glioblastoma—a systematic review and meta-analysis. Cancer Manag Res. 2019;11:6741–53. Published 2019 Jul 18. https://doi.org/10.2147/CMAR.S206033.
28. Melincovici CS, Boşca AB, Şuşman S, et al. Vascular endothelial growth factor (VEGF)—key factor in normal and pathological angiogenesis. Romanian J Morphol Embryol. 2018;59(2):455–67.
29. Buruiană A, Florian ŞI, Florian AI, et al. The roles of miRNA in glioblastoma tumor cell communication: diplomatic and aggressive negotiations. Int J Mol Sci. 2020;21(6):1950. Published 2020 Mar 12. https://doi.org/10.3390/ijms21061950.
30. Yasargil MG. Microneurosurgery, volume IVB. Stuttgart: Georg Thieme Verlag; 1996. p. 344–63.
31. Florian IS, Tomuleasa C, Soritau O, et al. Cancer stem cells and malignant gliomas. From pathophysiology to targeted molecular therapy. J BUON. 2011;16(1):16–23.
32. Abrudan C, Florian IS, Baritchii A, et al. Assessment of temozolomide action encapsulated in chitosan and polymer nanostructures on glioblastoma cell lines. Romanian Neurosurg. 2014;XXI 1:18–29.

33. Aldea M, Florian IA, Kacso G, et al. Nanoparticles for targeting intratumoral hypoxia: exploiting a potential weakness of glioblastoma. Pharm Res. 2016;33(9):2059–77. https://doi.org/10.1007/s11095-016-1947-8.
34. Sharma V, Kedia R, Narang KS, Jha AN. Enhanced resection of primary high-grade gliomas using a combination of intraoperative magnetic resonance imaging and intraoperative fluorescence (5-aminolevulinic acid): a single-centre experience. Neurol India. 2018;66(3):747–52. https://doi.org/10.4103/0028-3886.232334.
35. Kakucs C, Florian IA, Ungureanu G, Florian IS. Fluorescein angiography in intracranial aneurysm surgery: a helpful method to evaluate the security of clipping and observe blood flow. World Neurosurg. 2017;105:406–11. https://doi.org/10.1016/j.wneu.2017.05.172.
36. Falco J, Cavallo C, Vetrano IG, et al. Fluorescein application in cranial and spinal tumors enhancing at preoperative MRI and operated with a dedicated filter on the surgical microscope: preliminary results in 279 patients enrolled in the FLUOCERTUM prospective study. Front Surg. 2019;6:49. Published 2019 Aug 13. https://doi.org/10.3389/fsurg.2019.00049.
37. Neira JA, Ung TH, Sims JS, et al. Aggressive resection at the infiltrative margins of glioblastoma facilitated by intraoperative fluorescein guidance. J Neurosurg. 2017;127(1):111–22. https://doi.org/10.3171/2016.7.JNS16232.
38. Stummer W. Factors confounding fluorescein-guided malignant glioma resections: edema bulk flow, dose, timing, and now: imaging hardware? Acta Neurochir. 2016;158(2):327–8. https://doi.org/10.1007/s00701-015-2655-6.
39. Duffau H, Taillandier L, Gatignol P, Capelle L. The insular lobe and brain plasticity: lessons from tumor surgery. Clin Neurol Neurosurg. 2006;108(6):543–8. https://doi.org/10.1016/j.clineuro.2005.09.004. Epub 2005 Oct 6. PMID: 16213653.
40. Cargnelutti E, Ius T, Skrap M, Tomasino B. What do we know about pre- and postoperative plasticity in patients with glioma? A review of neuroimaging and intraoperative mapping studies. Neuroimage Clin. 2020;28:102435. https://doi.org/10.1016/j.nicl.2020.102435.
41. Majos A, Bryszewski B, Kośla KN, Pfaifer L, Jaskólski D, Stefańczyk L. Process of the functional reorganization of the cortical centers for movement in GBM patients: fMRI study. Clin Neuroradiol. 2017;27(1):71–9. https://doi.org/10.1007/s00062-015-0398-7.
42. Lacroix M, Abi-Said D, Fourney DR, Gokaslan ZL, Shi W, DeMonte F, et al. A multivariate analysis of 416 patients with glioblastoma multiforme: prognosis, extent of resection, and survival. J Neurosurg. 2001;95:190–8.
43. Sanai N, Polley MY, McDermott MW, Parsa AT, Berger MS. An extent of resection threshold for newly diagnosed glioblastomas. Clinical article. J Neurosurg. 2011;115:3–8.
44. Abrudan C, Cocis A, Dana C, Suciu B, Cheptea M, St. Florian I. Surgery of high grade gliomas—pros in favor of maximal cytoreductive surgery. Romanian Neurosurg. 2011;XVIII 1:38–53.
45. Almenawer SA, Badhiwala JH, Alhazzani W, et al. Biopsy versus partial versus gross total resection in older patients with high-grade glioma: a systematic review and meta-analysis. Neuro Oncol. 2015;17(6):868–81. https://doi.org/10.1093/neuonc/nou349.
46. McGirt MJ, Chaichana KL, Gathinji M, et al. Independent association of extent of resection with survival in patients with malignant brain astrocytoma. J Neurosurg. 2009;110(1):156–62. https://doi.org/10.3171/2008.4.17536.
47. Almeida JP, Chaichana KL, Rincon-Torroella J, Quinones-Hinojosa A. The value of extent of resection of glioblastomas: clinical evidence and current approach. Curr Neurol Neurosci Rep. 2015;15(2):517. https://doi.org/10.1007/s11910-014-0517-x.
48. Chowdhury T, Gray K, Sharma M, Mau C, McNutt S, Ryan C, Farou N, Bergquist P, Caldwell C, Uribe AA, Todeschini AB, Bergese SD, Bucher O, Musto G, Azazi EA, Zadeh G, Tsang DS, Mansouri SA, Kakumanu S, Venkatraghavan L. Brain cancer progression: a retrospective multicenter comparison of awake craniotomy versus general anesthesia in high-grade glioma resection. J Neurosurg Anesthesiol. 2022;34(4):392–400. https://doi.org/10.1097/ANA.0000000000000778. PMID: 34001816.
49. Howell WS. The empathic communicator. Bellmont, CA: Wadsworth; 1982.

50. Sadideen H, Alvand A, Saadeddin M, Kneebone R. Surgical experts: born or made? Int J Surg. 2013;11:773–8. https://doi.org/10.1016/j.ijsu.2013.07.001.
51. Cowan JA, Dimick JB, Thompson BG, Stanley JC, Upchurch GR Jr. Surgeon volume as an indicator of outcomes after carotid endarterectomy: an effect independent of specialty practice and hospital volume. J Am Coll Surg. 2002;195:814–21.
52. Schaverien MV. Development of expertise in surgical training. J Surg Educ. 2010;67:37–43.
53. Gallagher AG, Smith CD, Bowers SP, et al. Psychomotor skills assessment in practicing surgeons experienced in performing advanced laparoscopic procedures. J Am Coll Surg. 2003;197:479–88.
54. Chowdhury MM, Dagash H, Pierro A. A systematic review of the impact of volume of surgery and specialization on patient outcome. Br J Surg. 2007;94(2):145–61. https://doi.org/10.1002/bjs.5714.
55. Boudourakis LD, Wang TS, Roman SA, Desai R, Sosa JA. Evolution of the surgeon-volume, patient-outcome relationship. Ann Surg. 2009;250(1):159–65. [published correction appears in Ann Surg. 2009 Dec;250(6):1046]. https://doi.org/10.1097/SLA.0b013e3181a77cb3.
56. Davies JM, Ozpinar A, Lawton MT. Volume-outcome relationships in neurosurgery. Neurosurg Clin N Am. 2015;26(2):207–8. https://doi.org/10.1016/j.nec.2014.11.015.

# Chapter 10
# Jugular Foramen Paragangliomas

Guilherme H. W. Ceccato and Luis A. B. Borba

## Contents




G. H. W. Ceccato
Department of Neurosurgery, Mackenzie Evangelical University Hospital,
Curitiba, PR, Brazil

L. A. B. Borba (✉)
Department of Neurosurgery, Mackenzie Evangelical University Hospital,
Curitiba, PR, Brazil

Department of Neurosurgery, Federal University of Paraná, Curitiba, PR, Brazil



© The Author(s), under exclusive license to Springer Nature
Switzerland AG 2024
C. Di Rocco (ed.), *Advances and Technical Standards in Neurosurgery*,
Advances and Technical Standards in Neurosurgery 49,
https://doi.org/10.1007/978-3-031-42398-7_10

## 10.1  Introduction

Jugular foramen (JF) pathologies are complex deep-seated lesions that demand profound knowledge of skull base anatomy. Theses lesions can extend between intraextradural or intra-extracranial spaces, disturb related venous drainage or arterial flow, also present complex relationships with cranial nerves. Their blood supply may come from the external/internal carotid arteries or vertebral system. Fortunately, along the end of past century advances of imaging and microsurgical techniques allowed to safely approach the jugular foramen area.

The most common tumor of jugular foramen is the paraganglioma in ~57% of cases [1, 2], with an incidence of 1 case per 1.3 million people per year or 0.07 cases per 100,000 people per year, occurring about 250 cases in USA each year [3].

The symptomatology among jugular foramen masses shares similarities due to local anatomical relationships [1, 2]. Common initial symptoms of jugulotympanic paragangliomas include hearing loss in 61.7% of cases, pulsatile tinnitus in 56.1%, cranial nerves deficits in 29.7%, hoarseness in 23%, dysphagia in 16.5%, and headache/neck or ear pain in 27.2% [3]. In some cases, tumor may be seen exteriorizing through external acoustic canal, and a retrotympanic mass may be identified in 91% of cases [4] (Fig. 10.1).

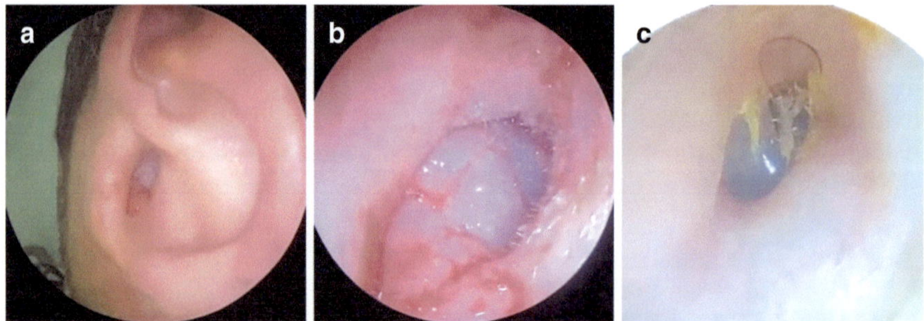

**Fig. 10.1** (**a**, **b**) Inspection of left external acoustic canal demonstrating tumor inside it. (**c**) Contralateral ear without pathological findings

## 10.2  Anatomy Highlights

Jugular foramen (JF) is considered one of the most complex cranial foramina, and it is in an oblique orientation between occipital bone posteromedial and temporal bone anterolaterally [1, 5] (Fig. 10.2). Intracranially, its boundaries are the bony labyrinth superiorly, carotid canal anteriorly, sigmoid groove posteriorly, occipital condyle/jugular tubercle medially, and mastoid air cells laterally [7]. From an extracranial perspective superiorly to JF, there is the external auditory canal/tympanic cavity; anteriorly the carotid ridge and anteromedially the rectus capitis anterior muscle; posteriorly lies the jugular process of occipital bone where rectus capitis lateralis muscle is attached; medially the occipital condyle/hypoglossal canal; and laterally the styloid process, mastoid/digastric groove, also the facial nerve [7]. The classic description of JF divides it into the pars nervosa anteromedially and pars venosa posterolaterally, using as landmark a fibrous septum connecting the intrajugular process of temporal bone to occipital bone; however, different classifications of jugular foramen divisions have been reported [8, 9] (Fig. 10.3). Pars nervosa contains the glossopharyngeal nerve, inferior petrosal sinus, and the meningeal branch of ascending pharyngeal artery. The pars venosa contains the sigmoid sinus, jugular bulb, vagus, and accessory nerves [10]. Glossopharyngeal nerve gives the Jacobson's nerve from its inferior ganglion, which runs through tympanic canaliculus in the medial aspect of carotid ridge toward middle fossa floor across tympanic cavity. Vagus nerve provides Arnold's nerve from its superior ganglion, which runs through mastoid canaliculus in the anterior part of pars venosa and exists through tympanomastoid suture [1, 10].

Arterial supply to the jugular foramen is provided mainly from the external carotid artery, by the occipital and ascending pharyngeal arteries. Regarding the lower cranial nerves, a key concept is that these nerves are covered by the medial wall of internal jugular vein from a lateral perspective [11] (Fig. 10.4).

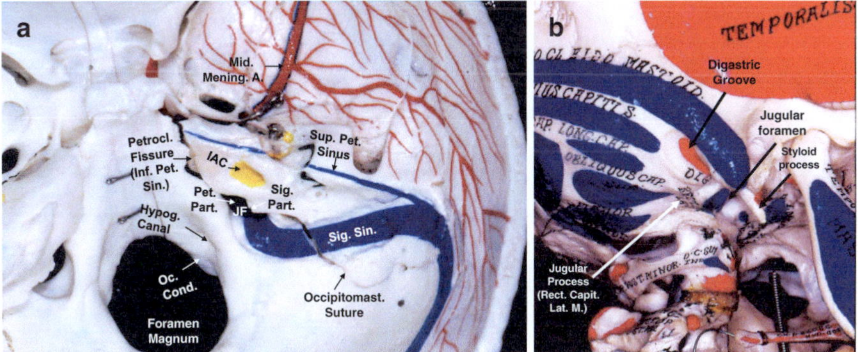


**Fig. 10.2** Bony relationships of jugular foramen. (**a**) Intracranial and (**b**) extracranial view. *Hypog. Canal* hypoglossal canal, *IAC* internal auditory canal, *Inf. Pet. Sin.* inferior petrosal sinus, *JF* jugular foramen, *Mid. Mening. A.* middle meningeal artery, *Oc. Cond.* occipital condyle, *Petrocl. Fissure* petroclival fissure, *Pet. Part* petrosal part, *Rect. Capit. Lat. M.* rectus capitis lateralis muscle, *Sig. Part* sigmoid part, *Sig. Sin.* sigmoid sinus, *Sup. Petr. Sin.* superior petrosal sinus. (A reuse with permission from Ceccato et al. [6])

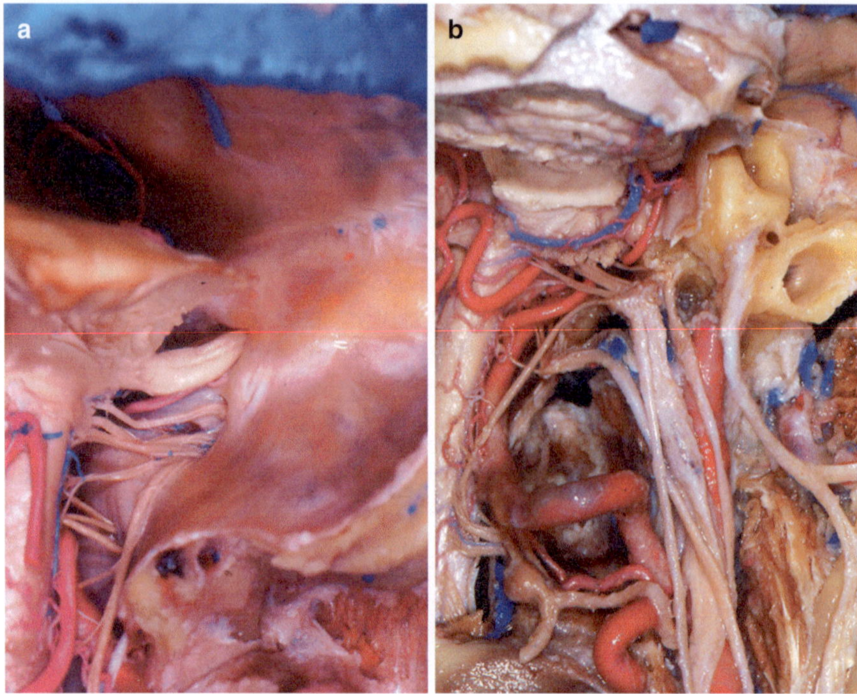

**Fig. 10.3** (**a**) Intradural view of jugular foramen area, depicting lower cranial nerves running to it. The fibrous septum is highlighted dividing the foramen into pars nervosa and pars venosa. Also, hypoglossal nerve roots are depicted, also seventh/eight nerve complex. (**b**) Intra to extradural trajectory of lower cranial nerves through jugular foramen and hypoglossal canal, with highlight to proximity with vertebral and internal carotid arteries, also to facial nerve

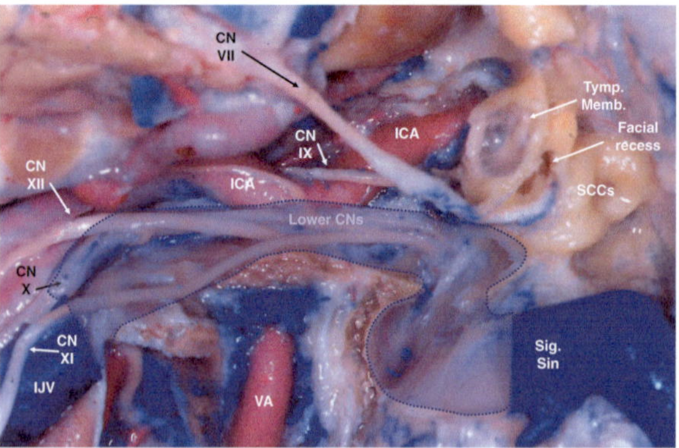


**Fig. 10.4** Neurovascular relationships of jugular foramen. Lower cranial nerves are covered by the anteromedial wall of internal jugular vein/jugular bulb. Proximity to internal carotid artery is depicted, also trajectory of facial nerve. *CN* cranial nerve, *ICA* internal carotid artery, *IJV* internal jugular vein, *SCCs* semicircular canals, *Tymp. Memb.* tympanic membrane, *VA* vertebral artery

## 10.3  Paraganglioma

Paragangliomas are an uncommon group of highly vascularized neuroendocrine tumors that arise from extra-adrenal neural crest remnants and contain chief cells associated with autonomic nervous system [12–14]. Head and neck paragangliomas (HNPGLs) comprise 0.6% of all head and neck neoplasms and present an overall incidence of 1/30.000 to 1/100.000 cases each year [15, 16]. Age of presentation is usually between 50 and 60 years and tumors are 3–6 times more common in females. The most common site of origin is from carotid body in up to 60% of situations, followed by jugulo-tympanic and vagus nerve tumors [13, 17, 18]; however, up to 20 sites of origin have already been reported [17, 19]. The majority of HNPGLs are benign, but between 6% and 19% of cases are malignant and can develop metastases, mainly to regional lymph nodes [12]. HNPGLs account for most of cases of paragangliomas (65–70% of cases), followed by abdominal tumors [12, 20]. HNPGLs are mainly related to parasympathetic system and rarely secrete catecholamines, while thoracic, abdomen and pelvic cases are more commonly related with sympathetic system and prone to be secretory [12]. Around 44% HNPGLs grow and usually they progress annually ~1 mm in its maximum diameter or present a volume increase of 13.6–18.6% in mm$^3$, with a doubling volume in 4.2–5.4 years in average [20, 21]; however, the features of growth are variable in the literature [16, 22]. Jugulotympanic tumors present an average tumor growth rate of 0.41 mm/year [22], and it is important to identify growing lesions to be candidates to intervention (Fig. 10.5).

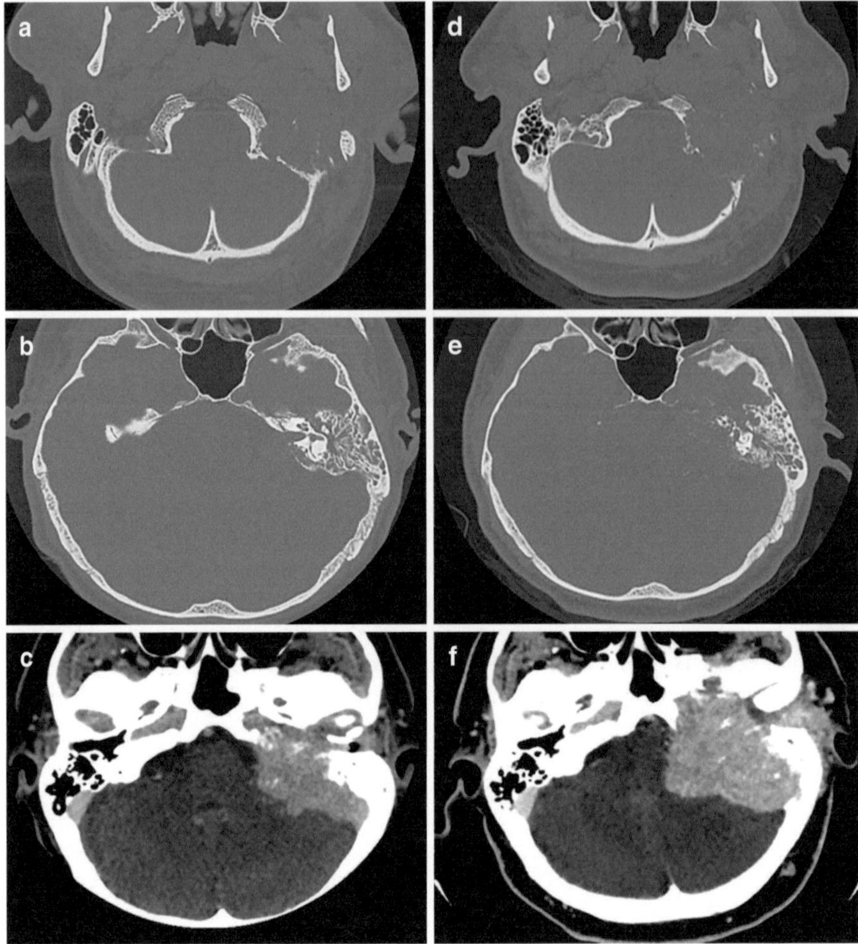

**Fig. 10.5** Demonstration of the growth of a jugular foramen paraganglioma. (**a–c**) Initial CT scans. Patient has chosen to wait-and-scan initially instead of intervention and lost follow-up. (**d–f**) Three years later, CT scan depicting progression of bone erosion and increase of the mass dimensions

## 10.4   Genetics

Almost 1/5 patients have an autosomal dominance inheritance with incomplete penetrance, usually associated with mutations in the subunit (A-D, AF2) of the succinate dehydrogenase (SHDx), most frequently involving subunit D, enzyme involved in the Krebs cycle. A germline mutation is identified in about 40% of cases, and in situations of multifocal tumors germline mutations are found in up to 70% of cases, also familial cases harbor a greater incidence of germline mutations [3, 19, 20, 23].

Genetic pathways for development of paragangliomas started to be highlighted in the last two decades. Observations of hyperplasia/dysplasia of carotid body cells in individuals chronic exposed to hypoxia, as high altitudes, or chronic pulmonary/cyanotic heart diseases, led to discover of SDHx mutations, initially described in 2000 and associated with development of HNPGL [24–26].

Familial disease of HNPGLs may be associated with syndromes like Von Hippel-Lindau in less than 10% of cases, neurofibromatosis type 1, and multiple endocrine neoplasia type 2A and type 2B [19, 23]. Around 20 genes were already described as hereditary susceptibility genes to the development of paragangliomas, and NF1 mutations are the most common in sporadic paragangliomas, identified in 25% of cases [27]. SDHx genes are considered tumor suppressor genes, and germline mutations associated with HNPGL are considered to affect cellular hypoxic response [19]. Also, there are reported five paraganglioma (PGL) syndromes, clinically differentiated by the proportion of phaeochromocytoma, thoracoabdominal or head/neck paragangliomas, renal cell carcinoma, or other associated tumors, also multifocality or malignancy [24]. HNPGLs are more commonly associated with PGL 1 and 2 syndromes, usually associated with SDHD and SDHAF2 mutations, respectively.

Penetrance of inherited pheochromocytoma/paragangliomas depends on parent origin (imprinting), with tumor development in 90–100% of individuals with paternal transmission of SDHD mutation, while maternal transmission rarely leads to tumor development [28]. Jugulotympanic tumors are more common in female patients, however, paradoxically in females they are more rarely associated with germline SDHx mutations (23.8% in women vs. 54.5% in men), suggesting another pathway for tumorigenesis beyond SDHx [29]. SDHx mutations are associated with carotid body and multiple HNPGLs, also larger lesions; however, in overall, less than 1/3 of jugulotympanic cases are associated with SDHx mutation [29].

## 10.5  Histopathology

Neuroendocrine cells of paraganglia contain chromaffin and chief cells, the first ones named this way due to its more abundant neurosecretory granules strongly reacting with chromate salts. However, both chromaffin and chief cells can synthetize and release catecholamines, but the second is usually associated with parasympathetic system. A common histological pattern observed is like an acinar/lobular/nest configuration, named *zellballen,* presenting functional cells surrounded by a fibrovascular stroma (Fig. 10.6).

Immunohistochemistry feature of these tumors is the presence of chromogranin-A and synaptophysin, also the confirmation of paraganglioma nature is by stain for tyrosine hydroxylase, enzyme involved in the cascade of catecholamine synthesis. Also, it is common the presence of positive S100 protein in the sustentacular

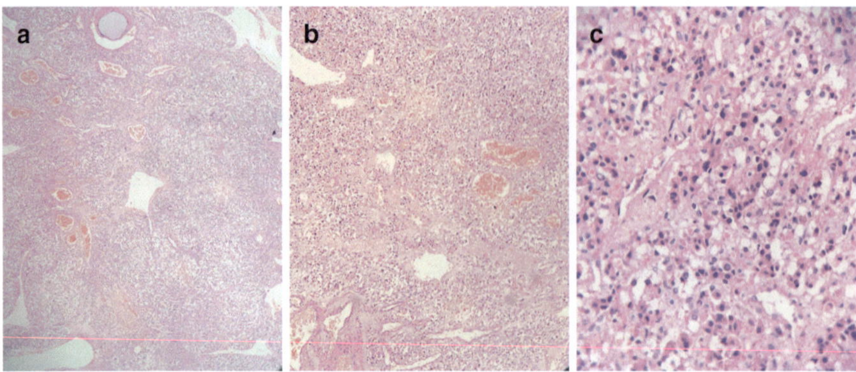

**Fig. 10.6** Histopathology of a jugular foramen paraganglioma, depicting many blood vessels and a *zellballen* arrangement

network [30]. Usually, chromogranin-A and tyrosine hydroxylase present weaker and more variable positivity in parasympathetic lesions.

## 10.6 Endocrine Function

Despite its neuroendocrine origin, only 1–3% of HNPGLs are secretory [3]. Especially in patients with apparent adrenergic symptoms is important to screen for other possible synchronic tumors, as HNPGLs are mostly associated with parasympathetic system, while thoracic, abdominal, and pelvic tumors are more likely linked with sympathetic system. It is interesting to comment that phenylethanolamine $N$-methyltransferase is the enzyme that converts norepinephrine in epinephrine, and it is largely restricted to adrenal medulla [31]. Biochemical screen should include plasmatic free and 24-h urinary metanephrines and catecholamines [32]. It is important to know that some drugs and dietary constituents may alter the level of catecholamines and its metabolites.

An important issue regarding secreting paragangliomas is the preoperative management. The surgical stress may lead to an intraoperative hypersecretion of catecholamines causing hypertensive crisis, while severe hypotension may occur after tumor resection due to an acute withdraw of catecholamines storage and production [33]. Anesthesia team must be prepared to floating levels of arterial blood pressure and have readily available rapid-acting vasopressors.

α-Blockers are the main drug for preoperative administration in adrenergic tumors. There are two types of alpha receptors: α1 and α2, the first one located in vascular smooth muscle leading to vasoconstriction when activated; the second located in the peripheral nerve ending and inhibiting release of norepinephrine [34]. Nonselective blockers as phenoxybenzamine cause blockage of both receptors, while selective α-blockers usually act over α1 receptors. Phenoxybenzamine binds covalently to the receptors leading to an irreversible blockage, better preventing a possible hypertensive crisis, however, with higher risk of postoperative hypotension and need for vasopressors and fluid resuscitation about 24–48 h postoperative [33]. Other α-blockers as doxazosin or prazosin provide a weaker connection to α-receptors, with higher risk of hypertensive crisis intraoperatively if their blockage is overload, but less risk of postoperative hypotension because their shorter half-life [33].

There are three β-receptors: β1 is located primarily in the heart mediating its activity, β2 in various organs and mediating vasodilation, while β3 presents less clinical significance as are involved in fat metabolism [35]. β-blockers should never be used alone in preoperative prepare for paraganglioma resection, because the non-opposed effect of α-receptors may lead to severe vasoconstriction leading to hypertensive crisis. As a side effect of complete α-blockage is reflex tachycardia, selective β1-blocker may be administered to reduce it [33].

Some authors also point the possibility to use calcium-channel blockers in preoperative prepare, as nicardipine or amlodipine. They have cardiac and renal protective effects, also may be used if intolerance to α-blockers, manifested by severe orthostatic hypotension, or as intraoperative adjunct if uncontrolled hypertension [28, 33]. Other possible drug to be used as an adjunct is metyrosine, a blocker of tyrosine hydroxylase. Preoperative time for prepare is not completely defined, usually initiating between 7 and 14 days before the procedure and increasing drug dosage until achieve blood pressure control [33]. Extrapolating from pheochromocytoma studies, risk factors for intraoperative hemodynamic instability may be higher serum concentration of norepinephrine, larger tumors, higher blood pressure before α-blockage, and more pronounced preoperative orthostatic hypotension following α-block [36].

Exclusively dopamine-secreting tumors are rare, with less than 40 cases reported in literature, and it is unclear its physiological impact [37]. However, about 30% of HNPGLs are suggestive for dopamine production, evaluated by increase of plasma 3-methoxytyramine [28, 29]. These tumors have median age of 48 years at diagnosis (range 18–76 years) and a male:female ratio of 1:1.5 [18]. Probably, there is a defect of the dopamine β-hydroxylase, which converts dopamine to norepinephrine [38]. Diagnostic tests include plasmatic and 24-h urine dopamine dosage, also its metabolites 3-methoxytyramine and homovanillic acid [14]. Plasma 3-methoxytyramine tends to be a more useful biomarker compared to its urinary dosage because urinary dopamine is derived almost exclusively from renal uptake and decarboxylation of circulating L-DOPA [28].

Usually exclusive dopamine-secreting tumors do not present sweating, headache, palpitation, or hypertension, as common in other tumors with catecholamine excess symptoms due to norepinephrine or epinephrine production, and many dopaminergic cases are even asymptomatic or have nonspecific symptoms. Symptomatology is nonspecific and usually diagnosis is delayed until tumor be large enough to cause mass effect [39] (Fig. 10.7).

Dopamine has a dose-dependent hemodynamic effect, and asymptomatic patients may present a low serum concentration and production rate of dopamine,

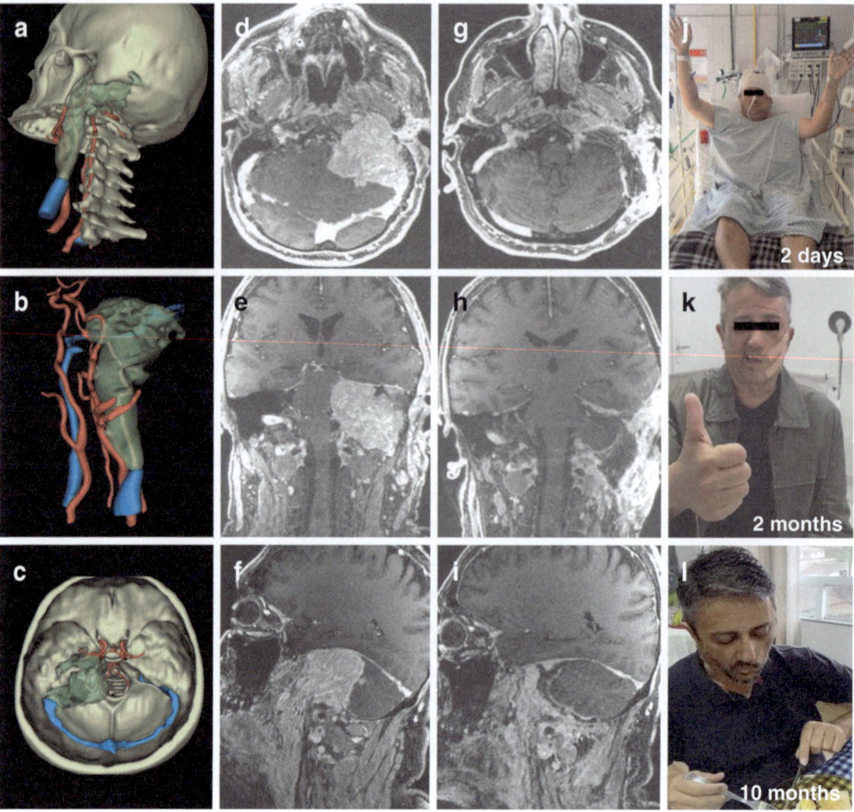



**Fig. 10.7** Giant jugular foramen paraganglioma, exclusively dopamine-secreting, in a 43-year-old male patient presenting with headache, hearing loss and tinnitus, also facial nerve palsy House-Brackmann V, hypoglossal nerve palsy and facial hypoesthesia; no preoperative dysphagia identified. Plasmatic dopamine dosage dropped from more than 2500 pg/mL preoperative to less than 30 pg/mL postoperatively, also postoperative 24-h urinary dosage of homovanillic acid was 3.7 mg, within normal range. (**a–c**) Preoperative 3D models, depicting a large lesion with occlusion of sigmoid sinus and extension inside internal jugular vein to neck, also significant intracranial component. (**d–f**) Preoperative MRI. (**g–i**) Postoperative MRI demonstrating complete resection. (**j–l**) Postoperative images of the patient during follow-up, with no new neurological deficits following the procedure

in a range which its effect is mainly vasodilatory [18]. Preoperative α or β receptors blockage is controversial in dopamine-secreting paragangliomas, as intraoperative and postoperatively hemodynamic changes can occur depending on the impact that a sudden dopamine withdraw or even release to bloodstream can produce, especially considering its dose-dependent effect [18]. However, it seems that dopamine-secreting tumors are more linked to hypotension scenarios, and preoperative α or β receptors blockage should be avoided and is not advised [28, 40].

## 10.7  Imaging

Imaging evaluation of paragangliomas should encompass since skull to the pelvis [28]. Functional imaging like PET-CT employing $^{68}$Ga radiolabelled somatostatin analogues or 6-[$^{18}$F] fluoro-3,4-dihydroxyphenylalanine ([$^{18}$F]-FDOPA) present high sensitivity detecting HNPGLs, and CT scan is essential to demonstrate bone involvement [28].

Jugulotympanic paragangliomas can present with important bone erosion surrounding jugular foramen toward middle ear in a "moth-eaten" pattern (Figs. 10.5 and 10.8). They usually spread along the path of least resistance as mastoid air cells, neural foramina, vascular channels, tympanic cavity, and eustachian tube, for example [41]. They are highly vascularized lesions, usually hypointense in T1WI and hyperintense in T2WI, presenting flow voids in the MRI, with a strong contrast enhancement. They may have a "salt-and-pepper" appearance in the MRI, with the salt appearance due to products from hemorrhage and pepper due to high vascularity [41].

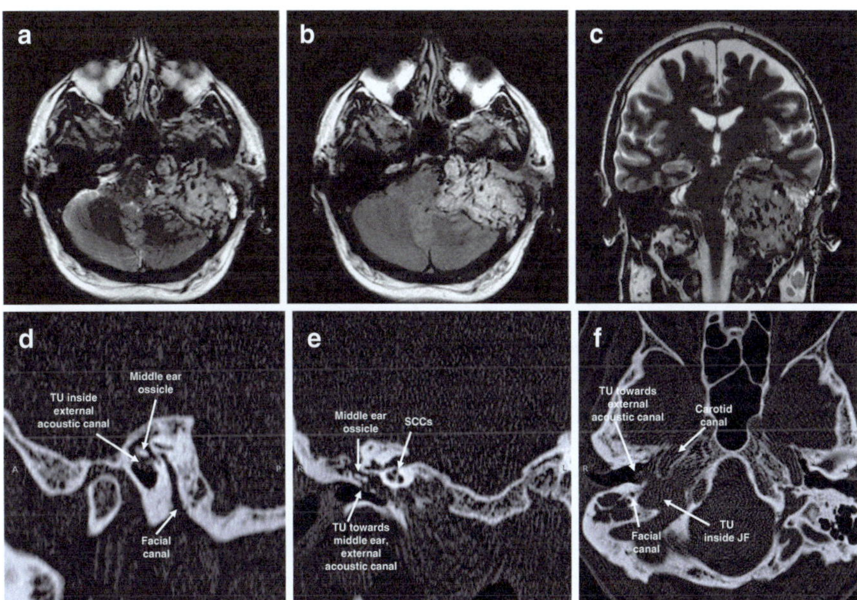


**Fig. 10.8** Imaging features of jugular foramen paraganglioma. (**a**) Axial T2-weighted image. (**b**) Axial FLAIR. (**c**) Coronal T2-weighted image demonstrating great number of flow-voids. (**d–f**) CT scan of a paraganglioma showing dilation and erosion of jugular foramen, with tumor extending toward middle ear and close to carotid canal. It is demonstrated preservation of facial canal. *JF* jugular foramen, *SCCs* semicircular canals, *TU* tumor

## 10.8   Classification

Jugulotympanic paragangliomas can be classified either by Fisch [42] or Jackson-Glasscock [43] system. Fisch description is more widely used to guide surgical strategy, and surgical approaches consist mainly in variations of the infratemporal fossa approaches described by him [42].

## 10.9   Blood Supply

Paragangliomas are highly vascularized lesions with their blood supply coming mainly from external carotid artery, usually from ascending pharyngeal or occipital arteries, or from caroticotympanic branches of internal carotid artery, and some cases vascularized by vertebrobasilar system [3] (Fig. 10.9). Some tumors can benefit from preoperative embolization, especially lesions highly vascularized and with multiple feeders, large ones above 3 cm in diameter, and with lower cranial nerves deficits; the last because the theoretical risk of simultaneous embolization of vasa nervorum of lower cranial nerves blood supply [28, 44] (Fig. 10.10). Balloon test occlusion is important to be performed if internal carotid artery may be at risk of injury/sacrifice during resection [28]. Angiography depicts an intense tumor blush and early venous drainage and may depict sub/occlusion of ipsilateral sigmoid sinus or jugular vein (Figs. 10.11 and 10.12).

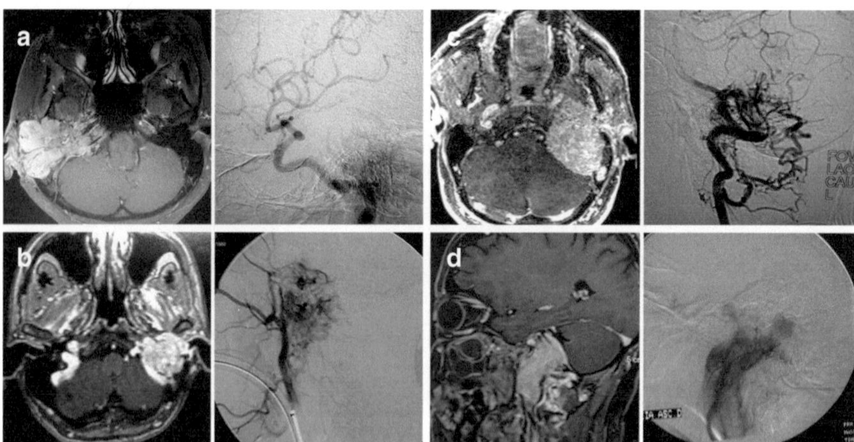

**Fig. 10.9** Angiographic features of jugulotympanic paragangliomas. It is depicted blood supply from internal carotid artery (**a**), external carotid artery (**b**), vertebrobasilar system (**c**). In (**d**) is demonstrated venous drainage of the tumor delineating it inside the internal jugular vein

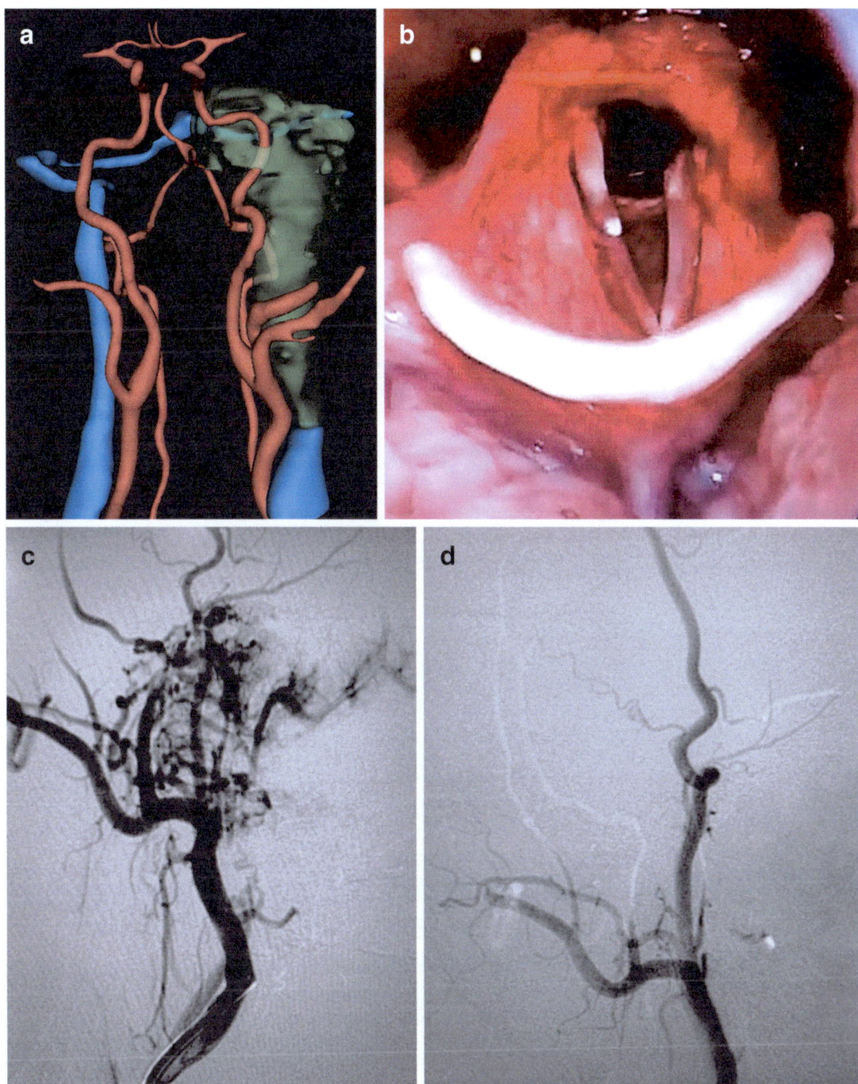

Fig. 10.10 (a) 3D model of a large jugular foramen paraganglioma. (b) Videolaryngoscopy depicts left vocal cord palsy. (c) Pre-embolization angiogram show a highly vascularized lesion. (d) Post-embolization angiogram depicts just superficial temporal artery filling distally

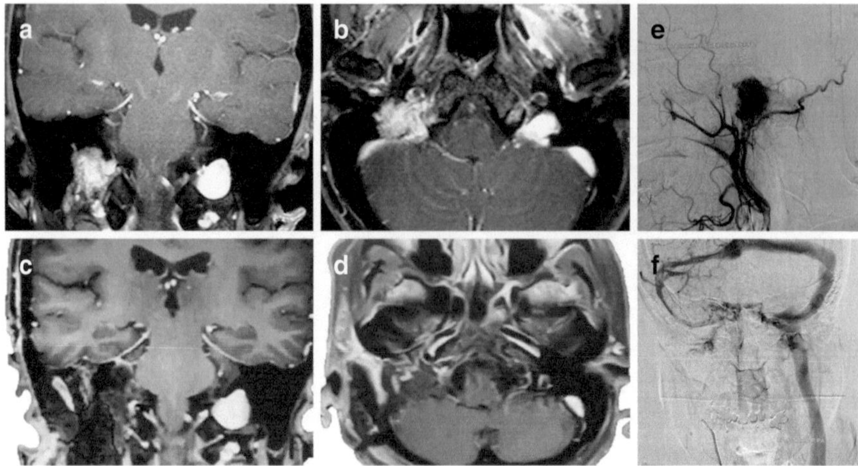

**Fig. 10.11** Patient with 64-year-old presenting hearing loss and tinnitus, also facial nerve palsy House-Brackmann VI. (**a, b**) Preoperative MRI demonstrates a right jugular foramen paraganglioma. (**c, d**) Postoperative imaging depicts complete tumor resection. (**e**) Angiography show intense blush from external carotid artery branches. (**f**) Signs of occlusion of right sigmoid sinus

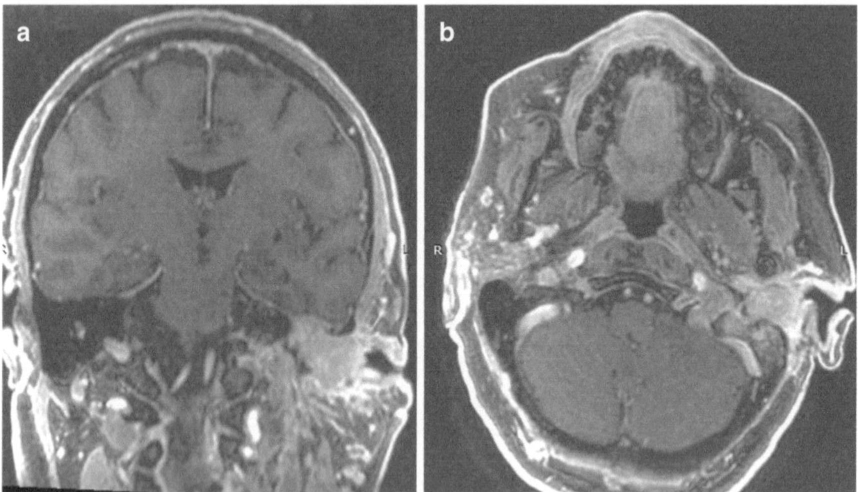

**Fig. 10.12** Patient with 62-year-old presenting hearing loss and tinnitus, also facial palsy House-Brackmann V. (**a, b**) Jugulotympanic paraganglioma with signs of extension to external auditory canal. (**c**) Angio-CT scan depicting patency of ipsilateral sigmoid sinus and internal jugular vein. (**d**) Angiography showing bilateral patency of sigmoid sinus, highlighting importance of preoperative vascular study

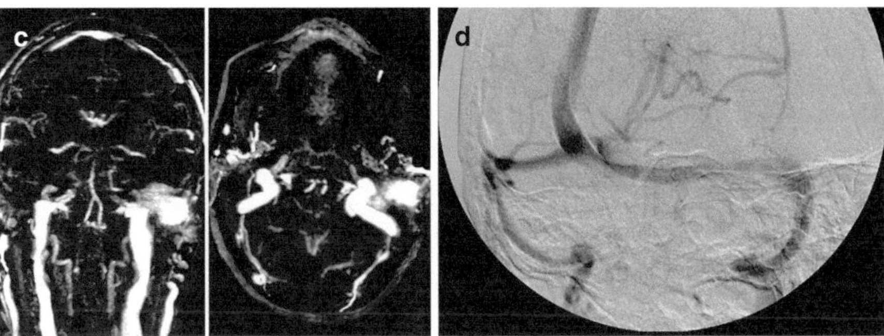

**Fig. 10.12** (continued)

## 10.10   Malignancy

About 6–24% of non-adrenal paragangliomas are malignant, while 1–5% of jugulo-tympanic cases have malignant features [3, 45]. Usually, metastases occur to cervical lymph nodes also to bone and less commonly to other sites as lung, liver, or thyroid [45]. Malignant paragangliomas tend to be more common in young patients, with multifocal and secreting tumors, usually harboring a SDHB mutation, while D subunit sometimes is involved.

## 10.11   Treatment Options

Microsurgical resection of jugular foramen lesions is usually preferred in cases of smaller tumors like Fisch A and B; larger tumors may have a more individualize therapeutic decision. Preoperative lower cranial nerves/facial nerve function should be evaluated, also tumor extensions and mass effect symptoms, associated with performance status, age and comorbidities of the patient, to choose between wait-and-scan, radiation, subtotal resection + radiation, or intended complete microsurgical resection [3].

Usually, patients without an urgent indication for treatment may benefit from an initial period of observation to better understand the biological behavior and evaluate evolution of symptoms. Especially older and debilitated patients may do not tolerate some cranial neuropathies, affecting swallowing and ventilatory capability, leading to an increased risk of dysphagia and aspiration [28]. Attention should be paid to avoid bilateral lower cranial nerves deficit, especially in bilateral lesions or previous treated ones, as it can lead to bilateral vocal cord palsy and need for tracheostomy, for example. Unilateral lesions gradually allow contralateral compensation; however, acute lower cranial nerves palsy uni/bilaterally may lead to deleterious consequences. This is especially important considering vagal paragangliomas and

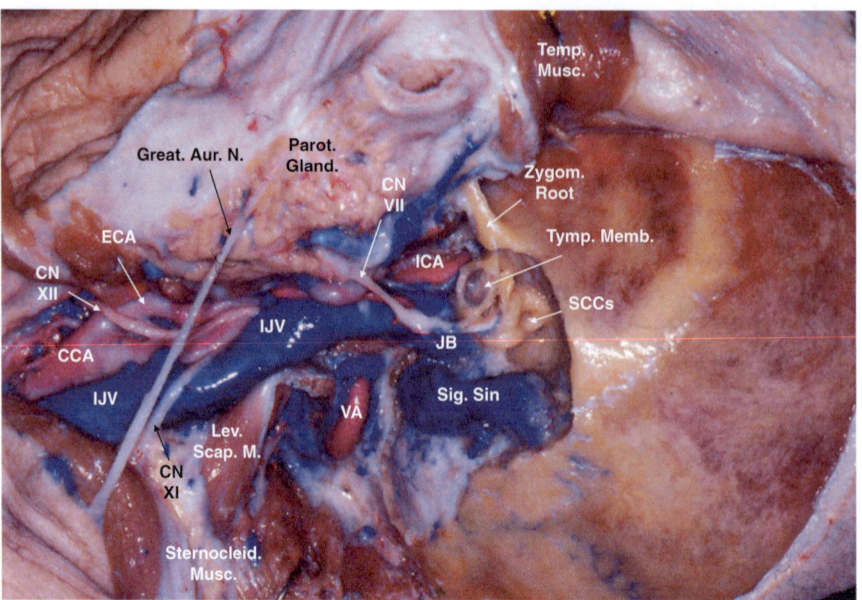



**Fig. 10.13** Overview of exposure following mastoidectomy and neck dissection of neurovascular structures. *CCA* common carotid artery, *CN* cranial nerve, *ECA* external carotid artery, *Great Aur. N.* great auricular nerve, *ICA* internal carotid artery, *IJV* internal jugular vein, *JB* jugular bulb, *Parot. Gland* parotid gland, *Lev. Scap. M.* levator scapulae muscle, *SCCs* semicircular canals, *Sig. Sin.* sigmoid sinus, *Sternocleid. Musc.* sternocleidomastoid muscle, *Temp. Musc.* temporalis muscle, *Tymp. Memb.* tympanic membrane, *VA* vertebra artery, *Zygom. Root* zygomatic root. (Reuse with permission from Ceccato et al. [6])

the inherent risk of nerve sacrifice during resection, usually waiting up to patient develop vocal cord palsy to treat [28].

Bilateral jugular foramen tumors should be operated on the less aggressive/smaller side or where there is already lower cranial nerves palsy. Contralateral tumor should be followed to properly indicate intervention if reasonable or underwent stereotactic radiosurgery.

Indications for microsurgical resection include compressive effect over head and neck structures, sustained/increasing rate of growth (Fig. 10.5), refractory pain, multiple cranial nerves deficits, catecholamine production, and low likelihood to postoperative cranial nerves impairment. Usually, surgery is preferred in young and healthy patients [28].

We employ variations of the infratemporal fossa (ITF) approach described by Fisch [42] and refined by Al-Mefty [46] (Fig. 10.13). Briefly [11]:

– ITFA: retrofacial infralabyrinthine approach. Preferred in cases of tumor without blood supply from internal carotid artery (ICA) and without anterior/superior extension.
– ITFB: infralabyrinthine pre- and retrofacial approach, without occlusion of external acoustic meatus and with preservation of middle ear structures. Indicated

in cases with blood supply from ICA, as it can be reached anterior to facial nerve. However, this approach is not intended for superior and anterior projections.
- ITFC: infralabyrinthine pre- and retrofacial approach with occlusion of external acoustic meatus and removal of middle ear structures. Facial nerve may be preserved within the facial canal. Tumors with blood supply from ICA and anterior/superior extensions can be reached.
- ITFD: classical infratemporal fossa approach with anterior transposition of facial nerve. Indicated for cases where facial canal is destroyed, and the nerve may be fixed to a new position.

## 10.12  Microsurgical Technique

Patient is placed supine with the head rotated to the contralateral side about 60°. Head is fixed in a three-point head holder, slightly extended until malar eminence be the highest point and tilted down obliquely to open space between mandible angle and neck [47]. It is important to leave prepared abdominal or thigh skin for fat or fascia harvesting if needed for closure in the end (Fig. 10.14).

An arciform incision is performed starting 2 cm above the pinna, running 2–3 cm behind the ear, extending inferiorly up to about 3–4 cm below mastoid tip, and crossing anteriorly the anterior border of sternocleidomastoid muscle for 3–4 cm.

Following anterior reflection of skin, temporalis fascia is dissected from the exposed temporalis muscle and kept attached to sternocleidomastoid muscle, which one is detached from the mastoid process and reflected inferior and posteriorly (Fig. 10.15). It is interesting to comment that in surgical approaches aiming a more posterior target as a far lateral transcondylar one, sternocleidomastoid muscle would be reflected anteriorly. During this step is important to identify the great auricular nerve running above sternocleidomastoid muscle, as it is of value if would be intended to decompress and graft facial nerve in case of preoperative facial nerve palsy. Great auricular nerve is cut in its anterior portion and reflected posteriorly [11, 48] Finally, digastric muscle is detached from the digastric groove and mobilized anteriorly (Fig. 10.16).

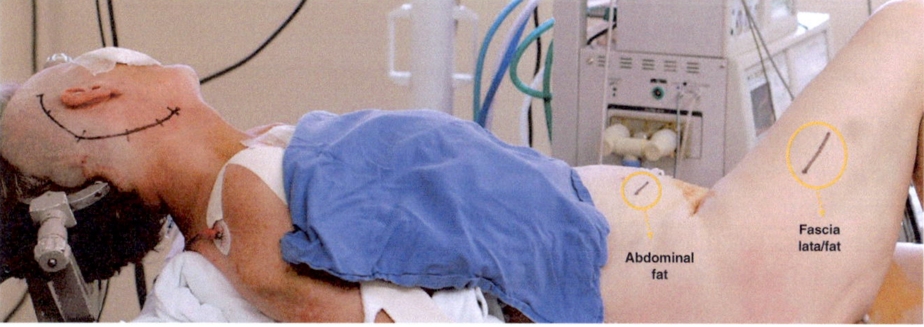


**Fig. 10.14** Patient positioning. Surgical skin incision is demonstrated, also highlighted the prepare for harvesting of abdominal fat or fascia lata/fat if necessary for closure

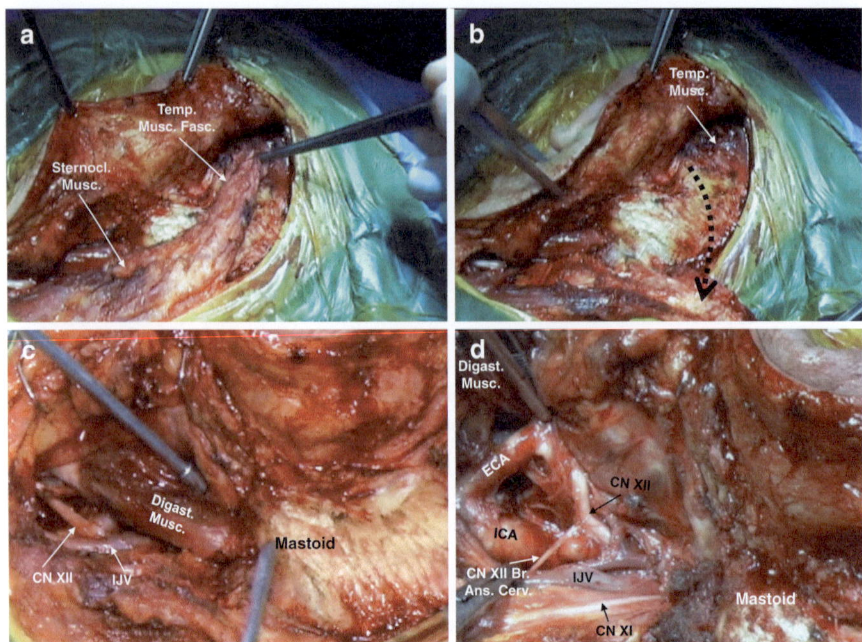



**Fig. 10.15** (**a**, **b**) Sternocleidomastoid muscle is reflected posteriorly attached to temporalis muscle fascia. (**c**) Digastric muscle is identified attached to digastric groove and will be mobilized anteriorly. (**d**) Neurovascular structures of neck dissected, better exposed following digastric muscle mobilization. *Br. Ans. Cerv.* branch to ansa cervicalis, *CN* cranial nerve, *Digast. Musc.* digastric muscle, *ECA* external carotid artery, *ICA* internal carotid artery, *IJV* internal jugular vein, *Sternocl. Muscl.* sternocleidomastoid muscle, *Temp. Musc.* temporalis muscle, *Temp. Musc. Fasc.* temporalis muscle fascia

Neurovascular structures in the upper cervical area are progressively dissected. Any identified arterial supply to the tumor is ligated/coagulated, usually composed by branches of posterior auricular, occipital, and ascending pharyngeal arteries. It is usually seen the glossopharyngeal nerve running anteriorly crossing over internal carotid artery and accessory nerve crossing posteriorly over internal jugular vein; vagus nerve runs between internal jugular vein and carotid artery inside carotid sheath. Hypoglossal nerve is better identified where it makes an anterior curve over carotid bifurcation and gives its branch to ansa cervicalis inferiorly.

If needed, posterior muscular layers including splenius capitis, semispinalis, and longissimus capitis muscles are reflected posteriorly exposing underneath the suboccipital triangle. If is intended to expose the vertebral artery for better vascular control, the suboccipital triangle may be opened detaching the superior oblique muscle from the inferior nuchal line and reflecting it inferiorly attached to lateral mass of atlas. The inferior oblique muscle is detached from C1 lateral mass/arch and reflected inferiorly also the rectus capitis posterior major, both kept attached to C2 spinous process. A sharp subperiosteal dissection along C1 arch detaching carefully the venous plexus surrounding vertebral artery may be performed to mobilize it after opening C1 foramen transversarium if needed.

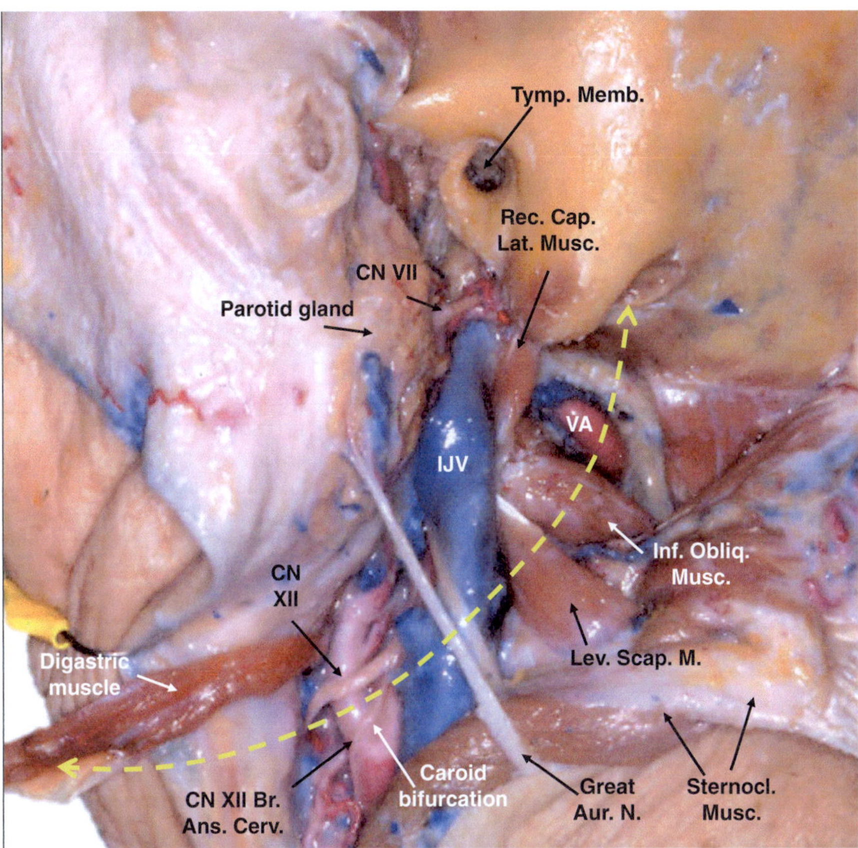


**Fig. 10.16** Soft tissues dissection depicting anterior mobilization of digastric muscle improving exposure toward lateral side of jugular foramen and allowing to advance anterior dissection to expose facial nerve leaving stylomastoid foramen. It is also important to observe the rectus capitis lateralis muscle as a posterior landmark of jugular foramen. *Br. Ans. Cerv.* branch to ansa cervicalis, *CN* cranial nerve, *Fac. Vein* facial vein, *Great Aur. N.* great auricular nerve, *IJV* internal jugular vein, *Inf. Obliq. Musc.* inferior oblique muscle, *Lev. Scap. M.* levator scapulae muscle, *Rec. Cap. Lat. Musc.* rectus capitis lateralis muscle, *Sternocleid. Musc.* sternocleidomastoid muscle, *Tymp. Memb.* tympanic membrane, *VA* vertebral artery. (Reuse with permission from Ceccato et al. [6])

After neck dissection of neurovascular structures, next step is the mastoidectomy (Fig. 10.17). Usually, a triangular aperture is performed with the base of triangle along a line parallel to zygomatic arch and other two lines connecting each other at the mastoid tip, with the anterior one running just posterior to external auditory canal. Then this cortical bony shell is removed followed by mastoid air cells removal and skeletonization of sigmoid sinus, semicircular canals, and facial canal. If there is no preoperative facial nerve palsy, the nerve is not exposed; however, if there is preoperative compromise the canal is opened, and the nerve just decompressed or grafted if invaded by tumor (Fig. 10.18). Digastric muscle must be detached from the digastric groove and mobilized anteriorly to be possible adequate mastoid exposure and expose extracranial course of facial nerve, also the rectus capitis lateralis

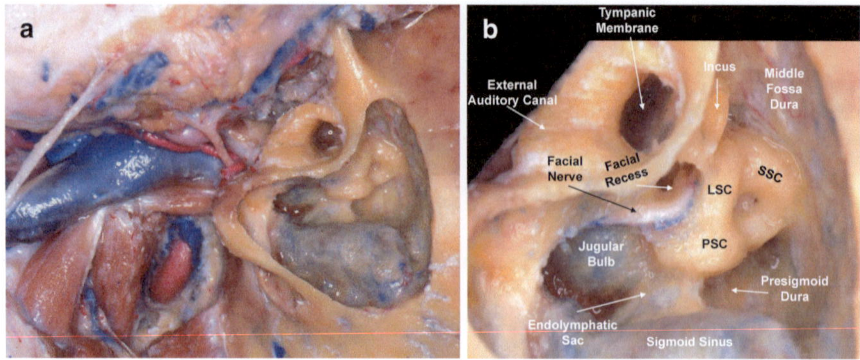



**Fig. 10.17** (**a**) Exposure following a mastoidectomy and upper cervical dissection, highlighting rectus capitis lateralis muscle posteriorly to internal jugular vein, also facial nerve close to stylomastoid artery. Proximity to suboccipital triangle is also demonstrated. (**b**) Close view after skeletonization of structures following mastoid air cells removal. Mastoid segment of facial nerve is demonstrated pointed by incus, and it is depicted the facial recess as a pathway toward tympanic cavity. Endolymphatic sac should be sectioned to allow increase in exposure of presigmoid dura. *LSC* lateral semicircular canal, *PSC* posterior semicircular canal, *SSC* superior semicircular canal. (Reuse with permission from Ceccato et al. [6])

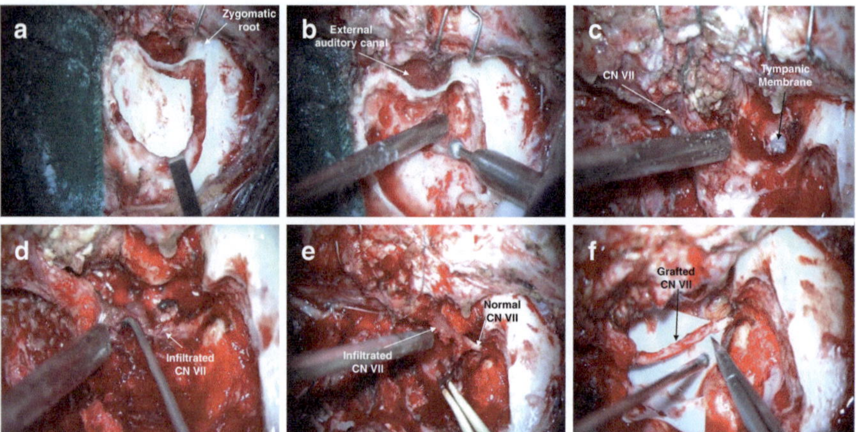



**Fig. 10.18** (**a**) Delineating a bony cortical shell during a mastoidectomy. (**b**) Removal of mastoid air cells and skeletonization of structures. (**c**) In this case, external acoustic canal was sectioned and bone removal progress toward middle ear structures; here, it is demonstrated deeply tympanic membrane. (**d**) Facial canal is opened, already eroded, and it is demonstrated infiltrated facial nerve by tumor. (**e**) Overview depicting a part of CN VII compromised and a healthy one. (**f**) Infiltrated segment of facial nerve is sectioned and removed, employing great auricular nerve as a nerve graft to replace the nerve sectioned. *CN* cranial nerve

muscle should be removed to expose the posterior border of jugular foramen. If needed, a posterior fossa craniotomy may be added if there is significant intradural extension, and in some cases also removal of part of occipital condyle.

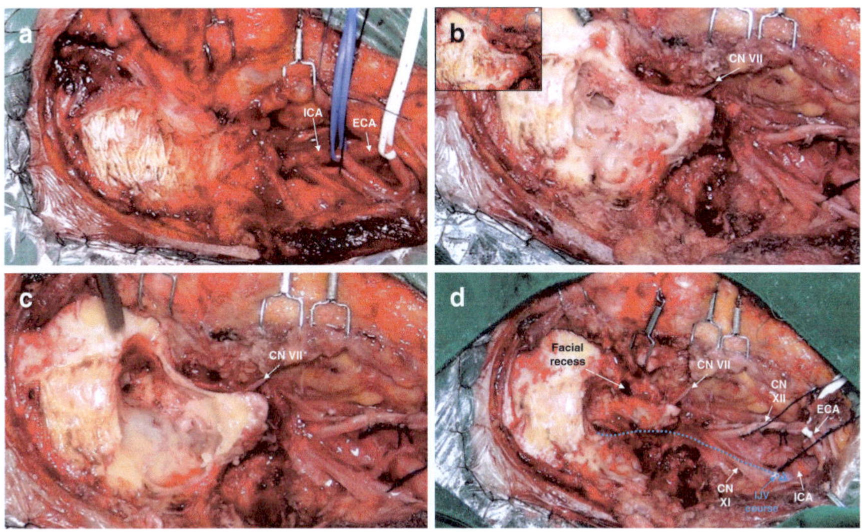



**Fig. 10.19** (**a**) Overview of exposure of mastoid and upper cervical area, highlighting carotid artery. (**b**, **c**) Mastoidectomy highlighting facial nerve leaving stylomastoid foramen, in (**b**) detail of inset image depicting delineation of a cortical bony shell to be removed at the beginning of mastoidectomy. (**d**) Global exposure following mastoidectomy and opening of jugular foramen exposing whole trajectory since sigmoid sinus up to internal jugular vein, also dissection of cervical neurovascular structures. *CN* cranial nerve, *ECA* external carotid artery, *ICA* internal carotid artery, *IJV* internal jugular vein

Sigmoid sinus is skeletonized up to jugular bulb, mastoid tip is removed, and jugular foramen is opened exposing the beginning of internal jugular vein, allowing an entire venous exposure in the surgical field (Fig. 10.19). During dissection, arterial branches running to the tumor are readily coagulated when visualized.

As jugular paragangliomas usually infiltrate into the lumen of jugular bulb and vein, also sigmoid sinus, preoperative vascular study is important to evaluate for the patency/occlusion of the sinus and vein. Intraoperatively the sigmoid sinus is ligated proximal and internal jugular vein is ligated distal to the tumor inside it. Sigmoid sinus blood leakage may be stopped packing hemostatic material inside it and ligating the sinus. The lateral wall of sigmoid sinus up to internal jugular vein may be incised and tumor inside it is removed (Figs. 10.20 and 10.21). If there is preoperative preservation of lower cranial nerves function, the anteromedial wall of internal jugular vein and bulb is preserved to avoid damage to these nerves, and it should be avoided excessive coagulation of the anteromedial wall of the vein. However, if there is preoperative lower cranial nerves palsy, this anteromedial wall may be removed together with the tumor. Especially in the jugular bulb care must be taken to avoid excessive bleeding from inferior petrosal sinus or condylar emissary vein while performing an intrabulbar resection [49] (Fig. 10.22). Tumor extending to middle ear and anteriorly may be reached employing a fallopian bridge technique keeping the facial nerve protected inside facial canal if preoperatively its function

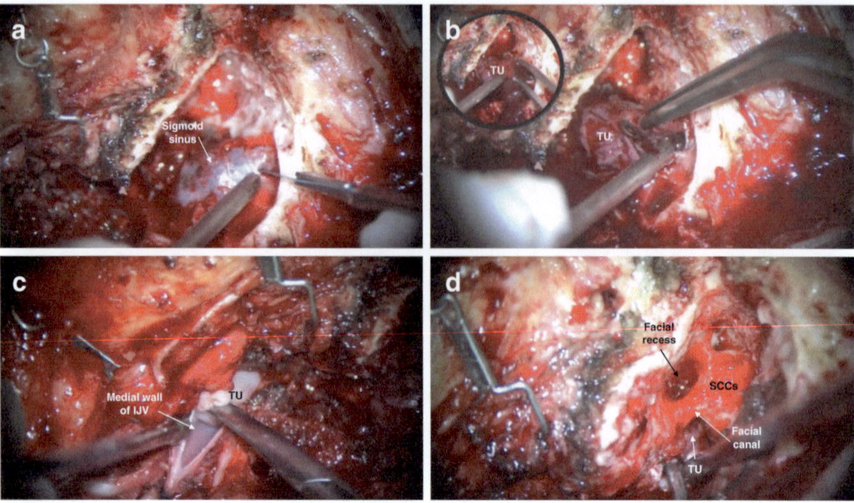

**Fig. 10.20** (**a**) Exposure of sigmoid sinus being incised following a mastoidectomy. (**b**) It is identified tumor inside the sinus, while significative venous blood leakage is demonstrated. (**c**) Following ligation of internal jugular vein below tumor extension its lateral wall is incised and tumor if removed from inside it, preserving the medial wall of the vein if there is preoperative lower cranial nerves function preservation. (**d**) Demonstration of fallopian bridge technique around facial canal, removing tumor extending toward middle ear. *CN* cranial nerve, *IJV* internal jugular vein, *SCCs* semicircular canals, *TU* tumor

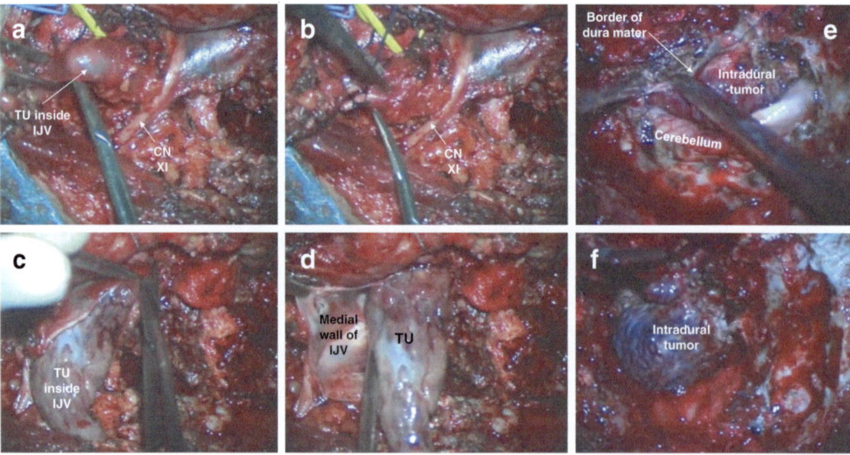

**Fig. 10.21** Intraoperative images of the case reported in Fig. 10.7. (**a**) Exposure of internal jugular vein presenting tumor inside it. (**b**) Ligation of IJV below tumor extension. (**c**) Opening of lateral of wall of IJV exposing tumor filling its lumen. (**d**) Demonstration of medial wall of internal jugular vein, which one should be preserved if there is preoperative preservation of lower cranial nerves function. (**e**, **f**) Demonstration of intradural tumor extension into posterior fossa. *CN* cranial nerve, *IJV* internal jugular vein, *TU* tumor

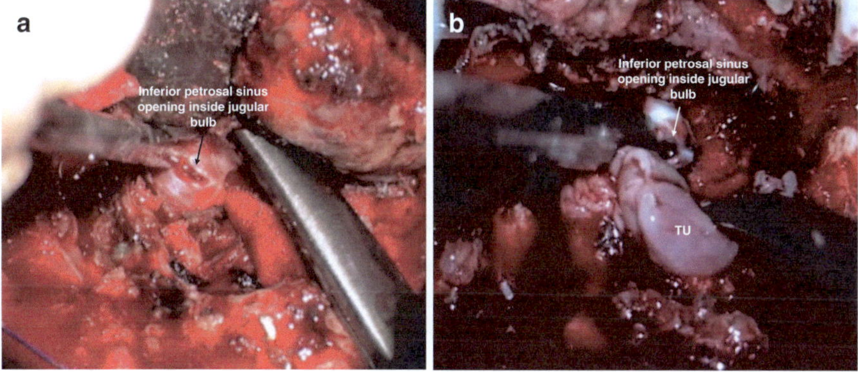

**Fig. 10.22** Intrabulbar resection is performed removing tumor inside jugular bulb. Care should be taken to control bleeding from venous channels draining to JB, as the inferior petrosal sinus. *JB* jugular bulb, *TU* tumor

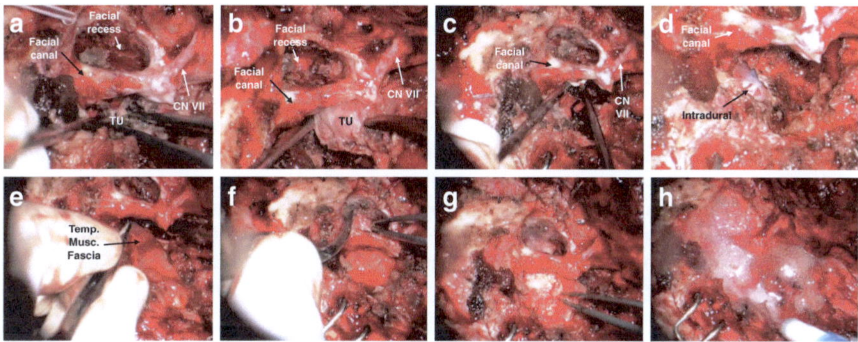

**Fig. 10.23** (**a–c**) Resection of tumor extending toward middle ear, removing a bigger piece of the mass underneath facial canal, also with a possible pathway through facial recess, in the way of a fallopian bridge technique. (**d**) Demonstration of extension of resection to intradural component. (**e–h**) Closure steps. Temporalis fascia attached to sternocleidomastoid muscle in a pedicled fashion is put all the way toward middle ear, covering dural opening. Also, Eustachian tube must be packed. Use of abdominal/thigh fat and if needed fascia lata is also employed and finally covered with fibrin glue. *CN* cranial nerve, *Temp. Musc. Fascia* temporalis muscle fascia, *TU* tumor

was preserved, and in this way opening middle ear through facial recess and removing tumor working around facial canal [5] (Figs. 10.20, 10.23, and 10.24). If facial nerve is preoperative damaged, it may be grafted and can be rerouted to increase exposure anteriorly (Fig. 10.25). It is important to remind that anterior dissection through facial recess occurs close to internal carotid artery (Fig. 10.26). If there is middle ear structures destruction, it is possible to during skin incision and soft tissues dissection to section the external auditory canal and close it in a closed sac fashion (Fig. 10.27).

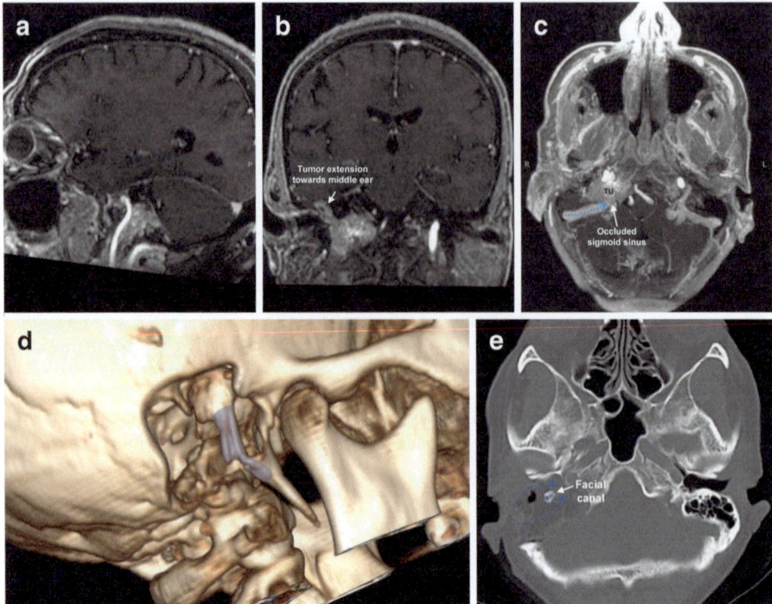

**Fig. 10.24** Case of a 68-year-old female patient with pain around the ear and hearing loss, presenting acute vocal cord palsy in adduction and need of urgent tracheostomy. (**a, b**) Right jugulotympanic tumor, depicting extension between middle ear and jugular foramen, also proximity with internal carotid artery. (**c**) Suggestive occlusion of sigmoid sinus is demonstrated by the presence of the mass in the topography of jugular foramen interrupting venous outflow. (**d, e**) Postoperative CT scan highlights the preservation of facial canal and depicts the working corridor around it in a fallopian bridge technique, as there was preoperative facial nerve function preservation. *TU* tumor

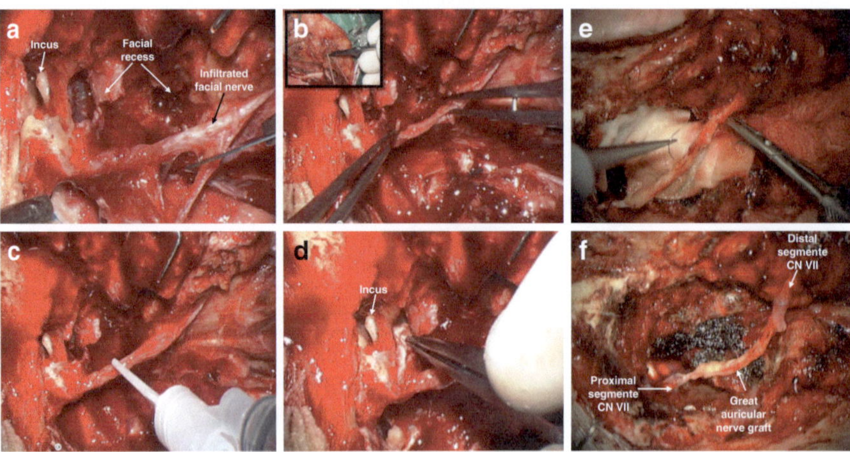

**Fig. 10.25** Technique of facial nerve reconstruction. (**a**) It is demonstrated facial nerve infiltrated by tumor. Tumor is dissected from the nerve, leaving a thin nerve. (**b, c**) Great auricular nerve is harvested and then put covering facial nerve aligning its extremities and then employed fibrin glue. (**d**) Packing of eustachian tube. (**e, f**) Case in which compromised facial nerve was sectioned and replaced by a graft of great auricular nerve, employing microsurgical termino-terminal suture. *CN* cranial nerve

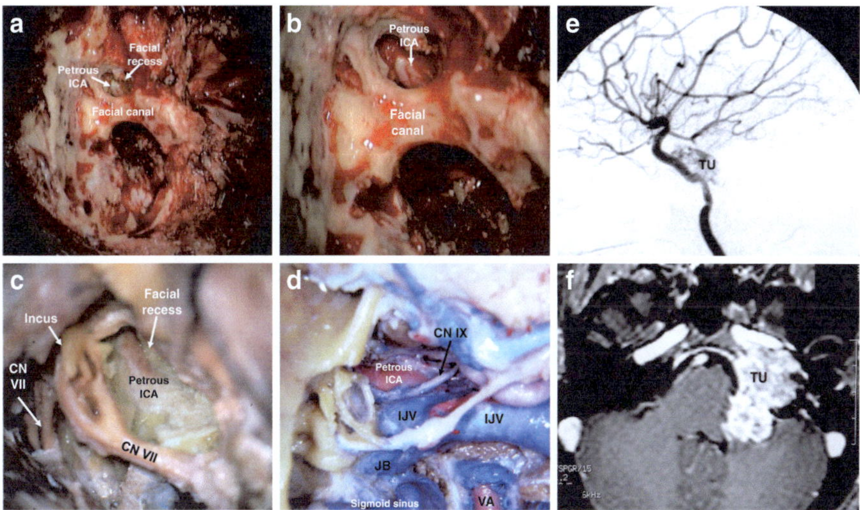



**Fig. 10.26** Relationship of jugulotympanic tumors with internal carotid artery. (**a, b**) Intraoperative and (**c, d**) anatomical images highlighting internal carotid artery reachable through facial recess. (**e, f**) Case of a jugulotympanic tumor with blood supply from caroticotympanic branches of internal carotid artery, which would require exposure of ICA through facial recess for an adequate vascular control. *CN* cranial nerve, *ICA* internal carotid artery, *IJV* internal jugular vein, *JB* jugular bulb, *TU* tumor, *VA* vertebral artery

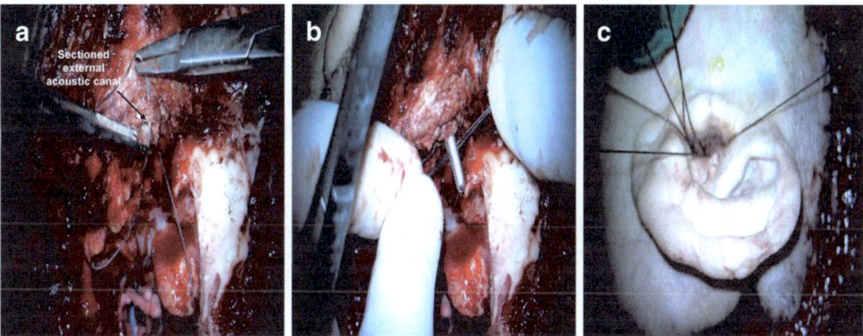



**Fig. 10.27** Demonstration of the suture to close the cartilaginous external acoustic canal. An everted suture is performed, in the way that pulling suture threads through external acoustic meatus would evert borders towards external side

Following extradural tumor removal, if there is an intradural extension of the mass, an infra/retrolabyrinthine presigmoid and suprajugular corridor is usually choose, adjusting it according to structures damaged by the lesion.

Closure is an important step to avoid at most postoperative CSF fistula. Usually, temporalis fascia attached to sternocleidomastoid muscle is used to cover mastoid air cells and dura-mater, and depending on the situation, fat graft of fascia lata may be used to help in closure, also fibrin glue. After working in middle ear, the

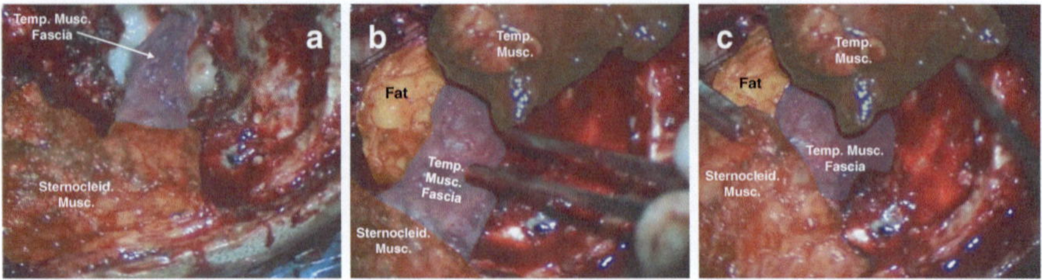


**Fig. 10.28** Demonstration of muscular layers closure. (**a**) Temporalis fascia is projected covering all the way dural opening, kept pedicled to sternocleidomastoid muscle. (**b**) Fat may be used to fill space above temporalis fascia. (**c**) Sternocleidomastoid and temporalis muscle are approximated and sutured. *Sternocleid. Musc.* sternocleidomastoid muscle, *Temp. Musc.* temporalis muscle

eustachian tube should be also packed to avoid CSF leak. Careful multilayer suture is tightly performed to adequately close skin and subcutaneous (Fig. 10.28).

## 10.13 Radiation

Radiotherapy is a possible adjunct therapy to induce vascular damage leading to tumor parenchymal fibrosis [3]. An extensive meta-analysis compared outcomes of radiosurgery and microsurgery, depicting a 3.5% of tumor growth in the radiosurgery group and 3.9% of recurrence rate in the microsurgical group, with 7.6% rate of complications using radiation against 29.6% of microsurgery [3]. Other review also depicted high rates of tumor control with radiosurgery between 79 up close to 100% [47]. Stereotactic radiosurgery as primary treatment to jugular paragangliomas may provide tumor control in 92% of patients, symptoms control in 93%, and complications in 8% [28]. This highlights the potential use of radiation in cases where microsurgical resection is not feasible due to patients with high surgical risks, advanced age, without lower cranial nerves palsy, large tumors, or residual ones; however, it is more effective in smaller lesions <3 cm [3, 28]. Also, in cases where just subtotal resection was achieved, radiation could be considered as an adjunct therapy [3]. However, microsurgical resection provides the chance for cure, symptomatic control and is preferred in young patients with smaller and more accessible tumors.

## References

1. Guinto G, Kageyama M, Trujillo-Luarca VH, Abdo M, Ruiz-Than A, Romero-Rangel A. Nonglomic tumors of the jugular foramen: differential diagnosis and prognostic implications. World Neurosurg. 2014;82(6):1283–90.
2. Ramina R, Maniglia JJ, Fernandes YB, Paschoal JR, Pfeilsticker LN, Neto MC, Borges G. Jugular foramen tumors: diagnosis and treatment. Neurosurg Focus. 2004;17(2):31–40.

3. Dharnipragada R, Butterfield JT, Dhawan S, Adams ME, Venteicher AS. Modern management of complex tympanojugular paragangliomas: a systematic review and meta-analysis. World Neurosurg. 2023;170:149–56.

4. Fayad JN, Keles B, Brackmann DE. Jugular foramen tumors: clinical characteristics and treatment outcomes. Otol Neurotol. 2010;31(2):299–305.

5. Pensak ML, Jackler RK. Removal of jugular foramen tumors: the fallopian bridge technique. Otolaryngol Head Neck Surg. 1997;117:586–91.

6. Ceccato GHW, Cândido DN. 32 Microsurgical anatomy of the jugular foramen. In: de Oliveira JG, Borba LA, editors. Microsurgical and endoscopic approaches to the skull base: anatomy, tactics, and techniques. New York: Thieme; 2021. p. 297.

7. Basma J, Michael LM II, Sorenson JM, Robertson JH. Deconstruction of the surgical approach to the jugular foramen region: anatomical study. J Neurol Surg B Skull Base. 2019;80(5):518–26.

8. Bond JD, Zhang M. Compartmental subdivisions of the jugular foramen: a review of the current models. World Neurosurg. 2020;136:49–57.

9. Bernard F, Zemmoura I, Cottier JP, Fournier HD, Terrier LM, Velut S. The interperiosteodural concept applied to the jugular foramen and its compartmentalization. J Neurosurg. 2017;129(3):770–8.

10. Tummala RP, Coscarella E, Morcos JJ. Surgical anatomy of the jugular foramen. Oper Tech Neurosurg. 2005;8(1):2–5.

11. Borba LA, Araújo JC, de Oliveira JG, Giudicissi Filho M, Moro MS, Tirapelli LF, Colli BO. Surgical management of glomus jugulare tumors: a proposal for approach selection based on tumor relationships with the facial nerve. J Neurosurg. 2010;112(1):88–98.

12. Sandow L, Thawani R, Kim MS, Heinrich MC. Paraganglioma of the head and neck: a review. Endocr Pract. 2023;29(2):141–7.

13. Taïeb D, Kaliski A, Boedeker CC, Martucci V, Fojo T, Adler JR Jr, Pacak K. Current approaches and recent developments in the management of head and neck paragangliomas. Endocr Rev. 2014;35(5):795–819.

14. Erickson D, Kudva YC, Ebersold MJ, Thompson GB, Grant CS, Van Heerden JA, Young WF Jr. Benign paragangliomas: clinical presentation and treatment outcomes in 236 patients. J Clin Endocrinol Metabol. 2001;86(11):5210–6.

15. Smith JD, Harvey RN, Darr OA, Prince ME, Bradford CR, Wolf GT, et al. Head and neck paragangliomas: a two-decade institutional experience and algorithm for management. Laryngoscope Investig Otolaryngol. 2017;2(6):380–9.

16. Tamaki A, Nyirjesy S, Cabrera CI, Lancione P, Hatef A, Rice R, et al. Treatment decision and estimation of growth of head and neck paragangliomas. Am J Otolaryngol. 2022;43(2):103357.

17. Lin EP, Chin BB, Fishbein L, Moritani T, Montoya SP, Ellika S, Newlands S. Head and neck paragangliomas: an update on the molecular classification, state-of-the-art imaging, and management recommendations. Radiol Imaging Cancer. 2022;4(3):e210088.

18. Pellitteri PK, Rinaldo A, Myssiorek D, Jackson CG, Bradley PJ, Devaney KO, et al. Paragangliomas of the head and neck. Oral Oncol. 2004;40(6):563–75.

19. Cleere EF, Martin-Grace J, Gendre A, Sherlock M, O'Neill JP. Contemporary management of paragangliomas of the head and neck. Laryngoscope Investig Otolaryngol. 2022;7(1):93–107.

20. Michałowska I, Ćwikła J, Michalski W, Wyrwicz LS, Prejbisz A, Szperl M, et al. Growth rate of paragangliomas related to germline mutations of the SDHX genes. Endocr Pract. 2017;23(3):342–52.

21. Jansen JC, van den Berg R, Kuiper A, van der Mey AG, Zwinderman AH, Cornelisse CJ. Estimation of growth rate in patients with head and neck paragangliomas influences the treatment proposal. Cancer. 2000;88(12):2811–6.

22. Jansen TT, Timmers HJ, Marres HA, Kunst HP. Feasibility of a wait-and-scan period as initial management strategy for head and neck paraganglioma. Head Neck. 2017;39(10):2088–94.

23. Pereira BC, Aznar JD, Zambon AL, de Melo DFC, Silva MN. Jugular Foramen's paraganglioma in a patient with Von Hippel-Lindau disease: case report. Arquivos Brasileiros de Neurocirurgia: Brazilian Neurosurgery. 2021;40(2):e200–6.
24. Benn DE, Robinson BG, Clifton-Bligh RJ. 15 years of paraganglioma: clinical manifestations of paraganglioma syndromes types 1–5. Endocr Relat Cancer. 2015;22(4):T91.
25. Baysal BE, Ferrell RE, Willett-Brozick JE, Lawrence EC, Myssiorek D, Bosch A, et al. Mutations in SDHD, a mitochondrial complex II gene, in hereditary paraganglioma. Science. 2000;287(5454):848–51.
26. Niemann S. Mutations in SDHC cause autosomal dominant paraganglioma. Nat Genet. 2000;26:141–50.
27. Guilmette J, Sadow PM. A guide to pheochromocytomas and paragangliomas. Surg Pathol Clin. 2019;12(4):951–65.
28. Taïeb D, Wanna GB, Ahmad M, Lussey-Lepoutre C, Perrier ND, Nölting S, et al. Clinical consensus guideline on the management of phaeochromocytoma and paraganglioma in patients harbouring germline SDHD pathogenic variants. Lancet Diabetes Endocrinol. 2023;11(5):345–61.
29. Richter S, Qiu B, Ghering M, Kunath C, Constantinescu G, Luths C, et al. Head/neck paragangliomas: focus on tumor location, mutational status and plasma methoxytyramine. Endocr Relat Cancer. 2022;29(4):213.
30. Hayashi T, Mete O. Head and neck paragangliomas: what does the pathologist need to know? Diagn Histopathol. 2014;20(8):316–25.
31. Grouzmann E, Tschopp O, Triponez F, Matter M, Bilz S, Brändle M, et al. Catecholamine metabolism in paraganglioma and pheochromocytoma: similar tumors in different sites? PLoS One. 2015;10(5):e0125426.
32. Shen Y, Cheng L. Biochemical diagnosis of pheochromocytoma and paraganglioma. Brisbane: Exon Publications; 2019. p. 23–39.
33. Fishbein L, Orlowski R, Cohen D. Pheochromocytoma/paraganglioma: review of perioperative management of blood pressure and update on genetic mutations associated with pheochromocytoma. J Clin Hypertens. 2013;15(6):428–34.
34. Nachawati D, Patel JB. Alpha blockers; 2020.
35. Farzam K, Jan A. Beta blockers. In: StatPearls. Treasure Island, FL: StatPearls Publishing; 2022.
36. Bruynzeel H, Feelders RA, Groenland THN, Van Den Meiracker AH, Van Eijck CHJ, Lange JF, et al. Risk factors for hemodynamic instability during surgery for pheochromocytoma. J Clin Endocrinol Metabol. 2010;95(2):678–85.
37. Miyamoto S, Yoshida Y, Ozeki Y, Okamoto M, Gotoh K, Masaki T, et al. Dopamine-secreting pheochromocytoma and paraganglioma. J Endocr Soc. 2021;5(12):bvab163.
38. Yi JW, Oh EM, Lee KE, Choi JY, Koo DH, Kim KJ, et al. An exclusively dopamine secreting paraganglioma in the retroperitoneum: a first clinical case in Korea. J Korean Surg Soc. 2012;82(6):389–93.
39. Foo SH, Chan SP, Ananda V, Rajasingam V. Dopamine-secreting phaeochromocytomas and paragangliomas: clinical features and management. Singapore Med J. 2010;51(5):e89.
40. Wu S, Chen W, Shen L, Xu L, Zhu A, Huang Y. Risk factors for prolonged hypotension in patients with pheochromocytoma undergoing laparoscopic adrenalectomy: a single-center retrospective study. Sci Rep. 2017;7(1):5897.
41. Vogl TJ, Bisdas S. Differential diagnosis of jugular foramen lesions. Skull Base. 2009;19(1):3–16.
42. Fisch U. Infratemporal fossa approach to tumours of the temporal bone and base of the skull. J Laryngol Otol. 1978;92(11):949–67.
43. Jackson CG, Glasscock ME, Harris PF. Glomus tumors: diagnosis, classification, and management of large lesions. Arch Otolaryngol. 1982;108(7):401–6.
44. Colli BO, Junior CGC, de Oliveira RS, Gondim GGP, Abud DG, Massuda ET, et al. Surgical management of embolized jugular foramen paragangliomas without facial nerve transposition: experience of a public tertiary hospital in Brazil. Surg Neurol Int. 2021;12:482.

45. Mediouni A, Ammari S, Wassef M, Gimenez-Roqueplo AP, Laredo JD, Duet M, et al. Malignant head/neck paragangliomas. Comparative study. Eur Ann Otorhinolaryngol Head Neck Dis. 2014;131(3):159–66.
46. Al-Mefty O, Fox JL, Rifai A, Smith RR. A combined infratemporal and posterior fossa approach for the removal of giant glomus tumors and chondrosarcomas. Surg Neurol. 1987;28(6):423–31.
47. Ceccato GHW, Cândido DN. 37 Infratemporal fossa approach to the jugular foramen. In: de Oliveira JG, Borba LA, editors. Microsurgical and endoscopic approaches to the skull base: anatomy, tactics, and techniques. New York: Thieme; 2021. p. 342.
48. Borba LA, Ale-Bark S, London C. Surgical treatment of glomus jugulare tumors without rerouting of the facial nerve: an infralabyrinthine. Neurosurg Focus. 2004;17(2):E8.
49. Al-Mefty O, Teixeira A. Complex tumors of the glomus jugulare: criteria, treatment, and outcome. Neurosurg Focus. 2004;17(2):1356–66.

# Chapter 11
# Contemporary Management of Pediatric Brainstem Tumors

Sheng-Che Chou, Yu-Ning Chen, Hsin-Yi Huang, Meng-Fai Kuo, Tai-Tong Wong, Sung-Hsin Kuo, and Shih-Hung Yang

## Contents




S.-C. Chou
Division of Neurosurgery, Department of Surgery, National Taiwan University Hospital, National Taiwan University College of Medicine, Taipei, Taiwan

Department of Traumatology, National Taiwan University Hospital, National Taiwan University College of Medicine, Taipei, Taiwan

Y.-N. Chen
Division of Neurosurgery, Department of Surgery, National Taiwan University Hospital Hsin-Chu Branch, Hsin-Chu County, Taiwan

H.-Y. Huang
Department of Pathology, National Taiwan University Hospital and National Taiwan University College of Medicine, Taipei, Taiwan

M.-F. Kuo · S.-H. Yang (✉)
Division of Neurosurgery, Department of Surgery, National Taiwan University Hospital, National Taiwan University College of Medicine, Taipei, Taiwan

T.-T. Wong
Division of Pediatric Neurosurgery, Department of Neurosurgery, Taipei Medical University Hospital, Taipei Medical University, Taipei, Taiwan

S.-H. Kuo
Department of Oncology, National Taiwan University Hospital, National Taiwan University College of Medicine, Taipei, Taiwan
e-mail: shkuo101@ntu.edu.tw



© The Author(s), under exclusive license to Springer Nature Switzerland AG 2024

C. Di Rocco (ed.), *Advances and Technical Standards in Neurosurgery*, Advances and Technical Standards in Neurosurgery 49, https://doi.org/10.1007/978-3-031-42398-7_11

# 11.1   Pediatric Brainstem Tumor

## 11.1.1   Epidemiology

Brainstem tumors account for 10–20% of all pediatric brain tumors and 20–30% of pediatric posterior fossa tumors [1–3]. About 85% of pediatric brainstem tumors are classified as high-grade glioma and the remaining are low-grade glioma [3]. The median age of pediatric brainstem tumors on diagnosis is 6.5 years, and the peak incidence is 3–10 years old, with males and females being equally affected [4]. The duration from symptom onset to diagnosis is shorter in high-grade glioma (HGG) than in low-grade glioma (LGG) patients [5]. Diagnostic latency of less than 2 months and diffuse lesions are poor prognostic factors for overall survival (OS) [6]. Only 3% of patients have concurrent type 1 neurofibromatosis (NF) [4]. In patients with type 1 NF and brainstem tumor, the average age of diagnosis is 7.2 years, with a slight male predominance (56%). Two-thirds of these tumors are located in the midbrain or medulla and more than half (54%) of these patients are asymptomatic [7].

A patient with a diffuse tumor has a 1-year survival rate lower than one with a focal tumor (23.4% vs. 75.0%) [6]. Among the pediatric brainstem tumors, diffuse intrinsic pontine glioma (DIPG) has the worst prognosis. Progression-free survival (PFS) is 25% at 1 year, and the median PFS is 7 months. Median survival is 11 months, and cerebrospinal fluid (CSF) dissemination occurs in 50% of DIPG patients prior to death [8].

Most (69.8%) brainstem HGGs are diagnosed using magnetic resonance imaging (MRI). The incidence of brainstem HGG is higher in young children (1–9 years) and Caucasians [9]. The overall age-adjusted prevalence rate of brainstem HGG is 1.49 per 100,000 [9]. The median OS of brainstem HGG is 10–15 months [9, 10], and the OS in HGG is 41% at 1 year, 15.3% at 2 years, and 7.3% at 3 years [11]. In HGG, histology, older age, and larger tumor size are significantly associated with worse cancer-specific survival (CSS) [10].

LGGs, such as pilocytic astrocytoma, have fair to good prognosis. In LGG, histology (diffuse astrocytic and oligodendroglial tumor, DAOT) and metastasis are associated with worse CSS, but ventricular extension is associated with better CSS [12]. The metastasis rate is 1.3% in LGG [12]. Tumors in patients with NF type 1 also exhibit indolent behavior, and intervention is thus preserved for those exhibiting rapid growth or significant clinical deterioration [13, 14].

## 11.1.2  *Clinical Features*

The clinical presentation is different in diffuse and focal brainstem tumors. Diffuse brainstem tumors, commonly arising from the pons, may present as a triad of signs: cranial neuropathy (particularly abducens or facial nerve palsy), long tract signs (hyperreflexia, Babinski sign, and motor weakness), and cerebellar deficits (ataxia, dysarthria, or dysmetria) [15]. The onset of symptoms is usually rapid, and the duration to diagnosis is about 1–2 months, which is longer than that in overall pediatric brain tumors (median, 24 days) [2, 15, 16]. In focal brainstem tumors, a focal neurological sign with insidious onset is common, such as isolated cranial neuropathy or motor weakness [15].

In DIPG, the first symptoms are usually esotropia and diplopia due to abducens nerve palsy, followed by facial asymmetry, limb weakness, and truncal imbalance [17]. In all pediatric brainstem tumors, 54% of patients present with abducens palsy [4]. Signs and symptoms of increased intracranial pressure secondary to obstructive hydrocephalus, such as headache, nausea, and vomiting, may occur when expansion of the tumor hinders CSF flow by compression of the cerebral aqueduct and the fourth ventricle from the floor. Hydrocephalus can be seen on neuroimaging in 41–46.2% of patients [4, 18, 19].

The nonenhancing computed tomography (CT) imaging of pediatric brainstem tumors usually presents as a hypodense lesion with brainstem enlargement and possible cyst formation inside the lesion. The contrast enhancement of the tumor is variable and depends on its pathology. Pilocytic astrocytomas (PA) are usually enhancing. MRI is the main diagnostic tool for pediatric brainstem tumors. The MRI provides information regarding location, extent, and pathological clues of the tumor [18]. The tumor usually appears as hypointense on T1-weighted imaging and hyperintense on T2-weighted imaging [4]. The tumor can be diffuse (63.6–90%) or focal (10–36.4%) on MRI and cysts can be present in 5% of patients [6, 18, 19]. Tumor hemorrhage (2%) or necrosis (9%) is not frequently seen. A diffuse brainstem tumor, such as DIPG, may present as an infiltrative, poorly enhanced and expansile lesion in most areas of the pons. The basilar artery is commonly engulfed by the DIPG, but the artery is not narrowed. In contrast, a focal brainstem tumor is usually well demarcated and enhanced [4, 15]. Displacement of white matter tract can be evaluated in diffusion tensor imaging (DTI) tractography and provide information for surgical planning. In DIPG, the white matter tracts are usually displaced or infiltrated. Lower apparent diffusion coefficient (ADC) values, higher relative cerebral blood volumes (rCBV), and higher choline to *N*-acetylaspartate (NAA) ratios on magnetic resonance spectroscopy (MRS) are associated with shorter survival time [20]. The differential diagnosis on imaging studies includes brainstem abscess, acute disseminated encephalomyelitis, osmotic demyelination syndrome, and cavernous malformation.

In positron emission tomography (PET), higher fluorodeoxyglucose (FDG) uptake is associated with shorter survival [21, 22]. Higher levels of negative PET-ADC correlation also lead to more unfavorable PFS [23].

### *11.1.3   Classification*

#### 11.1.3.1   Anatomical Location and Growth Pattern

Numerous classification systems have been proposed to classify brainstem tumors by location (midbrain, pons, or medulla), growth pattern (intrinsic or exophytic), focality (diffuse or focal), and associated features (hemorrhage, necrosis, or hydrocephalus, etc.) [24]. However, with the advancement of molecular diagnosis, prognosis can be better predicted by molecular classification.

More than half (54.5–84%) of the tumors are located in the pons, 7–30.3% in the midbrain or tectum and 9–18% in the medulla [4, 6, 18]. According to the anatomical location, brainstem gliomas can be simply classified into DIPG, medullary glioma, and midbrain (including tectal) glioma [4, 16]. However, the tumor usually invades adjacent structures (62.5%) [19].

DIPG exhibits a diffuse and poorly demarcated pattern. It usually causes expansion of the pons and the fourth ventricle can be compressed, resulting in hydrocephalus. The basilar artery is usually anteriorly displaced and engulfed by the lesion. Tumor extension into the midbrain (66%), medulla (56%), peduncle (79%), or cerebellum (49%) is frequent [18].

The midbrain (including tectal) glioma is usually focal and tumor growth tends to cause obstruction of the cerebral aqueduct and obstructive hydrocephalus. Tumor growth can also extend into the third ventricle or involve the thalamus [18] or pons (50%) [18].

The medullary glioma exhibits a variable pattern, including focal, diffuse, or exophytic. Its extension into the pons (63%) or cervical cord (63%) is frequent [18]. An exophytic medullary glioma can block fourth ventricle outflow and cause obstructive hydrocephalus [25].

#### 11.1.3.2   Pathology

Most pediatric brainstem tumors are World Health Organization (WHO) grade 1–4 gliomas. HGG (WHO grade 3 and 4) accounts for the majority of the pediatric brainstem tumors and most others are LGG (WHO grade 1 and 2). Ganglioglioma (GG), oligodendroglioma, and pilomyxoid astrocytoma are rare [26, 27].

Pilocytic astrocytoma (WHO grade 1) is usually an enhancing, discrete lesion, arising from the dorsal medulla or midbrain and most are exophytic. GG (WHO grade 1) is rare and usually arise from the cervicomedullary junction. BRAF V600E mutation is seen in 15.4% of pediatric brainstem LGG, while higher mutation rates (38%) are seen in pediatric brainstem GG. Although the BRAF V600E mutation has a worse 10-year PFS rate than that in the wild type (27% vs. 60.2%), the mutant gene can be a therapeutic target to improve clinical outcomes [28, 29]. WHO grade 2 astrocytomas can arise from anywhere in the brainstem, but a diffuse pontine grade 2 astrocytoma behaves more aggressively than those in other locations [30].

High-grade (WHO grade 3 and 4) pediatric brainstem tumors include WHO grade 3 anaplastic astrocytoma, WHO grade 4 glioblastoma, WHO grade 4 atypical teratoid rhabdoid tumor (ATRT), and WHO grade 4 embryonal tumor with multi-layered rosettes (ETMR). High-grade tumors outside of the pons arise mostly from the middle cerebellar peduncle junction, pontomedullary junction, and midbrain [31].

The LGG can become an HGG via malignant transformation, especially when it contains the BRAF V600E mutation and CDKN2A deletion [32]. The H3K27M mutation has poor prognosis regardless of histological grade [33]. In autopsy cases, H3K27M mutation is found in 87% of previously diagnosed DIPGs, which were reclassified as H3K27M-mutated diffuse midline glioma, and all long-term survivors had no H3K27M mutation [34]. In addition to H3K27 mutation, isocitrate dehydrogenase (IDH) wild type and EGFR mutations also have poor prognosis. However, the IDH mutant is rare in pediatric brainstem tumors [35]. In contrast, a low grade diffuse astrocytoma with alterations in MYB or MYBL1 has good prognosis and the 10-year PFS and OS rates are 89.6% and 95.2%, respectively [36].

## 11.2 Contemporary Surgical Treatment for Pediatric Brainstem Tumors

### 11.2.1 Diffuse Intrinsic Pontine Glioma

Diffuse brainstem tumor belongs to the category of diffuse midline glioma, which consists of all grades of tumors with H3K27M and other H3 altered gene mutations in the thalamus, brainstem, or spinal cord [37]. The most common pediatric brainstem tumor is DIPG, which accounts for 75–80% of all tumors in the brainstem region [16]. The histopathology consists mainly of anaplastic astrocytoma (grade 3) and glioblastoma (grade 4), and occasionally of diffuse astrocytoma (grade 2). The prognosis is poor for DIPG irrespective of the pathological grade, with a mean survival time of less than 12 months [38]. For high-grade glioma in the cerebrum or cerebellum, maximally safe resection is considered an essential part of neuro-oncological treatment, as a greater extent of resection is associated with a better outcome. However, radical surgical excision is not appropriate in the management of DIPG, as the tumor diffusely infiltrates the bulbar nuclei and white matter fiber tracts [39]. While operative extirpation is not a therapeutic option for DIPG currently, surgical biopsy may play a certain role in the diagnosis and clinical trials for this dismal disease.

Indication for surgical biopsy of brainstem tumors is evolving along the timeline. In the pre-MRI era, when differentiation of DIPG from other brainstem tumors by CT scan was not reliable, tumor biopsy was performed for definitive diagnosis in some centers [40, 41]. Following the introduction of MRI into clinical practice, characteristic imaging findings are considered sufficient for the diagnosis of DIPG by the majority of clinicians, thus obviating the need for tissue sampling [42]. While most DIPG tumors exhibit typical imaging findings as infiltrating T1-hypointense and T2-hyperintense masses involving at least 50% of the ventral pons on cross-sectional MRI image, some DIPGs show atypical radiographic features of eccentric location, exophytic growth pattern, well-defined margins, or avid enhancement. Chiang reported that up to 30% of atypical DIPGs were WHO grade 1 tumors [43]. Therefore, surgical biopsy is recommended for pathological verification of atypical DIPGs, as proposed by the Consensus Conference on Pediatric Neurosurgery (CPN2011) held in Paris, France, in 2011 [44]. In addition, biopsy for typical DIPGs is also justified when the patient is enrolled in an ethically approved clinical trial in which the tissue obtained will be used to investigate or inform the role of biological markers after treatment selection or molecular tumor grading [45].

Surgical approaches for diagnostic biopsy of DIPG include open craniotomy and stereotactic procedures. Craniotomy is occasionally indicated for directly accessible tumors, e.g., atypical DIPG tumor with a ventral exophytic component (Fig. 11.1). Stereotactic biopsy is much often performed, either frame-based or framelessly, by CT/MRI navigation or robotic guidance [46], via suboccipital transcerebellar or supratentorial transfrontal route according to tumor characteristics and neurosurgeons' preferences [47]. The diagnostic yield is greater than 90%, with the morbidity rate between 0% and 20% and the mortality rate below 1% in modern series [48–53]. The Necker series was the largest one to date, with 130 cases of DIPG receiving transcerebellar biopsy [54]. The diagnostic yield was 100%. The morbidity and mortality rates were 3.9% and 0%, respectively. As a safe and effective procedure, biopsy for DIPG is expected to be increasingly indicated for differential diagnosis of atypical tumors, as well as clinical trials to search for novel treatment strategies to reverse tumor progression.

## 11.2.2   *Focal Brainstem Tumors*

Focal brainstem tumors are well-defined lesions of the midbrain, pons, and medulla. The growth pattern may be intrinsic or exophytic, depending on the epicenter location on the surface or deep part of the brainstem. Common pathological entities include glioma, ependymoma, cavernoma, and hemangioblastoma. The majority of focal brainstem tumors are gliomas, of which histopathology is usually pilocytic

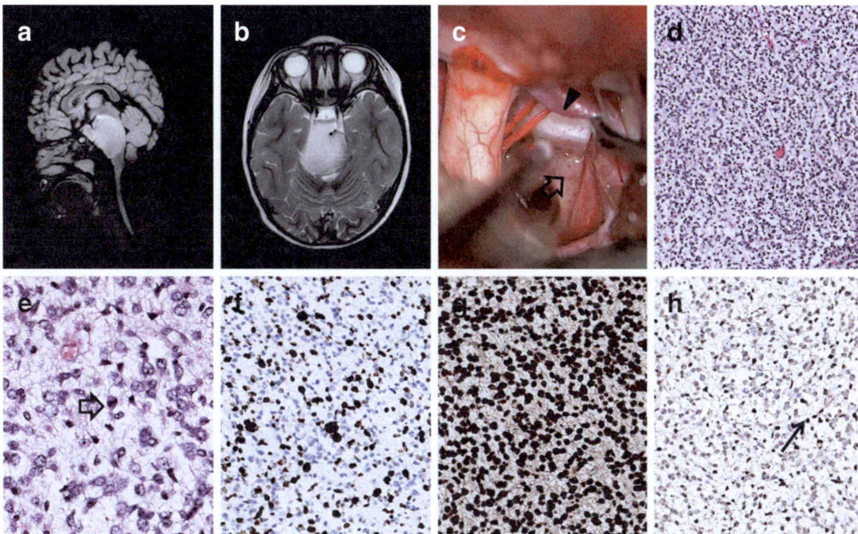

**Fig. 11.1** Diffuse intrinsic pontine glioma (DIPG) with ventral exophytic growth in a 3-year-old girl, (**a**) preoperative MRI, FLAIR image, sagittal view, (**b**) preoperative MRI, T2-weighted image, axial view, (**c**) intraoperative photo during open biopsy via right pterional approach, tumor (black open arrow) exposed behind dorsum sella (black arrow head), viewing from optico-carotid window, (**d**) H&E staining revealing an infiltrative and hypercellular neoplasm, (**e**) pleomorphic tumor nuclei and occasional mitosis (*black open arrow*), (**f**) high Ki-67 proliferative in this case, (**g**) histone H3 K27M mutation confirmed with the immunohistochemical stain for the mutant protein, (**h**) immunohistochemical staining for histone H3 lysine 27 trimethylation (H3K27me3) showing a marked loss of nuclear expression in tumor cells in contrast to preserved expression in non-neoplastic cells (*black arrow*)

astrocytoma, ganglioglioma, or other low-grade astrocytomas [53]. According to the growth pattern, focal brainstem gliomas can be classified as focal intrinsic, dorsal exophytic, and cervicomedullary tumors [55]. These lesions are amenable to operative intervention, owing to their circumscribed nature; however, surgery should be weighed against operative risks, which may result in significant morbidities or mortality, as the brainstem is a critically vital structure. Also, the rate of tumor progression should be taken into consideration. For example, brainstem tumors in neurofibromatosis type 1 patients may remain stable for years or even spontaneously regress, warranting a watchful waiting policy for the management of such lesions [7]. Nevertheless, regular imaging follow-up is necessary, as some seemingly indolent lesions may progress as the children grow up and demand neurosurgical intervention [56].

Focal midbrain tumors can occur in the cerebral peduncle, periaqueductal region, or tectum/quadrigeminal plate. Surgical decision will depend on tumor biology. For tectal and periaqueductal tumors in the midbrain, the size of the lesion tends to remain stationary for years [57]. The management of such lesions is conservative, and only CSF diversion for tumor associated hydrocephalus is sufficient (Fig. 11.2).

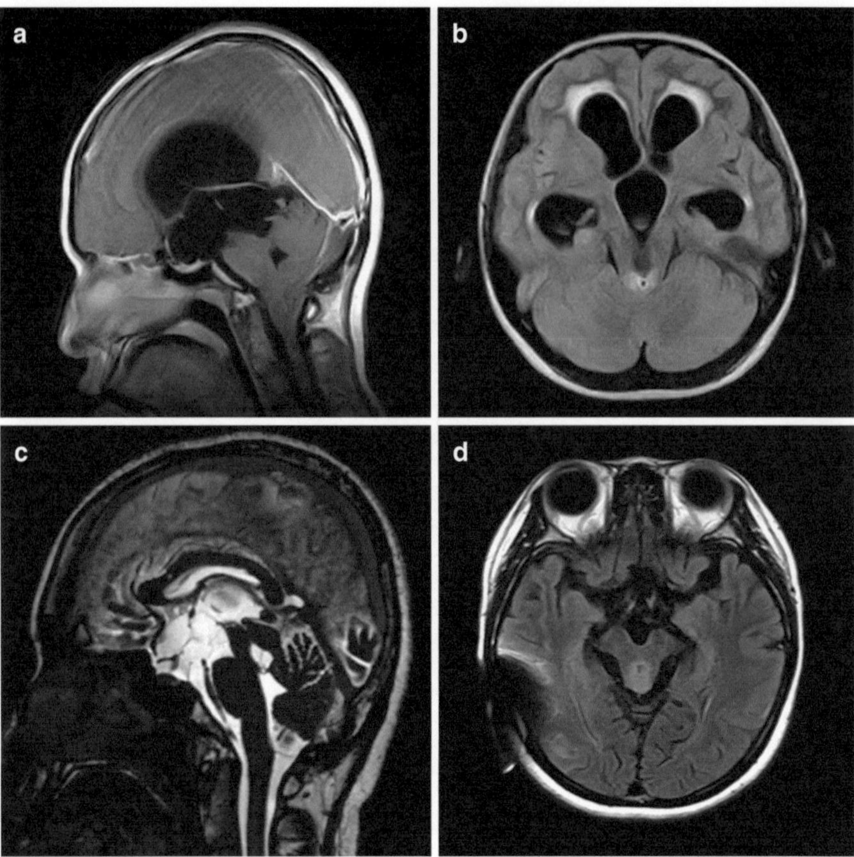

**Fig. 11.2** Midbrain tumor in the peri-aqueductal region with obstructive hydrocephalus in a 16-year-old girl, (**a**) preoperative MRI, T1-weighted image with contrast enhancement, (**b**) preoperative MRI, FLAIR image, (**c**) postoperative MRI, T2-weighted image, (**d**) postoperative MRI, FLAIR image, 12 years after CSF shunting surgery, showing stationary tumor size and normal ventricular dimension

When surgery is indicated for tumor progression, the surgical approach should be tailored to the location of the tumor. Peduncular tumors can be accessed anterolaterally via pterional, orbitozygomatic, or subtemporal trajectory. Endoscopic skull base surgery has evolved so that ventral midbrain tumors are also accessible by transsphenoidal transclival approach [58]. Periaqueductal tumors and peduncular tumors with thalamic extension (thalamopeduncular tumor) can be reached via the anterior transcortical/transcallosal transventricular corridor from above, and tumors in the lower aqueductal region via the telovelar or transvermian corridor from below. Tectal region tumors can be reached either supratentorially via the posterior transcortical/transcallosal transventricular or occipital transtentorial route, or infratentorially via the supracerebellar route (Fig. 11.3), depending on the direction of tumor extension.

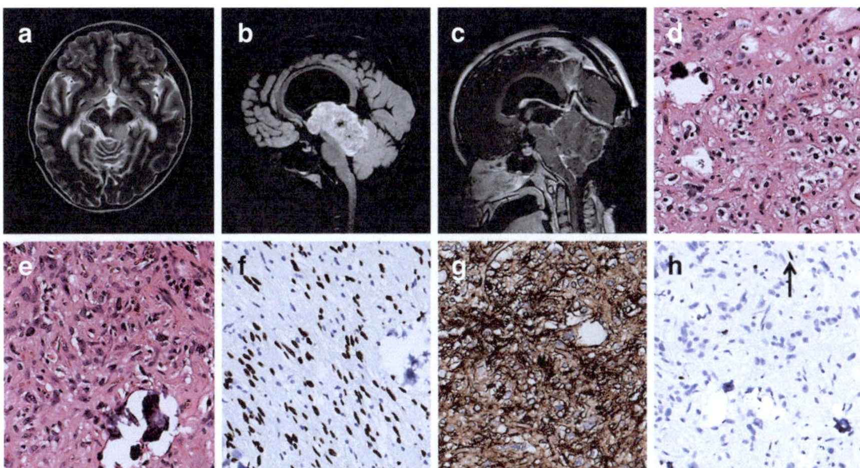

**Fig. 11.3** Midbrain tumor in the tectal region in a 5-year-old boy, (**a**) initial MRI, T2-weighted, (**b**) follow-up MRI at 8-year-old, FLAIR image, showing tumor progression and hydrocephalus, (**c**) intraoperative MRI, T1-weighted image with contrast enhancement, showing total tumor excision via the supracerebellar infratentorial corridor, (**d**) H&E staining revealing oligodendroglioma-like morphology with calcification in part of the tumor, (**e**) presence of a second tumor component with pleomorphic astrocytic nuclei, (**f**) tumor cells immunoreactive to the glial cell marker OLIG2, (**g**) diffuse and strong CD34 immunoreactivity, characteristic of polymorphous low-grade neuroepithelial tumor of the young (PLNTY), (**h**) low Ki-67 proliferative index in the tumor, which also harbored BRAF V600E mutation

Focal pontine tumors have a geographic preference in the dorsal pons, compared to the diffuse pontine tumors located in the ventral pons. It may present as an intrinsic lesion or a dorsal exophytic mass extending into the fourth ventricle (Fig. 11.4) [59]. Therefore, many pontine tumors (e.g., cavernoma and glioma) are amenable to resection by entering the fourth ventricle. Tumor location and the surgeon's preference dictate the selection of surgical path, either telovelar, subvermian, or transvermian. Dorsal intrinsic pontine tumors will require opening of the floor of the fourth ventricle, where many cranial nerve nuclei and white matter tracts reside. Safe entry zone has been described based on the anatomical topography; however, surface anatomy may be distorted, and intraoperative neurophysiological monitoring is essential to guide the selection of the least eloquent region to approach the lesion [60, 61]. For lateral pontine tumors, presigmoid transpetrosal and retrosigmoid routes are workhorse approaches. Lesions in the ventral pons can be accessed by anterior and anterolateral trajectories described in the previous paragraph of midbrain tumor approaches [58].

Focal medullary tumors are either confined to the medulla or extended to neighboring regions, e.g., cervicomedullary tumor [62]. Surgical access to this region is less demanding than approaches to the midbrain and pons. Two access routes are commonly utilized. The median suboccipital route with opening of the posterior foramen magnum can expose the posterior medullary surface by subvermian or

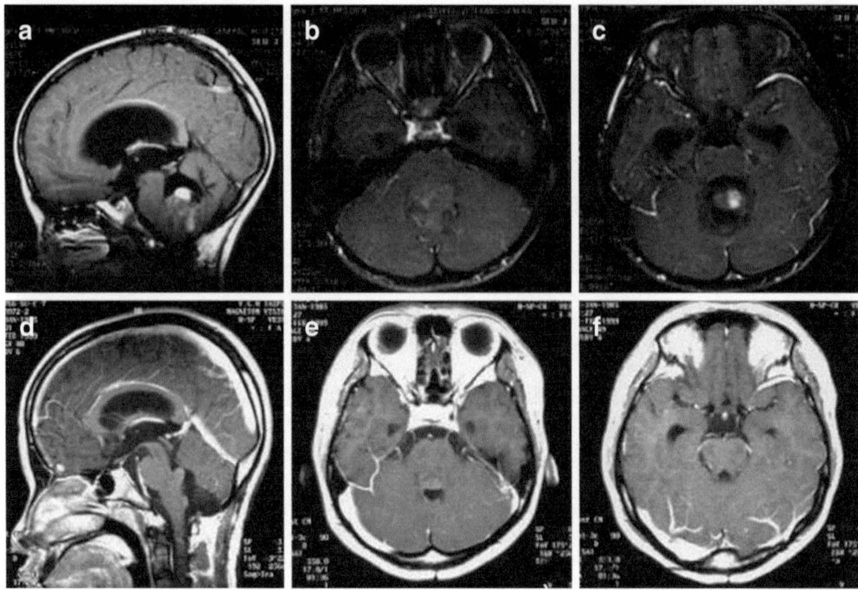

**Fig. 11.4** Dorsal exophytic pilocytic astrocytoma of the pons in an 8-year-old girl. Preoperative MRI, T1-weighted image with contrast enhancement, (**a**) sagittal view, (**b**) axial view at lower pontine level, (**c**) axial view at upper pontine level; postoperative MRI, T1-weighted image, (**d**) sagittal view, (**e**) axial view at lower pontine level, (**f**) axial view at upper pontine level, demonstrating stable residual tumor 6 years after nearly total resection without radiotherapy or chemotherapy

telovelar approach, and the lateral suboccipital route plus a transcondylar or paracondylar approach can reach the anterolateral medulla. For cervicomedullary tumor, the median approach will extend down to the cervical spine region (Fig. 11.5). En-bloc cervical laminectomy can expose the surface of posterior spinal cord. Repositioning of the laminae with miniplates and screws are recommended to prevent or reduce deformity of the cervical spine [63]. For anterolateral medullary lesions, the far lateral approach with resection of more than 50% of the condylar joint requires occipito-cervical fusion to prevent instability of the craniovertebral junction [64].

Many focal brainstem tumors are clinically asymptomatic and stationary, and a conservative approach is sufficient. When these lesions progress or become symptomatic, surgery is indicated. The surgical principle is maximally safe resection to reduce tumor burden and avoid neurological damage. In this highly eloquent region, special attention is directed to observe the junction of the lesion and the brain parenchyma. The demarcation is most obvious in cavernomas, and quite discernible in most low-grade tumors, such as pilocytic astrocytoma, yet ambiguous in high-grade tumors like glioblastoma. Neurosurgery has evolved over the years to enable surgeons to improve the surgical outcome. Modern neurosurgeons can plan an appropriate surgical corridor to perform brainstem operation with the aid of high-resolution

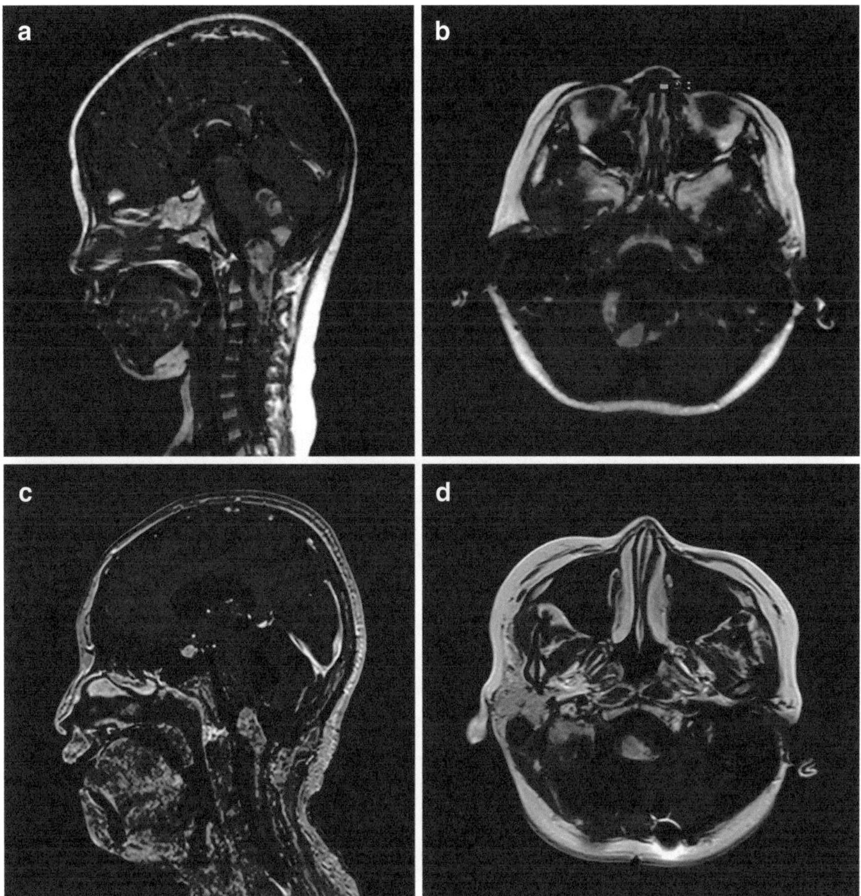

**Fig. 11.5** Cervicomedullary pilocytic astrocytoma in a 3-year-old girl. Preoperative MRI, T1-weighted image with contrast enhancement, (**a**) sagittal view, (**b**) axial view. Post-operative MRI, T1-weighted image with contrast enhancement, (**c**) sagittal view, (**d**) axial view, showing stable residual tumor in the medulla and spinal cord, 13 years after partial tumor excision and adjuvant chemotherapy

microscope or endoscope, cavitron ultrasonic surgical aspirator (CUSA), intraoperative neurophysiological monitoring, real-time neuronavigation, fluorescence-guidance, intraoperative MR imaging control, and so on [65]. Several surgical series of focal brainstem tumors reported favorable outcome. Among 34 cases of focal pediatric brainstem gliomas, 31 patients had grossly total or nearly total (>90%) tumor resection. There was no surgical mortality, and the progression-free survival (PFS) and overall survival (OS) were 75% and 66%, respectively [66]. In another long-term follow-up study of 52 focal brainstem tumors, 25 patients received surgical extirpation as the primary treatment, and the 10-year event-free survival and OS were 52% and 90%, respectively [67]. A study of 48 children with histologically proven low-grade glioma demonstrated that the PFS of DIPG and non-DIPG were 1.8 and 11.1 years, respectively. In this cohort, 27% of the patients had DIPG [30].

### 11.2.3  Hydrocephalus Secondary to Brainstem Tumor

In brainstem tumor patients, hydrocephalus results from obstruction of the cerebro-spinal fluid (CSF) circulation pathway by the tumor. The incidence of hydrocepha-lus varies among different tumor locations. While most patients with midbrain tumors in the tectum or aqueductal region present with hydrocephalus, only 22% of DIPG patients had hydrocephalus in a cohort of 51 patients [68]. Treatment of obstructive hydrocephalus follows a hierarchy of (1) removal of the obstructive lesion, (2) internal CSF diversion (endoscopic third ventriculostomy, i.e., ETV), and (3) CSF diversion to other body compartments (CSF shunt). The first priority is tumor removal, which may be applicable in select cases, e.g., pure aqueductal tumor as well as other focal brainstem tumors [69]. However, this treatment policy for hydrocephalus is not possible for diffuse brainstem tumors, or is not effective for incompletely resected focal brainstem tumors. In these cases, ETV can create a new outlet for CSF to bypass the obstruction in the cerebral aqueduct or the fourth ven-tricle. ETV is the treatment of choice for hydrocephalus due to tectal glioma, which usually remains dormant for years and requires neither biopsy nor excision. In a cohort of tectal tumors with hydrocephalus, a total of 18 patients received ETV. The procedures were successful in all patients and 16 patients (89%) remained shunt free [70]. However, certain tumors in the midbrain or pons may distort the regional anatomy, pushing the basilar artery ventrally and decreasing the subarachnoid space between the brainstem and clival bone. Despite the unfavorable surgical condition, ETV might be successfully performed [71, 72]. When the ETV fails or is deemed unsuitable to carry out, a CSF shunt can provide relief of hydrocephalus associated with brainstem tumors. However, peritoneal seeding of diffuse pontine tumor via the ventriculoperitoneal shunt has been reported [73], making CSF shunt surgery the last priority for hydrocephalus treatment in brainstem tumors patients.

## 11.3  Contemporary Radiation Treatment for Pediatric Brainstem Tumor

The modalities of contemporary radiation therapy (RT) for pediatric brainstem tumors include photon therapy, proton therapy, and stereotactic radiosurgery. For brainstem tumors, RT can play an important role as the primary or adjuvant treat-ment post-surgery, depending on the pathology and anatomical location of the lesion. Because the brainstem is a highly eloquent neural structure, both surgery and RT require meticulous evaluation and planning. The technology used in RT has progressed rapidly in recent years. New techniques, such as intensity-modulated radiation therapy (IMRT) or volumetric-modulated arc therapy (VMAT), can further improve the precision of radiation delivery and decrease radiation exposure to the surrounding tissue [74]. We believe these new techniques will further improve therapeutic and neurological outcomes of pediatric brainstem tumors in the future.

## *11.3.1   Radiation Therapy*

Based on the radiation source, RT can be classified into photon therapy, brachytherapy, and proton therapy. Photon therapy can also be further categorized as external-beam radiation therapy (EBRT) or brachytherapy, depending on the method used for radiation delivery.

### 11.3.1.1   Photon Therapy

Photon therapy utilizes electromagnetic radiation, such as X-ray, to damage the DNA structures in cells and subsequently kill tumor cells. For brainstem lesions, the conventional EBRT dose is 1.8–2 Gy per fraction for 25–30 fractions (total dose of 45–60 Gy) [75, 76]. With this dosage, most patients can tolerate the toxicity well. More severe acute toxic side effects, Common Terminology Criteria for Adverse Event (CTCAE) grade 3–5, have rarely been reported. The most common side effects are skin erythema and scaling, especially in the post-auricular area [75]. However, long-term side effects of RT are a concern, especially in pediatric patients. Many long-term complications in children, such as compromised school performance, neuroendocrine deficits, and hearing impairment, have been reported [77].

EBRT is often the treatment of choice for diffuse intrinsic pontine glioma (DIPG) because surgical resection of this tumor can cause severe neurological deficits and is usually not feasible. In patients with DIPG, the conventionally fractionated RT has been shown to provide a median progression-free survival (PFS) of 9 months and median overall survival (OS) of 12 months, although EBRT can dramatically relieve symptoms resulting from the original lesions [75]. Some studies have also used hypofractionated or hyperfractionated RT to try to improve clinical outcomes and decrease side effects of RT for DIPG. However, when compared to conventionally fractionated RT, there were no significant differences in PFS, OS, and toxicities found in patients with DIPG who were treated with either hypofractionated or hyperfractionated RT [75, 76]. These studies indicate that conventionally fractionated RT is still the standard treatment for newly diagnosed DIPG. However, most patients with DIPG developed progression within 1 year after completion of RT. Several studies have addressed the impact of reirradiation on these patients and found that reirradiation following DIPG progression may provide some benefit [78, 79]. In a single institute experience of five patients with histologically proven DIPG who received reirradiation, the authors showed that median OS was 116 days after completing reirradiation, and 16.3 months after initial diagnosis [79]. In a meta-analysis reviewing 90 cases throughout 7 different studies, reirradiation for patients with DIPG was performed 11.8–14 months after initial RT [80]. Reirradiation provided clinical improvement in 87% of the patients, with OS values of 6.2 and 18.0 months after reirradiation and initial diagnosis, respectively [80].

For low-grade brainstem glioma (LGBSG), complete surgical resection provides the best survival outcomes [81]. RT has been commonly administered in unresectable or residual tumors, but there is still some debate as to its efficacy [82]. A large series of 104 cases from the Hospital for Sick Children reported no significant survival benefits in patients receiving adjuvant RT compared to patients who were under initial observation only [83]. Another recent retrospective study using Surveillance Epidemiology and End Results (SEER) database also implied that the efficacy of RT in LGBSG is still vague [81]. Furthermore, because these patients have high long-term survival rates, the lasting side effects of RT need to be considered. Thus, it may be worthwhile to postpone therapy, either until the child can tolerate the side effects or the tumor recurs [82].

Brachytherapy is another modality of RT that has been applied to a few selected patients with LGBSG. Stereotactic implantation of $^{125}$I seed to the focal brainstem tumor has been administered as primary, adjunct, or salvage therapy [84, 85]. In the largest case series with brachytherapy, which included 26 children and 21 adults, 5- and 10-year PFS rates were reported as 81.2% and 62.0%, respectively. Fifty-one percent of the cases reported improved neurological symptoms at the last follow-up. The rates of transient and permanent neurological deficits were 12.8% and 4.3%, respectively [85]. However, because of improved safety in brainstem surgery and other forms of RT, the role of brachytherapy may be limited. In the future, it may be considered in select cases as adjunct or salvage rather than primary therapy.

### 11.3.1.2 Proton Therapy

The proton is a positively charged, heavy particle. Compared to photon therapy, proton therapy delivers less radiation to the surrounding normal tissue when administering an equivalent dose. Therefore, proton therapy can potentially result in fewer instances of radiation necrosis, cognitive deterioration, and endocrine complications in long-term follow-up. Thus, this treatment is especially suitable for pediatric patients [86].

However, because the prognosis of DIPG is dismal and long-term survival is rare, the lasting benefits of proton therapy have yet to be observed in these patients. In a recent retrospective study using proton therapy with 54 Gy (relative biological effectiveness) at 30 fractions to treat 12 pediatric patients with DIPG, the authors found that this treatment provided a median OS of 9 months and median PFS of

5 months [87]. These survival rates were not significantly different from those in patients receiving conventional RT. In this study, there was also no significant difference in acute toxicity between proton therapy and RT [87]. On the other hand, proton therapy may be considered for reirradiation in order to lower radiation exposure to the surrounding tissue and improve safety [87]. In the future, if the prognosis of DIPG is improved and long-term survival becomes more common, the benefits of proton therapy will be more evident.

In LGBSG, which are rare, only a small number of cases receiving proton therapy have been reported. A recent clinical study reviewed patients with low-grade gliomas of the central nervous system undergoing proton therapy, of which 28 cases were brainstem lesions. In these patients, the 5-year PFS and OS rates were 55% and 85%, respectively [88].

### 11.3.2 Stereotactic Radiosurgery

Stereotactic radiosurgery (SRS) delivers a large dose of radiation (12–35 Gy) per fraction and consists of 1–5 fractions per treatment course. The radiation is highly focused on the target lesion and thus radiation exposure to the surrounding tissue is significantly decreased. However, the usage of SRS is generally limited by lesion size (<3 cm in diameter) [89, 90].

For DIPG, because the tumor diameter is usually more than 3 cm and the tumor is usually diffused throughout the brainstem, SRS is usually not applicable.

A recent systemic review of compared SRS and RT in patients with LGBSG. The authors of this study found that SRS may provide better partial or complete response rates. They reported better, but not significant, survival outcomes in 5-year OS (97% vs. 93%) and PFS (92% vs. 79%) rates between the SRS and RT groups. It is worth noting that SRS induced significantly higher rates of treatment-related imaging changes (TRICs) than RT did, but most of the patients with TRICs reported no or mild and transient symptoms [89].

## 11.4 Contemporary Oncological Management for Pediatric Brainstem Tumors

### 11.4.1 Chemotherapy

The most common pediatric brainstem tumor is glioma. For high-grade glioma in the cerebrum, the combination of procarbazine, lomustine, and vincristine, so-called PCV regimen used in the last century, was modestly effective in adult patients. Temozolomide, a DNA alkylating agent that is active against anaplastic astrocytoma and glioblastoma, has become the standard treatment as initial concomitant chemoradiotherapy (CCRT) after operation and subsequent adjuvant chemotherapy, since the beginning of the twenty-first century. Therefore, clinicians undertook clinical investigation of these chemotherapeutic agents in the treatment of pediatric brainstem tumors. However, the results were disappointing in that the positive treatment results in adult malignant gliomas did not translate equally into pediatric diffuse gliomas in the brainstem [91]. In a retrospective study of the therapeutic efficacy of temozolomide in 18 children with DIPG, the outcome was no different for the group of patients undergoing CCRT with temozolomide plus adjuvant temozolomide versus the group of patients receiving radiotherapy plus adjuvant temozolomide [92]. A prospective randomized trial that recruited 35 DIPG patients did not show any survival benefits of temozolomide therapy [93]. Adjuvant therapy or CCRT with temozolomide had no impact on the outcome of children with DIPG. However, for malignant pediatric brainstem gliomas other than DIPG, the treatment efficacy may be similar to that of adult malignant gliomas.

## *11.4.2 Targeted Therapy*

Bevacizumab, a monoclonal antibody against vascular endothelial growth factor (VEGF), shows antineoplastic effects by inhibiting the growth of new tumor blood vessels in a wide range of human cancers, e.g., colon cancer, renal cell carcinoma, lung cancer, and glioblastoma. To investigate whether bevacizumab could enter DIPG tumor cells, researchers gave seven patients radioisotope-labeled bevacizumab, of which five had positive uptake [94]. Treatment response was evaluated in patients receiving a combination of bevacizumab with various agents, e.g., temozolomide, irinotecan, cetuximab, and valproic acid [95–99]. This agent seemed to be safe for pediatric DIPG patients and showed promising effects in open arm trials. Validation of its therapeutic efficacy awaits future randomized trials.

Several other targeted therapies were studied in pediatric DIPG cases. Unfortunately, superior outcomes are yet to be observed in clinical trials with drugs and monoclonal antibodies against specific targets, including epidermal growth factor receptor (EGFR), platelet derived growth factor receptor (PDGFR), vascular epidermal growth factor receptor 2 (VEGFR-2), and protein kinase C-PI3K-Akt pathways [100–105]. One potential target, the histone mutation H3K27M, seen in 80% of DIPG, may be subject to panobinostat, a histone deacetylase inhibitor, for reversal of epigenic dysregulation, and is under active investigation [106, 107]. As more DIPG patients undergo tumor biopsy for the purpose of clinical trials, future identification of novel therapeutic targets using a personalized approach may lead to better prognosis [108–110].

### *11.4.3 Immunotherapy and Miscellaneous*

Immunotherapy provides a new strategy against human cancer. For tumors like DIPG with limited therapeutic strategies, researchers began to study the feasibility of immunotherapy against this lethal disease. Pilot studies using dendritic cell therapy, immune checkpoint inhibition, and tumor vaccine showed potential tumoricidal effects [111–113]. The H3K27M mutated cells in DIPG and other diffuse midline gliomas highly expressed disialoganglioside GD2. A recent clinical study showed clinical and radiographic improvement in three of the four patients undergoing anti-GD2-CAR T-cell therapy [114]. The clinical efficacy will be elucidated in the coming years.

Many drugs with treatment efficacies in preclinical studies have failed to translate into outcome improvement in clinical trials, and this discrepancy might result from poor drug penetrance through the blood–brain barrier (BBB). One way to enhance drug delivery is to open the BBB by mannitol infusion intra-arterially [115] or focused ultrasound delivered transcranially [116]. Another way is convection enhanced delivery (CED) by direct drug administration via a catheter under slow and continuous pressure [117]. Other novel approaches include transcriptional regulation, microenvironmental manipulation, and so on. A multimodal therapeutic approach consisting of surgical biopsy, radiotherapy, chemotherapy, immunotherapy, and targeted therapy may be able to control disease progression for children with brainstem tumors in the future.

## 11.5 Conclusion

Brainstem tumors in children pose special challenges for pediatric neurosurgeons. The location and pathology of tumors in this location are heterogenous. From a neurosurgical perspective, different operative strategies should be applied for diffuse and focal brainstem tumors. For diffuse brainstem tumors, mostly DIPG, radical tumor excision is not indicated. Due to the poor outcome of DIPG despite standard treatment with radiotherapy, stereotactic tumor biopsy is indicated in the setting of clinical trials for typical DIPG. Another indication of biopsy is DIPG with atypical features. For focal brainstem tumors, radical excision should be attempted with tailored operative corridor according to the location of the tumor, and the assistance of intraoperative neurophysiological monitoring, as well as other surgical adjuncts if available. Radiotherapy is the main treatment for diffuse brainstem tumors and provides tumor control for remnant or recurrent focal tumor. Adjuvant treatment with chemotherapy, targeted therapy, and immunotherapy continue to evolve and is becoming an essential part of multimodal therapy for pediatric brainstem tumors. An algorithm for management of pediatric brainstem tumor is proposed for the readers' reference (Fig. 11.6).

**Acknowledgments** The authors would like to thank Dr. Tiffany Y. Hu for her help with critical editing of this chapter.

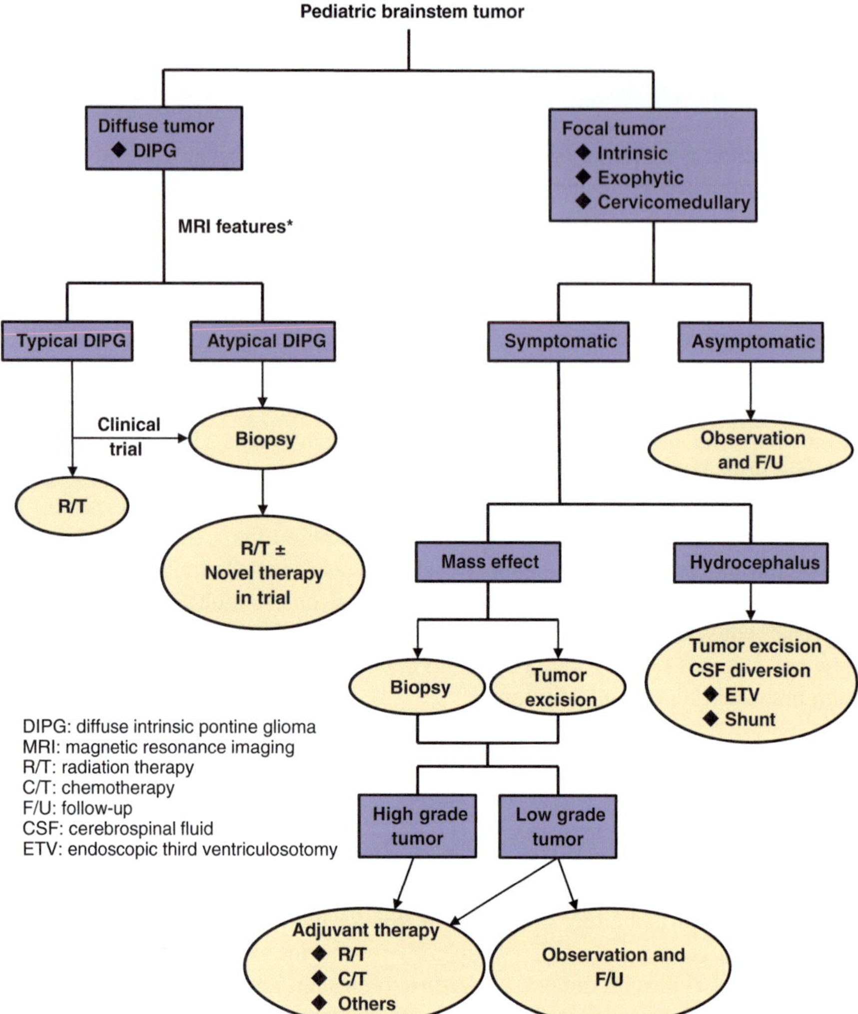



**Fig. 11.6** Algorithm for contemporary management of pediatric brainstem tumor

# References


1. Smith MA, Freidlin B, Ries LA, Simon R. Trends in reported incidence of primary malignant brain tumors in children in the United States. J Natl Cancer Inst. 1998;90(17):1269–77.
2. Reulecke BC, Erker CG, Fiedler BJ, Niederstadt TU, Kurlemann G. Brain tumors in children: initial symptoms and their influence on the time span between symptom onset and diagnosis. J Child Neurol. 2008;23(2):178–83.
3. Chamdine O, Elhawary GAS, Alfaar AS, Qaddoumi I. The incidence of brainstem primitive neuroectodermal tumors of childhood based on SEER data. Childs Nerv Syst. 2018;34(3):431–9.

4. Fisher PG, Breiter SN, Carson BS, Wharam MD, Williams JA, Weingart JD, et al. A clinico-pathologic reappraisal of brain stem tumor classification. Identification of pilocystic astrocytoma and fibrillary astrocytoma as distinct entities. Cancer. 2000;89(7):1569–76.
5. Fangusaro J. Pediatric high-grade gliomas and diffuse intrinsic pontine gliomas. J Child Neurol. 2009;24(11):1409–17.
6. Sun T, Wan W, Wu Z, Zhang J, Zhang L. Clinical outcomes and natural history of pediatric brainstem tumors: with 33 cases follow-ups. Neurosurg Rev. 2013;36(2):311–9; discussion 9–20.
7. Mahdi J, Shah AC, Sato A, Morris SM, McKinstry RC, Listernick R, et al. A multi-institutional study of brainstem gliomas in children with neurofibromatosis type 1. Neurology. 2017;88(16):1584–9.
8. Massimino M, Spreafico F, Biassoni V, Simonetti F, Riva D, Trecate G, et al. Diffuse pontine gliomas in children: changing strategies, changing results? A mono-institutional 20-year experience. J Neuro Oncol. 2008;87(3):355–61.
9. Patil N, Kelly ME, Yeboa DN, Buerki RA, Cioffi G, Balaji S, et al. Epidemiology of brainstem high-grade gliomas in children and adolescents in the United States, 2000-2017. Neuro Oncol. 2021;23(6):990–8.
10. Maxwell R, Luksik AS, Garzon-Muvdi T, Yang W, Huang J, Bettegowda C, et al. Population-based study determining predictors of cancer-specific mortality and survival in pediatric high-grade brainstem glioma. World Neurosurg. 2018;119:e1006–15.
11. Hassan H, Pinches A, Picton SV, Phillips RS. Survival rates and prognostic predictors of high grade brain stem gliomas in childhood: a systematic review and meta-analysis. J Neuro Oncol. 2017;135(1):13–20.
12. Liu Z, Feng S, Li J, Cao H, Huang J, Fan F, et al. The epidemiological characteristics and prognostic factors of low-grade brainstem glioma: a real-world study of pediatric and adult patients. Front Oncol. 2020;10:391.
13. Molloy PT, Bilaniuk LT, Vaughan SN, Needle MN, Liu GT, Zackai EH, et al. Brainstem tumors in patients with neurofibromatosis type 1: a distinct clinical entity. Neurology. 1995;45(10):1897–902.
14. Pollack IF, Shultz B, Mulvihill JJ. The management of brainstem gliomas in patients with neurofibromatosis 1. Neurology. 1996;46(6):1652–60.
15. Donaldson SS, Laningham F, Fisher PG. Advances toward an understanding of brainstem gliomas. J Clin Oncol. 2006;24(8):1266–72.
16. Grimm SA, Chamberlain MC. Brainstem glioma: a review. Curr Neurol Neurosci Rep. 2013;13(5):346.
17. Hennika T, Becher OJ. Diffuse intrinsic pontine glioma: time for cautious optimism. J Child Neurol. 2016;31(12):1377–85.
18. Barkovich AJ, Krischer J, Kun LE, Packer R, Zimmerman RA, Freeman CR, et al. Brain stem gliomas: a classification system based on magnetic resonance imaging. Pediatr Neurosurg. 1990;16(2):73–83.
19. Morais BA, Solla DJF, Matushita H, Teixeira MJ, Monaco BA. Pediatric intrinsic brainstem lesions: clinical, imaging, histological characterization, and predictors of survival. Childs Nerv Syst. 2020;36(5):933–9.
20. Poussaint TY, Vajapeyam S, Ricci KI, Panigrahy A, Kocak M, Kun LE, et al. Apparent diffusion coefficient histogram metrics correlate with survival in diffuse intrinsic pontine glioma: a report from the Pediatric Brain Tumor Consortium. Neuro Oncol. 2016;18(5):725–34.
21. Padma MV, Said S, Jacobs M, Hwang DR, Dunigan K, Satter M, et al. Prediction of pathology and survival by FDG PET in gliomas. J Neuro Oncol. 2003;64(3):227–37.
22. Zukotynski KA, Fahey FH, Kocak M, Alavi A, Wong TZ, Treves ST, et al. Evaluation of 18F-FDG PET and MRI associations in pediatric diffuse intrinsic brain stem glioma: a report from the Pediatric Brain Tumor Consortium. J Nucl Med. 2011;52(2):188–95.
23. Zukotynski KA, Vajapeyam S, Fahey FH, Kocak M, Brown D, Ricci KI, et al. Correlation of (18)F-FDG PET and MRI apparent diffusion coefficient histogram metrics with survival in

diffuse intrinsic pontine glioma: a report from the Pediatric Brain Tumor Consortium. J Nucl Med. 2017;58(8):1264–9.

24. Recinos PF, Sciubba DM, Jallo GI. Brainstem tumors: where are we today? Pediatr Neurosurg. 2007;43(3):192–201.

25. Kakkar C, Kakkar S, Saggar K, Goraya JS, Ahluwalia A, Arora A. Paediatric brainstem: a comprehensive review of pathologies on MR imaging. Insights Imaging. 2016;7(4):505–22.

26. Fukuoka K, Yanagisawa T, Watanabe Y, Suzuki T, Shirahata M, Adachi J, et al. Brainstem oligodendroglial tumors in children: two case reports and review of literatures. Childs Nerv Syst. 2015;31(3):449–55.

27. Sadighi ZS, Curtis E, Zabrowksi J, Billups C, Gajjar A, Khan R, et al. Neurologic impairments from pediatric low-grade glioma by tumor location and timing of diagnosis. Pediatr Blood Cancer. 2018;65(8):e27063.

28. Donson AM, Kleinschmidt-DeMasters BK, Aisner DL, Bemis LT, Birks DK, Levy JM, et al. Pediatric brainstem gangliogliomas show BRAF(V600E) mutation in a high percentage of cases. Brain Pathol. 2014;24(2):173–83.

29. Lassaletta A, Zapotocky M, Mistry M, Ramaswamy V, Honnorat M, Krishnatry R, et al. Therapeutic and prognostic implications of BRAF V600E in pediatric low-grade gliomas. J Clin Oncol. 2017;35(25):2934–41.

30. Ahmed KA, Laack NN, Eckel LJ, Orme NM, Wetjen NM. Histologically proven, low-grade brainstem gliomas in children: 30-year experience with long-term follow-up at Mayo Clinic. Am J Clin Oncol. 2014;37(1):51–6.

31. Klimo P Jr, Nesvick CL, Broniscer A, Orr BA, Choudhri AF. Malignant brainstem tumors in children, excluding diffuse intrinsic pontine gliomas. J Neurosurg Pediatr. 2016;17(1):57–65.

32. Mistry M, Zhukova N, Merico D, Rakopoulos P, Krishnatry R, Shago M, et al. BRAF mutation and CDKN2A deletion define a clinically distinct subgroup of childhood secondary high-grade glioma. J Clin Oncol. 2015;33(9):1015–22.

33. Khuong-Quang DA, Buczkowicz P, Rakopoulos P, Liu XY, Fontebasso AM, Bouffet E, et al. K27M mutation in histone H3.3 defines clinically and biologically distinct subgroups of pediatric diffuse intrinsic pontine gliomas. Acta Neuropathol. 2012;124(3):439–47.

34. Mikaela Porkholm AR, Vainionpää R, Salonen T, Hernesniemi J, Valanne L, Satopää J, Karppinen A, Oinas M, Tynninen O, Pentikäinen V, Kivivuori S-M. Molecular alterations in pediatric brainstem gliomas. Pediatr Blood Cancer. 2018;65(1):e26751.

35. Chang EK, Smith-Cohn MA, Tamrazi B, Ji J, Krieger M, Holdhoff M, et al. IDH-mutant brainstem gliomas in adolescent and young adult patients: report of three cases and review of the literature. Brain Pathol. 2021;31(4):e12959.

36. Chiang J, Harreld JH, Tinkle CL, Moreira DC, Li X, Acharya S, et al. A single-center study of the clinicopathologic correlates of gliomas with a MYB or MYBL1 alteration. Acta Neuropathol. 2019;138(6):1091–2.

37. Louis DN, Perry A, Reifenberger G, von Deimling A, Figarella-Branger D, Cavenee WK, et al. The 2016 World Health Organization classification of tumors of the central nervous system: a summary. Acta Neuropathol. 2016;131(6):803–20.

38. Khatua S, Moore KR, Vats TS, Kestle JR. Diffuse intrinsic pontine glioma-current status and future strategies. Childs Nerv Syst. 2011;27(9):1391–7.

39. Epstein F, McCleary EL. Intrinsic brain-stem tumors of childhood: surgical indications. J Neurosurg. 1986;64(1):11–5.

40. Coffey RJ, Lunsford LD. Diagnosis and treatment of brainstem mass lesions by CT-guided stereotactic surgery. Appl Neurophysiol. 1985;48(1–6):467–71.

41. Thomas DG, Bradford R, Gill S, Davis CH. Computer-directed stereotactic biopsy of intrinsic brain stem lesions. Br J Neurosurg. 1988;2(2):235–40.

42. Albright AL, Packer RJ, Zimmerman R, Rorke LB, Boyett J, Hammond GD. Magnetic resonance scans should replace biopsies for the diagnosis of diffuse brain stem gliomas: a report from the Children's Cancer Group. Neurosurgery. 1993;33(6):1026–9; discussion 9–30.

43. Chiang J, Diaz AK, Makepeace L, Li X, Han Y, Li Y, et al. Clinical, imaging, and molecular analysis of pediatric pontine tumors lacking characteristic imaging features of DIPG. Acta Neuropathol Commun. 2020;8(1):57.
44. Walker DA, Liu J, Kieran M, Jabado N, Picton S, Packer R, et al. A multi-disciplinary consensus statement concerning surgical approaches to low-grade, high-grade astrocytomas and diffuse intrinsic pontine gliomas in childhood (CPN Paris 2011) using the Delphi method. Neuro Oncol. 2013;15(4):462–8.
45. Gupta N, Goumnerova LC, Manley P, Chi SN, Neuberg D, Puligandla M, et al. Prospective feasibility and safety assessment of surgical biopsy for patients with newly diagnosed diffuse intrinsic pontine glioma. Neuro Oncol. 2018;20(11):1547–55.
46. Gupta M, Chan TM, Santiago-Dieppa DR, Yekula A, Sanchez CE, Elster JD, et al. Robot-assisted stereotactic biopsy of pediatric brainstem and thalamic lesions. J Neurosurg Pediatr. 2021;27(3):317–24.
47. Dellaretti M, Reyns N, Touzet G, Dubois F, Gusmao S, Pereira JL, et al. Stereotactic biopsy for brainstem tumors: comparison of transcerebellar with transfrontal approach. Stereotact Funct Neurosurg. 2012;90(2):79–83.
48. Wang ZJ, Rao L, Bhambhani K, Miller K, Poulik J, Altinok D, et al. Diffuse intrinsic pontine glioma biopsy: a single institution experience. Pediatr Blood Cancer. 2015;62(1):163–5.
49. Rajshekhar V, Moorthy RK. Status of stereotactic biopsy in children with brain stem masses: insights from a series of 106 patients. Stereotact Funct Neurosurg. 2010;88(6):360–6.
50. Pirotte BJ, Lubansu A, Massager N, Wikler D, Goldman S, Levivier M. Results of positron emission tomography guidance and reassessment of the utility of and indications for stereotactic biopsy in children with infiltrative brainstem tumors. J Neurosurg. 2007;107(5 Suppl):392–9.
51. Pincus DW, Richter EO, Yachnis AT, Bennett J, Bhatti MT, Smith A. Brainstem stereotactic biopsy sampling in children. J Neurosurg. 2006;104(2 Suppl):108–14.
52. Phi JH, Chung HT, Wang KC, Ryu SK, Kim SK. Transcerebellar biopsy of diffuse pontine gliomas in children: a technical note. Childs Nerv Syst. 2013;29(3):489–93.
53. Dellaretti M, Touzet G, Reyns N, Dubois F, Gusmao S, Pereira JL, et al. Correlation among magnetic resonance imaging findings, prognostic factors for survival, and histological diagnosis of intrinsic brainstem lesions in children. J Neurosurg Pediatr. 2011;8(6):539–43.
54. Puget S, Beccaria K, Blauwblomme T, Roujeau T, James S, Grill J, et al. Biopsy in a series of 130 pediatric diffuse intrinsic pontine gliomas. Childs Nerv Syst. 2015;31(10):1773–80.
55. Jallo GI, Biser-Rohrbaugh A, Freed D. Brainstem gliomas. Childs Nerv Syst. 2004;20(3):143–53.
56. Mohme M, Fritzsche FS, Mende KC, Matschke J, Löbel U, Kammler G, et al. Tectal gliomas: assessment of malignant progression, clinical management, and quality of life in a supposedly benign neoplasm. Neurosurg Focus. 2018;44(6):E15.
57. Robertson PL, Muraszko KM, Brunberg JA, Axtell RA, Dauser RC, Turrisi AT. Pediatric midbrain tumors: a benign subgroup of brainstem gliomas. Pediatr Neurosurg. 1995;22(2):65–73.
58. Julian JAS, Álvarez PS, Lloret PM, Ramirez EP, Borreda PP, Asunción CB. Full endoscopic endonasal transclival approach: meningioma attached to the ventral surface of the brainstem. Neurocirugia. 2014;25(3):140–4.
59. Rady MR, Enayet AE, Refaat A, Taha H, Said W, Maher E, et al. Management and outcome of pediatric brainstem and cerebellar peduncular low-grade gliomas: a retrospective analysis of 62 cases. Childs Nerv Syst. 2022;38(3):565–75.
60. Cavalcanti DD, Preul MC, Kalani MY, Spetzler RF. Microsurgical anatomy of safe entry zones to the brainstem. J Neurosurg. 2016;124(5):1359–76.
61. Sala F, Lanteri P, Bricolo A. Motor evoked potential monitoring for spinal cord and brain stem surgery. Adv Tech Stand Neurosurg. 2004;29:133–69.
62. Oka H, Utsuki S, Tanizaki Y, Hagiwara H, Miyajima Y, Sato K, et al. Clinicopathological features of human brainstem gliomas. Brain Tumor Pathol. 2013;30(1):1–7.

63. Chou SC, Kuo MF, Lai DM, Chen CM, Xiao F, Tsuang FY, et al. Contemporary management of pediatric spinal tumors: a single institute's experience in Taiwan in the modern era. J Neuro Oncol. 2020;146(3):501–11.
64. Bejjani GK, Sekhar LN, Riedel CJ. Occipitocervical fusion following the extreme lateral transcondylar approach. Surg Neurol. 2000;54(2):109–15; discussion 15–6.
65. Sabbagh AJ, Alaqeel AM. Focal brainstem gliomas. Advances in intra-operative management. Neurosciences (Riyadh). 2015;20(2):98–106.
66. Teo C, Siu TL. Radical resection of focal brainstem gliomas: is it worth doing? Childs Nerv Syst. 2008;24(11):1307–14.
67. Klimo P Jr, Pai Panandiker AS, Thompson CJ, Boop FA, Qaddoumi I, Gajjar A, et al. Management and outcome of focal low-grade brainstem tumors in pediatric patients: the St. Jude experience. J Neurosurg Pediatr. 2013;11(3):274–81.
68. Roujeau T, Di Rocco F, Dufour C, Bourdeaut F, Puget S, Rose CS, et al. Shall we treat hydrocephalus associated to brain stem glioma in children? Childs Nerv Syst. 2011;27(10):1735–9.
69. Serra C, Ture U. The extreme anterior interhemispheric transcallosal approach for pure aqueduct tumors: surgical technique and case series. Neurosurg Rev. 2022;45(1):499–505.
70. Li KW, Roonprapunt C, Lawson HC, Abbott IR, Wisoff J, Epstein F, et al. Endoscopic third ventriculostomy for hydrocephalus associated with tectal gliomas. Neurosurg Focus. 2005;18(6A):E2.
71. Kobayashi N, Ogiwara H. Endoscopic third ventriculostomy for hydrocephalus in brainstem glioma: a case series. Childs Nerv Syst. 2016;32(7):1251–5.
72. Souweidane MM, Morgenstern PF, Kang S, Tsiouris AJ, Roth J. Endoscopic third ventriculostomy in patients with a diminished prepontine interval. J Neurosurg Pediatr. 2010;5(3):250–4.
73. Barajas RF Jr, Phelps A, Foster HC, Courtier J, Buelow BD, Gupta N, et al. Metastatic diffuse intrinsic pontine glioma to the peritoneal cavity via ventriculoperitoneal shunt: case report and literature review. J Neurol Surg Rep. 2015;76(1):e91–6.
74. Citrin DE. Recent developments in radiotherapy. N Engl J Med. 2017;377(11):1065–75.
75. Gallitto M, Lazarev S, Wasserman I, Stafford JM, Wolden SL, Terezakis SA, et al. Role of radiation therapy in the management of diffuse intrinsic pontine glioma: a systematic review. Adv Radiat Oncol. 2019;4(3):520–31.
76. Zaghloul MS, Eldebawy E, Ahmed S, Mousa AG, Amin A, Refaat A, et al. Hypofractionated conformal radiotherapy for pediatric diffuse intrinsic pontine glioma (DIPG): a randomized controlled trial. Radiother Oncol. 2014;111(1):35–40.
77. Clark KN, Ashford JM, Pai Panandiker AS, Klimo P, Merchant TE, Billups CA, et al. Cognitive outcomes among survivors of focal low-grade brainstem tumors diagnosed in childhood. J Neuro Oncol. 2016;129(2):311–7.
78. Janssens GO, Gandola L, Bolle S, Mandeville H, Ramos-Albiac M, van Beek K, et al. Survival benefit for patients with diffuse intrinsic pontine glioma (DIPG) undergoing re-irradiation at first progression: a matched-cohort analysis on behalf of the SIOP-E-HGG/DIPG working group. Eur J Cancer. 2017;73:38–47.
79. Zamora PL, Miller SR, Kovoor JJ. Single institution experience in re-irradiation of biopsy-proven diffuse intrinsic pontine gliomas. Childs Nerv Syst. 2021;37(8):2539–43.
80. Lu VM, Welby JP, Mahajan A, Laack NN, Daniels DJ. Reirradiation for diffuse intrinsic pontine glioma: a systematic review and meta-analysis. Childs Nerv Syst. 2019;35(5):739–46.
81. Liu Z, Feng S, Li J, Cao H, Huang J, Fan F, et al. The survival benefits of surgical resection and adjuvant therapy for patients with brainstem glioma. Front Oncol. 2021;11:566972.
82. Upadhyaya SA, Koschmann C, Muraszko K, Venneti S, Garton HJ, Hamstra DA, et al. Brainstem low-grade gliomas in children-excellent outcomes with multimodality therapy. J Child Neurol. 2017;32(2):194–203.
83. Fried I, Hawkins C, Scheinemann K, Tsangaris E, Hesselson L, Bartels U, et al. Favorable outcome with conservative treatment for children with low grade brainstem tumors. Pediatr Blood Cancer. 2012;58(4):556–60.

84. Ruge MI, Kickingereder P, Simon T, Treuer H, Sturm V. Stereotactic iodine-125 brachytherapy for treatment of inoperable focal brainstem gliomas of WHO grades I and II: feasibility and long-term outcome. J Neuro Oncol. 2012;109(2):273–83.
85. Watson J, Romagna A, Ballhausen H, Niyazi M, Lietke S, Siller S, et al. Long-term outcome of stereotactic brachytherapy with temporary Iodine-125 seeds in patients with WHO grade II gliomas. Radiat Oncol. 2020;15(1):275.
86. Mizumoto M, Murayama S, Akimoto T, Demizu Y, Fukushima T, Ishida Y, et al. Long-term follow-up after proton beam therapy for pediatric tumors: a Japanese national survey. Cancer Sci. 2017;108(3):444–7.
87. Muroi A, Mizumoto M, Ishikawa E, Ihara S, Fukushima H, Tsurubuchi T, et al. Proton therapy for newly diagnosed pediatric diffuse intrinsic pontine glioma. Childs Nerv Syst. 2020;36(3):507–12.
88. Indelicato DJ, Rotondo RL, Uezono H, Sandler ES, Aldana PR, Ranalli NJ, et al. Outcomes following proton therapy for pediatric low-grade glioma. Int J Radiat Oncol Biol Phys. 2019;104(1):149–56.
89. Gagliardi F, De Domenico P, Snider S, Pompeo E, Roncelli F, Barzaghi LR, et al. Gamma knife radiosurgery as primary treatment of low-grade brainstem gliomas: a systematic review and metanalysis of current evidence and predictive factors. Crit Rev Oncol Hematol. 2021;168:103508.
90. Ekşi M, Yılmaz B, Akakın A, Toktaş ZO, Kaur AC, Demir MK, et al. Gamma knife treatment of low-grade gliomas in children. Childs Nerv Syst. 2015;31(11):2015–23.
91. Jakacki RI, Siffert J, Jamison C, Velasquez L, Allen JC. Dose-intensive, time-compressed procarbazine, CCNU, vincristine (PCV) with peripheral blood stem cell support and concurrent radiation in patients with newly diagnosed high-grade gliomas. J Neuro Oncol. 1999;44(1):77–83.
92. Chiang KL, Chang KP, Lee YY, Huang PI, Hsu TR, Chen YW, et al. Role of temozolomide in the treatment of newly diagnosed diffuse brainstem glioma in children: experience at a single institution. Childs Nerv Syst. 2010;26(8):1035–41.
93. Izzuddeen Y, Gupta S, Haresh KP, Sharma D, Giridhar P, Rath GK. Hypofractionated radiotherapy with temozolomide in diffuse intrinsic pontine gliomas: a randomized controlled trial. J Neuro Oncol. 2020;146(1):91–5.
94. Jansen MH, Veldhuijzen van Zanten SEM, van Vuurden DG, Huisman MC, Vugts DJ, Hoekstra OS, et al. Molecular drug imaging: (89)Zr-bevacizumab PET in children with diffuse intrinsic pontine glioma. J Nucl Med. 2017;58(5):711–6.
95. McCrea HJ, Ivanidze J, O'Connor A, Hersh EH, Boockvar JA, Gobin YP, et al. Intraarterial delivery of bevacizumab and cetuximab utilizing blood-brain barrier disruption in children with high-grade glioma and diffuse intrinsic pontine glioma: results of a phase I trial. J Neurosurg Pediatr. 2021;28(4):371–9.
96. El-Khouly FE, Veldhuijzen van Zanten SEM, Jansen MHA, Bakker DP, Sanchez Aliaga E, Hendrikse NH, et al. A phase I/II study of bevacizumab, irinotecan and erlotinib in children with progressive diffuse intrinsic pontine glioma. J Neuro Oncol. 2021;153(2):263–71.
97. Su JM, Murray JC, McNall-Knapp RY, Bowers DC, Shah S, Adesina AM, et al. A phase 2 study of valproic acid and radiation, followed by maintenance valproic acid and bevacizumab in children with newly diagnosed diffuse intrinsic pontine glioma or high-grade glioma. Pediatr Blood Cancer. 2020;67(6):e28283.
98. Crotty EE, Leary SES, Geyer JR, Olson JM, Millard NE, Sato AA, et al. Children with DIPG and high-grade glioma treated with temozolomide, irinotecan, and bevacizumab: the Seattle Children's Hospital experience. J Neuro Oncol. 2020;148(3):607–17.
99. Hummel TR, Salloum R, Drissi R, Kumar S, Sobo M, Goldman S, et al. A pilot study of bevacizumab-based therapy in patients with newly diagnosed high-grade gliomas and diffuse intrinsic pontine gliomas. J Neuro Oncol. 2016;127(1):53–61.
100. Kilburn LB, Kocak M, Decker RL, Wetmore C, Chintagumpala M, Su J, et al. A phase 1 and pharmacokinetic study of enzastaurin in pediatric patients with refractory primary

central nervous system tumors: a Pediatric Brain Tumor Consortium study. Neuro Oncol. 2015;17(2):303–11.

101. Broniscer A, Baker SD, Wetmore C, Pai Panandiker AS, Huang J, Davidoff AM, et al. Phase I trial, pharmacokinetics, and pharmacodynamics of vandetanib and dasatinib in children with newly diagnosed diffuse intrinsic pontine glioma. Clin Cancer Res. 2013;19(11):3050–8.

102. Pollack IF, Stewart CF, Kocak M, Poussaint TY, Broniscer A, Banerjee A, et al. A phase II study of gefitinib and irradiation in children with newly diagnosed brainstem gliomas: a report from the Pediatric Brain Tumor Consortium. Neuro Oncol. 2011;13(3):290–7.

103. Geoerger B, Hargrave D, Thomas F, Ndiaye A, Frappaz D, Andreiuolo F, et al. Innovative therapies for children with cancer pediatric phase I study of erlotinib in brainstem glioma and relapsing/refractory brain tumors. Neuro Oncol. 2011;13(1):109–18.

104. Broniscer A, Baker JN, Tagen M, Onar-Thomas A, Gilbertson RJ, Davidoff AM, et al. Phase I study of vandetanib during and after radiotherapy in children with diffuse intrinsic pontine glioma. J Clin Oncol. 2010;28(31):4762–8.

105. Pollack IF, Jakacki RI, Blaney SM, Hancock ML, Kieran MW, Phillips P, et al. Phase I trial of imatinib in children with newly diagnosed brainstem and recurrent malignant gliomas: a Pediatric Brain Tumor Consortium report. Neuro Oncol. 2007;9(2):145–60.

106. Vitanza NA, Biery MC, Myers C, Ferguson E, Zheng Y, Girard EJ, et al. Optimal therapeutic targeting by HDAC inhibition in biopsy-derived treatment-naïve diffuse midline glioma models. Neuro Oncol. 2021;23(3):376–86.

107. Homan MJ, Franson A, Ravi K, Roberts H, Pai MP, Liu C, et al. Panobinostat penetrates the blood-brain barrier and achieves effective brain concentrations in a murine model. Cancer Chemother Pharmacol. 2021;88(3):555–62.

108. Warren KE, Killian K, Suuriniemi M, Wang Y, Quezado M, Meltzer PS. Genomic aberrations in pediatric diffuse intrinsic pontine gliomas. Neuro Oncol. 2012;14(3):326–32.

109. Grill J, Puget S, Andreiuolo F, Philippe C, MacConaill L, Kieran MW. Critical oncogenic mutations in newly diagnosed pediatric diffuse intrinsic pontine glioma. Pediatr Blood Cancer. 2012;58(4):489–91.

110. Zarghooni M, Bartels U, Lee E, Buczkowicz P, Morrison A, Huang A, et al. Whole-genome profiling of pediatric diffuse intrinsic pontine gliomas highlights platelet-derived growth factor receptor alpha and poly (ADP-ribose) polymerase as potential therapeutic targets. J Clin Oncol. 2010;28(8):1337–44.

111. Cacciotti C, Choi J, Alexandrescu S, Zimmerman MA, Cooney TM, Chordas C, et al. Immune checkpoint inhibition for pediatric patients with recurrent/refractory CNS tumors: a single institution experience. J Neuro Oncol. 2020;149(1):113–22.

112. Benitez-Ribas D, Cabezón R, Flórez-Grau G, Molero MC, Puerta P, Guillen A, et al. Immune response generated with the administration of autologous dendritic cells pulsed with an allogenic tumoral cell-lines lysate in patients with newly diagnosed diffuse intrinsic pontine glioma. Front Oncol. 2018;8:127.

113. Mueller S, Taitt JM, Villanueva-Meyer JE, Bonner ER, Nejo T, Lulla RR, et al. Mass cytometry detects H3.3K27M-specific vaccine responses in diffuse midline glioma. J Clin Invest. 2020;130(12):6325–37.

114. Majzner RG, Ramakrishna S, Yeom KW, Patel S, Chinnasamy H, Schultz LM, et al. GD2-CAR T cell therapy for H3K27M-mutated diffuse midline gliomas. Nature. 2022;603(7903):934–41.

115. Doolittle ND, Muldoon LL, Culp AY, Neuwelt EA. Delivery of chemotherapeutics across the blood-brain barrier: challenges and advances. Adv Pharmacol. 2014;71:203–43.

116. Chen KT, Chai WY, Lin YJ, Lin CJ, Chen PY, Tsai HC, et al. Neuronavigation-guided focused ultrasound for transcranial blood-brain barrier opening and immunostimulation in brain tumors. Sci Adv. 2021;7(6):eabd0772.

117. Souweidane MM, Kramer K, Pandit-Taskar N, Zhou Z, Haque S, Zanzonico P, et al. Convection-enhanced delivery for diffuse intrinsic pontine glioma: a single-centre, dose-escalation, phase 1 trial. Lancet Oncol. 2018;19(8):1040–50.

# Chapter 12
# Surgery for Central Nervous System Tuberculosis in Children

**Dattatraya Muzumdar, Puru Bansal, Survender Rai, and Kushal Bhatia**

## Contents




D. Muzumdar (✉) · P. Bansal · S. Rai · K. Bhatia
Department of Neurosurgery, Seth Gordhandas Sunderdas Medical College and King Edward
VII Memorial Hospital, Mumbai, India



© The Author(s), under exclusive license to Springer Nature
Switzerland AG 2024
C. Di Rocco (ed.), *Advances and Technical Standards in Neurosurgery*,
Advances and Technical Standards in Neurosurgery 49,
https://doi.org/10.1007/978-3-031-42398-7_12

## 12.1  Introduction

Tuberculosis (TB) is a chronic granulomatous disease caused by acid-fast bacilli, of the *Mycobacterium tuberculosis* complex. The incidence of TB is on the decline in developed world, but the emergence of multi-drug resistant form of tuberculosis (MDR TB) is a worrisome threat due to its enhanced morbidity and mortality. Tuberculous meningitis and its sequelae, viz. vasculitis, arachnoiditis, direct parenchymal injury, and raised intracranial pressure, are responsible for its poor outcome [1, 2]. Extrapulmonary TB accounts for 10–15% of all TB cases in HIV negative patients, while it is 40–50% in HIV positive patients [3]. Musculoskeletal TB accounts for nearly 10% of extrapulmonary TB of which spinal TB is found in 50% of cases. Involvement of the spinal vertebrae, also known as Pott's disease, accounts for 1–2% of the world spinal deformity [4–6]. It can also result in complications, such as spinal arachnoiditis, intramedullary tuberculoma, and spinal cord compression from epidural abscess. The management algorithm for CNS tuberculosis is specific to the geographic area or institution. There are no specific international guidelines or studies that demonstrate the superiority of one treatment protocol over another.

## 12.2  Epidemiology

The global epidemiology of CNS-TB still remains unknown. Central nervous system (CNS-TB) has high morbidity and mortality. Low immunity, malnutrition, and overcrowding are the principal contributing factors in the developing world. The CNS-TB morbidity was influenced mainly by country's TB burden, Human Development Index, and prevalence of HIV. The estimated global prevalence of CNS-TB in the general population is 2 cases per 100,000 inhabitants and 8% in hospitalized patients. About 15% of the cases are extrapulmonary. Children less than 5 years of age and those under immunosuppression have also a high risk of CNS-TB Tuberculous meningitis is the most common reported presentation is TB meningitis (ranging from 3% to 14%). The prevalence of TB meningitis in patients with meningitis of 14.63%, especially from high- and upper-middle-income countries who have relatively low TB burden. Tuberculoma is reported in few studies with a frequency of <1% [7].

## 12.3  Pathogenesis

*Mycobacterium tuberculosis* commonly causes CNS TB, although in immunocompromised patients other species may be involved. Following initial pulmonary infection, the tuberculous bacteria may enter the systemic circulation and subsequently reach the CNS, which is rich in oxygen establishing itself in the meninges, subpial, or subependymal regions of the brain or the spinal cord. It is known as the Rich focus, which may rupture into the subarachnoid space or ventricular system leading to meningitis. Alternatively, the meninges can be involved due to rupture of a tuberculoma into a vessel in the subarachnoid space, or rupture of miliary tubercles in disseminated TB. The brain can rarely be involved following contiguous spread of infection from the skull or paranasal sinuses. It forms dense, gelatinous, inflammatory exudates along the basal surface of the brain. In advanced cases, it may involve the leptomeninges over the cerebral convexities and extend into the ventricular system causing ependymitis and choroid plexitis [1, 2]. Several risk factors for CNS tuberculosis have been identified. Both children and HIV co-infected patients are at high risk for developing CNS tuberculosis. Other risk factors include malnutrition and recent measles in children and alcoholism, malignancies, and the use of immunosuppressive agents in adults studies conducted in developed countries have also identified that foreign-born individuals (individuals born outside of developed countries) are overrepresented among CNS tuberculosis cases [8].

## 12.4  Clinical Presentation

Central nervous system tuberculosis has varied clinical manifestations. The most common signs of brain tuberculosis include fever, headache, vomiting, and an altered sensorium. Neck rigidity and cranial nerve palsies are commonly seen [1, 2, 4–6, 9]. Variable degrees of encephalitis, hydrocephalus, and infarction are responsible for altered sensorium in patients with tuberculous meningitis (TBM). In contrast to TBM, patients with brain tuberculomas without TBM most often do not have fever. Focal deficits may occur in the forms of mild to total weakness of the limbs or varying degrees of cranial nerve paresis. Among the cranial nerves, the abducens and oculomotor nerves are frequently involved. Patients with tuberculomas usually present with headache, seizures, focal neurologic deficit, and features of raised intracranial tension. Infratentorial tuberculomas may present with brainstem syndromes, cerebellar symptoms, and multiple cranial nerve palsies [10]. Fever is not a prominent symptom. Hydrocephalus has been described as a marker of visual impairment. Tuberculous abscesses have an acute clinical presentation and a more rapidly deteriorating course than tuberculomas, with symptoms of fever, headache, and focal neurologic signs. Calvarial TB commonly presents as a scalp swelling with or without a discharging sinus and pain. Rarely the patient may present with seizures or motor deficit. Spinal cord tuberculosis presents as tuberculous radiculomyelopathy due to adhesive arachnoiditis or tuberculous myelitis. It may also present with features of syringomyelia with dissociative sensory loss and multilevel flaccid paresis.

## 12.5 Clinical Subtypes

### 12.5.1 *Calvarial Tuberculosis*

Calvarial tuberculosis is rare, even in areas where tuberculosis is endemic because of paucity of lymphatics in the calvarial bone [11, 12]. Younger population is at higher risk to develop calvarial tuberculosis, and it is rare in infancy. The disease might be limited or there may be widespread destruction of the inner table with abundant extradural granulation tissue in the form of pachymeningitis externa [13, 14]. The most common sites of involvement are frontal and parietal bones as both the bones have large amount of cancellous bone [13–17]. In circumscribed and sclerotic type, there is marked thickening of the bone because of lack of blood supply to the diseased bone.

Plain X-ray of the skull can be helpful. Areas of rarefaction are seen early in the disease, which develop into punched-out defects with a central sequestrum later on [15]. Both osteolytic and osteoblastic areas may be seen. Rarely, sclerosis may be seen and indicates secondary infection. CT scan of the brain is helpful in assessing the extent of bone destruction, scalp swelling, and degree of intracranial involvement (Fig. 12.1) [15, 16, 18]. Another infection of the skull, namely, melioidosis caused by *Burkholderia pseudomallei,* can cause symptoms and signs having radiological features similar to that of calvarial tuberculosis. Other differential diagnoses include eosinophilic granuloma and unusual tumors such as Ewing's sarcoma.

Combination of surgical excision and anti-tubercular therapy is the preferred treatment. Surgery is indicated to establish the diagnosis, obtain pus and tissue for culture and sensitivity studies, to remove thick extradural granulation tissue and necrotic bone and in patients with sinus discharge, intracranial extensions and large collections of caseating material causing mass effect [11–17].

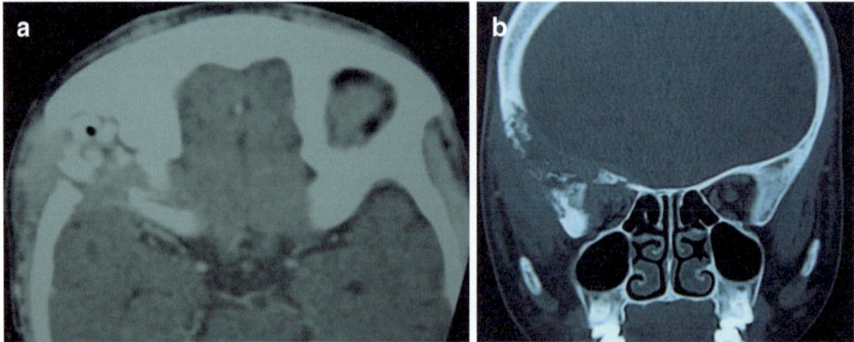

**Fig. 12.1** Erosion of the right lesser and greater wings of sphenoid bone associated with overlying scalp swelling suggestive of Calvarial Koch. (**a**) Axial T1-weighted contrast image. (**b**) Coronal bone window reconstruction image

## 12.5.2  Tuberculous Meningitis

TBM in developing countries is more common among infants and children. TBM is the most lethal manifestation of extrapulmonary tuberculosis, which accounts for hospital mortality up to 50% in those treated for drug susceptible TBM and 5-year mortality rate of 58% [19, 20]. The basal exudates cause abnormal meningeal enhancement and obstruction to cerebrospinal fluid (CSF) flow, causing hydrocephalus. It can also result in obliterative vasculitis due to occlusion of blood vessels at the base of the brain [21, 22]. The complications of meningitis include infarction, vasculitis, hydrocephalus, hyponatremia, cranial nerve involvement, and associated multiple tuberculomas [22]. On clinical suspicion of TBM, cerebrospinal fluid (CSF) examination is the initial modality of investigation [22]. Diagnosis of TBM is categorized as definite or probable. Definitive diagnosis of TBM depends upon the detection of the tubercle bacilli in the CSF, either by smear examination or by bacterial culture [9, 23, 24]. The predominance of cerebrospinal fluid lymphocytosis (>50% of the cells) is highly suggestive of TBM. It is seen in 80–83% of patients with TBM. Low levels of cerebrospinal fluid glucose and elevated levels of protein are also seen. TBM is a paucibacillary disease and yield of culture studies are low. AFB may be seen in 20–90% of cases when centrifuged CSF is tested. The polymerase chain reaction (GeneXpert test) allows for a rapid and specific diagnosis of TBM [23]. The yield of positive mycobacterial cultures from CSF in TBM varies from 19% to 70% [9, 24, 25].

Molecularly based techniques include commercially available nucleic acid amplification (NAA) methods and other polymerase chain reaction (PCR) based methods, antibody detection, antigen detection, or chemical assays such as adenosine deaminase (ADA) and tuberculostearic acid measurements [26]. Commercial nucleic acid amplification (NAA) assays for the diagnosis of TBM are 56% sensitive and 98% specific and the diagnostic yield of NAA increases when large volumes of CSF are processed. The sensitivity of CSF microscopy and culture falls rapidly after the start of treatment, whereas mycobacterial DNA may remain detectable within the CSF until 1 month after the start of treatment. The measured sensitivities and specificities of ADA in the CSF range from 44% to 100% and 71% to 100%, respectively. Standardized cutoffs of ADA values for the diagnosis of TBM have not been established, and the values used in various studies ranged from >5.0 to >15 IU/L. It is helpful in predicting poor neurological outcomes among pediatric TBM cases [27, 28]. A raised ADA activity in the CSF of patients with CNS TB lacks specificity. CSF ADA activity is not recommended as a routine diagnostic test for CNS tuberculosis. Tuberculostearic acid has good sensitivity, but requirement of expensive equipment has limited its clinical use [28]. The diagnostic utility of skin testing has been reported to be positive for CNS tuberculosis in 10–50% of patients with TBM.

Contrast enhanced computed tomography (CT) is the investigation of choice since it is easily available and can be quickly performed. It can depict the presence of hydrocephalus, infarcts, and basal exudates (classical "spider web" appearance seen in the suprasellar cisterns) [29]. The presence of periventricular lucency in isolation can suggest ischemia but along with a rounded third ventricle is suggestive of interstitial edema and raised intracranial pressure syndrome. In some series, a normal CT scan has been reported in up to 5% of cases.

Hydrocephalus is a frequent accompaniment of TBM with the incidence varying between 50% and 80%. CT cannot predict the level of CSF block in TBM because both types of hydrocephalus can present with panventricular dilatation [29]. The presence of basal enhancement, hydrocephalus, tuberculoma, and infarction were more common in TBM than in children with pyogenic meningitis (Figs. 12.2, 12.3, and 12.4). They reported that basal enhancement, tuberculomas, or both were 100% specific and 89% sensitive for the diagnosis of TBM. Andronikou and colleagues suggested nine criteria for the diagnosis of TBM on computed tomography (CT). Przybojewski and colleagues evaluated these 9 criteria and showed high specificity for all the criteria, and 100% specificity for 4 individual criteria [29]. It has been shown that sensitivity was improved when more than one criterion was present. Presence of hyperdensity on precontrast scans in the basal cisterns might be the specific sign of TBM in children. The reported incidence of infarcts on CT varies from 20.5% to 38%.

Magnetic resonance (MR) imaging has been shown to be superior to CT in evaluating patients with suspected meningitis and its associated complications [30–32]. Noncontrast MR imaging shows little or no evidence of meningitis in early stages of the disease. Contrast-enhanced MR imaging shows abnormal meningeal enhancement in the basal cisterns and sylvian fissures (Fig. 12.3). The cerebral convexities show enhancement in severe and late-stage TBM. Tentorial and cerebellar meningeal involvement is less common. There could be minimal or absent meningeal enhancement in immunocompromised patients although some reports show no significant difference. The flow around fourth ventricle may not be easily appreciated. MR ventriculography has been used to evaluate CSF flow dynamics and in patients with hydrocephalus. MR imaging depicts hemorrhagic transformation of infarcts better. Multiple infarcts in the anterior circulation territory favored tuberculous etiology.

MR angiogram reveals small segmental narrowing, uniform narrowing of large segments, irregular beaded appearance of vessels, or complete occlusion with contrast enhanced MR being more sensitive to detect smaller vessels. The infarcts mostly involve thalamus, basal ganglia, and internal capsule regions. Diffusion-weighted MR imaging helps in early detection and delineating extent of infarction (Fig. 12.4). Magnetization transfer (MT) MR imaging is considered superior to conventional MR imaging for showing abnormal meninges [33]. It also helps in differentiating TBM from other causes of meningitis. The abnormal meninges appearing hyperintense on precontrast T1-weighted (T1W) MT images strongly suggest TBM. Radiograph/CT pneumoencephalography or contrast-enhanced cisternography may help in differentiating communicating and noncommunicating hydrocephalus [29–33].

**Fig. 12.2** Axial
postcontrast T1-weighted
image showing extensive
basal enhancement along
basal cisterns and cortical
subarachnoid spaces in
both hemispheres. There is
moderate hydrocephalus

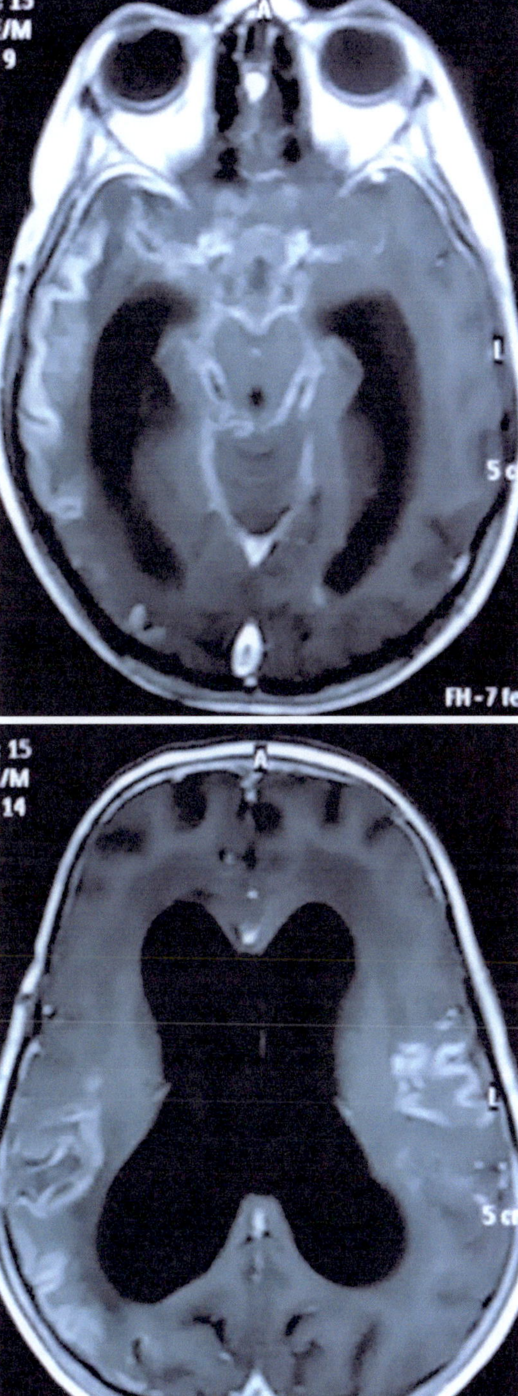

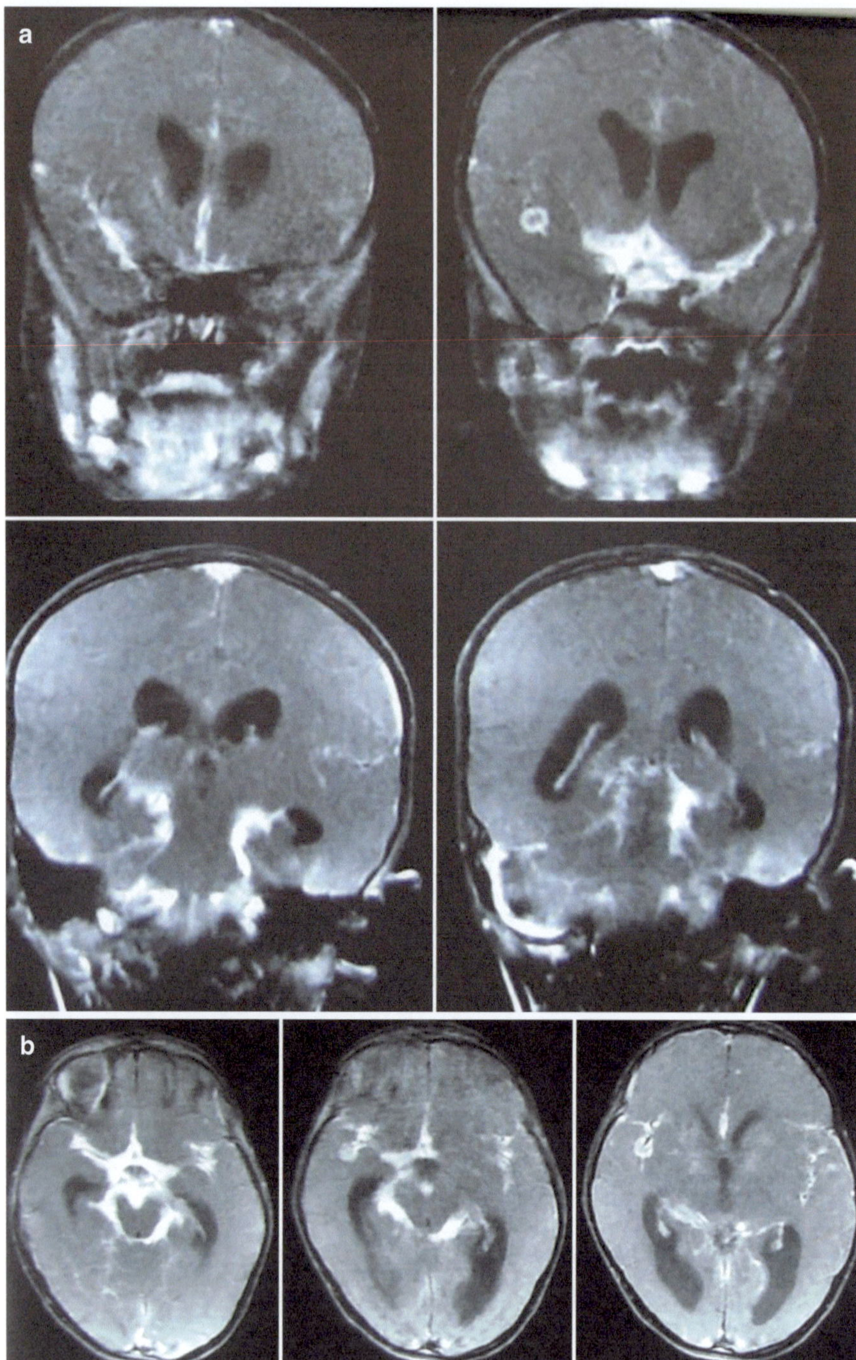

**Fig. 12.3** T1-weighted MR images showing basal exudates associated with tuberculoma. (**a**) Coronal MR image. (**b**) Axial MR image

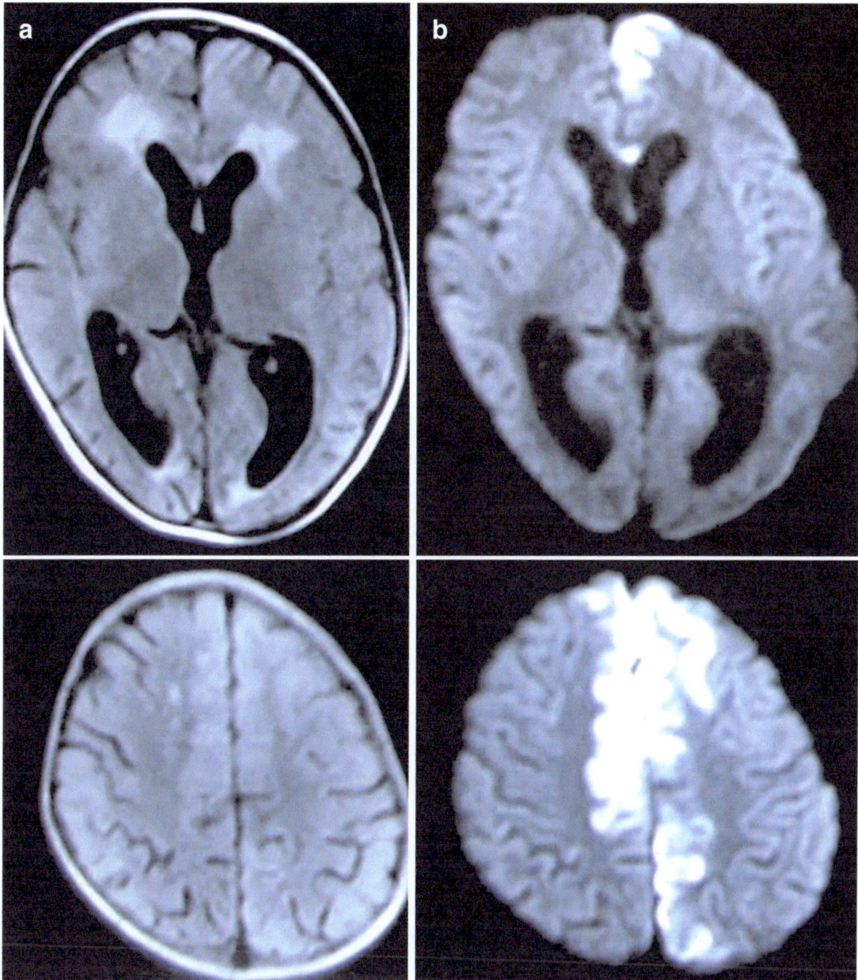

**Fig. 12.4** MR images showing infarction in bilateral parafalcine region. (**a**) Axial T2-Flair image. (**b**) Axial diffusion-weighted image showing restriction in bilateral parafalcine region

## 12.5.3 Treatment

The primary line of treatment for TBM is medical therapy with antituberculous multidrug chemotherapy [2, 9, 21, 23–25, 28, 34]. The primary drugs include rifampicin (10 mg/kg), isoniazid (5 mg/kg), ethambutol (20 mg/kg), streptomycin (20 mg/kg), or pyrazinamide (25 mg/kg) (3 or 4 drugs) for 3 months followed by isoniazid and rifampicin daily for the next 15 months. The therapy is prolonged and is continued for 18 months [2, 9, 21, 23–25, 34]. In certain situations like relapse, therapy can be continued for one more year. All patients with TBM may receive adjunctive corticosteroids regardless of disease severity at presentation [9, 21, 23–25, 28, 34].

Children can be given prednisolone 4 mg/kg/24 h (or equivalent dose dexamethasone: 0.6 mg/kg/24 h) for 4 weeks, followed by a tapering course over 4 weeks. It has been shown to significantly improve survival rate. They are withheld if the patient has also manifested with lung tuberculosis. Patients with multidrug-resistant (MDR) tuberculosis are administered second and third line of antituberculous drugs including kanamycin or ethionamide. Linezolid with high penetration of cerebrospinal fluid in short-term use has shown improved clinical outcome with two clinical trials (NCT03927313, NCT04021121) underway [35, 36]. Bedaquiline which has shown encouraging results in drug-resistant pulmonary TB, but its role in TBM is uncertain considering high protein binding of this drug which will limit its ability to cross blood brain barrier [37]. The liver and renal functions are closely monitored during the course of therapy. Visual charting is performed to detect abnormality with color vision. TBM carries very high risk of death 25% at 12 months after treatment of TBM. While TBM with HIV-positive status has mortality rate of 59% and those treated for drug-resistant TBM is 67% [38]. In spite of intensified regimens and use of newer drug mortality rate for those undergoing treatment for MDR-TBM ranges from 67% to 100% in literature [39, 40]. In short treatment of TBM remains suboptimal in spite of better newer drugs and diagnostic adjuncts/facilities.

### 12.5.3.1  Hyponatremia

Hyponatremia is common in TBM and is independently associated with worse outcome. In conjunction with raised intracranial pressure, it may contribute to poor outcome through worsening cerebral edema, and its surveillance and prevention are of paramount importance. It manifests either as syndrome of inappropriate ADH secretion (SIADH) or cerebral salt wasting syndrome (CSW) [22]. CSW is most often the cause of the hyponatremia [41]. It usually results from hypothalamic injury or inflammation. The mainstay of treatment for SIADH has been based on fluid restriction unless patients are severely symptomatic, in which case hypertonic saline is used. Diuretics and urea have been used. Demeclocycline has been used in chronic SIADH. The treatment of CSW revolves around fluid and sodium replacement because these patients develop hyponatremia in the setting of volume depletion [42, 43]. Most patients will respond within 3 days to therapy with fluid and sodium replacement. Central venous pressure monitoring can help guide the diagnosis and management of hyponatremia with natriuresis [42]. Fludrocortisone or hypertonic saline has yielded good results. Correction of chronic hyponatremia should be performed very slowly (<0.5 mM/h) to prevent central pontine myelinolysis [2, 22]. If hyponatremia is severe, it requires longer correction time affecting the prognosis of TBM patients.

### 12.5.3.2 Hydrocephalus

Hydrocephalus is a sequalae or complication of TBM [1, 2, 21, 22]. The inflammatory basal exudates cause obstruction to the CSF flow resulting in a communicating type of hydrocephalus in about 80% of the cases (Figs. 12.2 and 12.5). Noncommunicating or obstructive hydrocephalus can occur either because of obstruction of fourth ventricular outlet foramina by the exudates or when there is obstruction of the aqueduct either due to a strangulation of the brain stem by exudates or by a subependymal tuberculoma. Trapped or loculated ventricle is also seen due to entrapment of a part of a ventricle by ependymitis. Sometimes, there is a combination of noncommunicating (obstructive) and communicating (defective absorption) hydrocephalus, which may be difficult to treat. Defective CSF absorption can be a cause of failure of endoscopic third ventriculostomy (ETV). About 50% of patients with TBM have evidence of active or healed pulmonary tuberculosis on chest radiographs; 10% have miliary disease, which is strongly associated with CNS involvement [21, 24].

Patients with symptomatic hydrocephalus or radiologically worsening hydrocephalus benefit from CSF diversion procedures. The Modified Vellore grading system is reproducible across different levels of clinical expertise and more reliable system. Both grading systems correlate well with outcome and prognostication.

Medical management with tapering doses of steroids and decongestants including acetazolamide (100 mg/kg) and frusemide (1 mg/kg) can be tried for a few days or a week in patients in grades I and II [44]. Grade II and grade III patients should be monitored closely during this period to detect any worsening or lack of improvement and a shunt should be promptly offered in case of failure of medical management. In good grade patients, prolonging medical therapy could be harmful and may lead to irreversible brain damage. Grade IV patients should undergo external ventricular drainage and shunt should be inserted if they show neurological improvement [44, 45]. Ventricular tap is sometimes indicated as an emergency measure to assess and reduce the CSF pressure and stabilize the neurological condition. It can also yield ventricular CSF for exam. Serial ventricular tap every 6–8 h can be done till definitive CSF diversion procedure is contemplated.

The initial choice of surgical procedure is ventriculoperitoneal (VP) shunt. Bhagwati et al. have observed that reduction in ICP and size of the ventricles is helpful to improve periventricular perfusion and enhance drug delivery to the tissues in a more effective manner [46, 47]. The complications of shunt surgery include shunt infection and shunt blockage requiring one or multiple revisions. Poor general condition of patient and high CSF protein and cellular content were responsible for frequent shunt blockages. Agrawal et al. reported shunt-related complications in 11 (30%) children and 3 of 37 children had to undergo multiple shunt revisions [48]. Palur et al. reported that 26 of 114 (22.8%) patients had to undergo one or more shunt revisions, 1 patient requiring more than 3 revisions [44]. Sil and Chatterjee reported a shunt infection rate of 15.6% and revision rate of 43.8% in their series of 37 children who underwent shunt surgery for TBM with hydrocephalus [49]. Multiple revisions were done in 18.7% of patients.

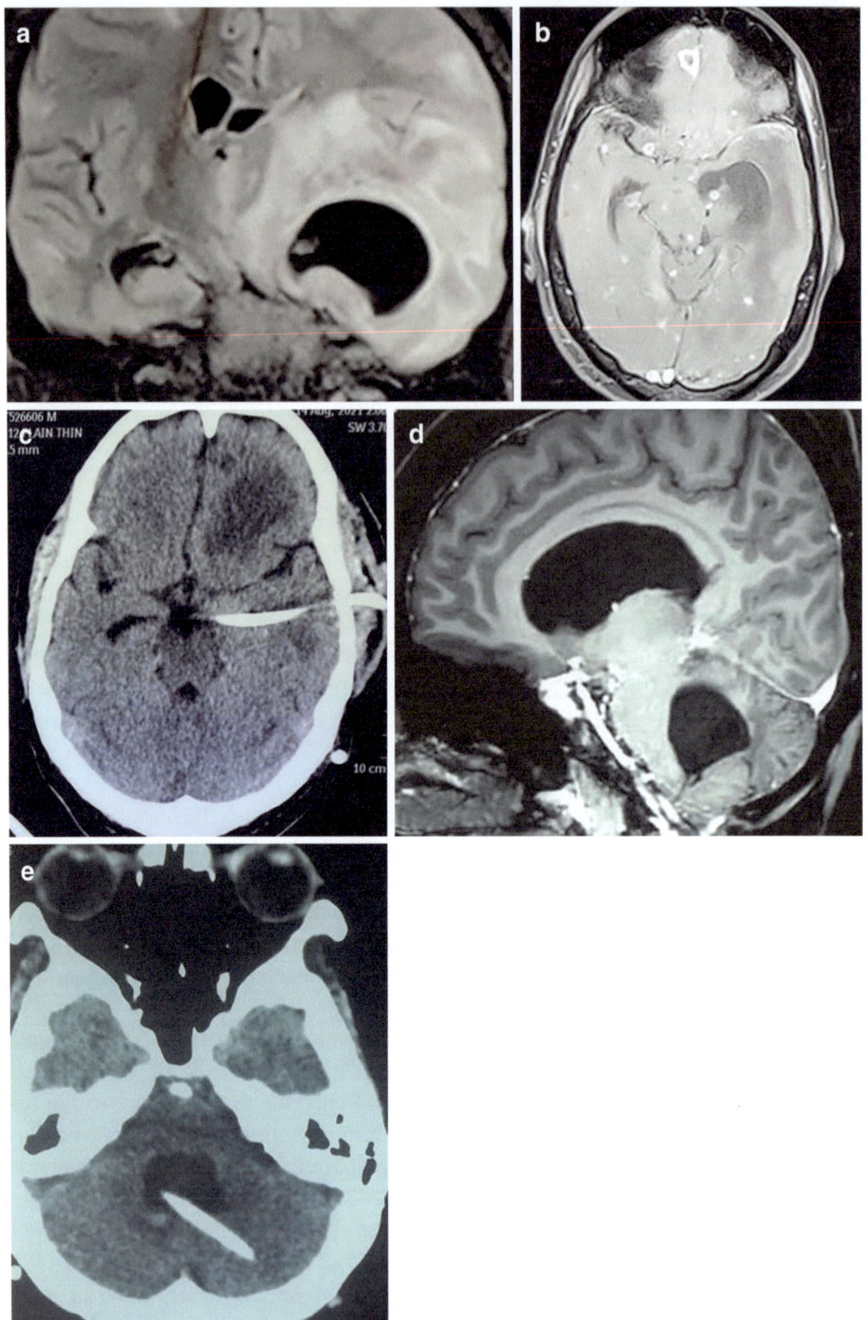

**Fig. 12.5** Entrapment of ventricular system causing trapped temporal horn and isolated fourth ventricle. (**a**) Coronal T1 Flair MR image showing trapped temporal horn and the perifocal edema in temporal brain and mass effect. (**b**) Axial T1-post contrast MR image showing multiple tiny tuberculosis with trapped temporal horn. (**c**) Axial plain CT brain showing ventricular catheter in the decompressed temporal horn. (**d**) Sagittal MR image showing enhancement along the clival dura and isolated fourth ventricle. (**e**) Axial plain CT brain showing ventricular catheter in decompressed fourth ventricle

Endoscopic third ventriculostomy is an option for patients who have completed at least 4 weeks of antituberculous therapy [50]. It is technically demanding and should be performed by a surgeon who is skilled in endoscopic procedures [50–55]. It is difficult to recognise anatomical landmarks since the floor of the third ventricle is frequently thick and the subarachnoid space is also likely to be obliterated by exudates in early stages of the disease [49, 56]. The basilar artery and its branches are at enhanced risk of injury. The tubercles and granulation tissue on the thick floor of third ventricle bleed when touched and obscure the endoscopic field. Patients with longer duration of symptoms and ATT were more likely to benefit from the ETV [51].

With the advent of effective antituberculous chemotherapy and steroids, the indication for surgery is infrequent [2, 9, 28]. Intrathecal hyaluronidase has been tried in children with communicating hydrocephalus but does not offer any particular advantage over shunt insertion in terms of regression of specific neurological deficit or overall functional improvement [57].

The factors contributing to poor outcome include cerebrovascular involvement with resultant cerebral ischemia, abscess formation, hydrocephalus and raised intracranial pressure, direct parenchymal injury, hyponatremia, seizures, and delayed diagnosis. The grade at presentation is the best and most consistent predictor of outcome following shunt surgery in patients with TBM. The presence of infarcts in the basal ganglia and internal capsule are also likely to indicate a poor outcome following shunting [2, 5, 9, 58–60].

### 12.5.3.3  Vasculitis

The inflammatory basal exudates are associated with vasculitis of the vessels in the subarachnoid spaces predominantly involving the small arterial branches of the arteries in the circle of Willis [27, 28]. The adventitia and media are affected initially and later the lumen of the vessel. It causes reactive subendothelial cellular proliferation leading to complete occlusion and thrombus formation. Middle cerebral and lenticulostriate arteries are the most common vessels involved.

### 12.5.3.4  Cranial Nerve Involvement

Cranial nerve involvement in TBM is variable and is seen in 17–70% of patients. It primarily occurs due to ischemia of the nerve or entrapment of the nerve in basal exudates causing neuritis or perineuritis or there may be a tuberculoma on the nerve within the subarachnoid course. The proximal portion of the nerve at root entry zone is usually affected. The brainstem nucleus of the nerve in proximity can be affected. Permanent loss of function can ensue in late stages due to fibrosis [1, 2, 4–6, 9].

### 12.5.3.5 Tuberculous Encephalitis and Encephalopathy

Tuberculous Encephalitis results from parenchymal inflammation adjacent to the meninges. It shows edema, perivascular infiltration, and a microglial reaction, known as border zone reaction. Tuberculous encephalopathy is a delayed type IV hypersensitivity reaction caused by tuberculous protein. It is a fulminant immunologic mechanism resulting in extensive damage to the white matter with perivascular demyelination. Infants and young children with pulmonary TB are commonly affected. There is a high incidence of mortality in these patients despite antituberculous medication [6, 9].

## 12.5.4 Tuberculous Pachymeningitis

Tuberculous pachymeningitis is rare in children. It is defined as a chronic inflammation causing focal or diffuse thickening of the dura mater resulting in fibrous constriction of the basal meninges [58, 61, 62]. It can cause obstructive hydrocephalus, venous hypertension, brain edema, and entrapment of lower cranial nerves. The clinical symptoms resemble migraine, including intense headaches, cranial nerve palsies, cerebellar symptoms, blindness, and optic neuropathy. MR imaging shows nodular or linear dural thickening with intense meningeal enhancement. Differential diagnosis would include connective tissue disorders or malignancies. Empirical antituberculous treatment can be considered in case of a positive history of tuberculosis elsewhere in the body. However in doubtful cases, a diagnostic biopsy would be helpful [58, 61]. Treatment options include antituberculous treatment and steroids with or without immunomodulating agents. The clinical outcome is variable and occasionally there may be steroid dependence [58, 61]. Surgical debulking is rarely needed [58, 61, 62].

### 12.5.4.1 Tuberculous Arachnoiditis

It is a known sequalae of tuberculous meningitis. It results due to organization of the exudates present in the interpeduncular, suprasellar, and sylvian cisterns. It is prominently seen in the optochiasmatic region, skull base, and spine [59, 60, 63]. High CSF protein content is often a risk factor for tuberculous arachnoiditis [3]. The treatment is challenging, and the response is generally unsatisfactory. Corticosteroids especially methyl prednisolone has been tried. Thalidomide and hyaluronidase have been used with variable success.

## *12.5.5 Post Tubercular Hydrocephalus*

The incidence of post tubercular hydrocephalus in children in most series ranges from 71% to 85% in children as compared to 12% in adults. It is usually of communicating type. According to Singh et al., the incidence of communicating hydrocephalus is 45.7% while non-communicating is 54.3%, while Sil et al. reported 78.1% communicating hydrocephalus and 21.9% noncommunicating type in their study [49, 56]. Bhagwati et al., in a study of 260 patients over a 10-year period, reported 80.6% incidence of communicating hydrocephalus [54].

The hydrocephalus in tuberculosis can be communicating or noncommunicating. The dense, thick basal exudates blocking the arachnoid cisterns can cause communicating hydrocephalus while the blockade of outlet of the fourth ventricle and the aqueduct can lead to obstructive hydrocephalus [64]. The inflammatory exudate extending to the ventricle may lead to choroid plexitis and cause increased CSF production. Secondary aqueductal obstruction can be caused by a strategically located tuberculoma or collar of exudates surrounding the brainstem leading to brainstem edema and displacement of the brainstem. A tuberculoma can cause fourth ventricular obstruction.

The diagnostic investigations include CT brain with contrast which is easily available, quick, avoiding the need for sedation or anesthetist, inexpensive, and can be performed even in unstable patients or patients with altered sensorium. An MRI brain with MR angiogram can depict abnormal meningeal enhancement in the basal cisterns and sylvian fissures as well as information about hydrocephalus (communicating and obstructive), tuberculomas, brainstem and basal ganglia vasculitis, edema, and infarcts (Figs. 12.2, 12.3 and 12.4). Cine MRI used as an adjunct with endoscopic procedures for TBH [53]. Dynamic invasive studies like air encephalography or CT ventriculogram or ICP monitoring are not widely used due to the invasiveness and poor correlation with clinical signs of raised ICP and degree of hydrocephalus [65].

The initial treatment options include pharmacotherapy of TB, steroids, and decongestants for raised intracranial pressure (ICP). It should be monitored closely and in event of progressive neurological deterioration and radiological progression, timely CSF diversion procedure is helpful in resolution of symptoms and determines long-term outcome. Post tubercular hydrocephalus can be complex and sometimes treatment can be frustrating.

## 12.6 Indications for Surgery

1. Grade I and II communicating hydrocephalus after adequate trial of medical therapy.
2. Rapid deterioration in patient's consciousness.
3. Radiological evidence of progressive enlargement of ventricles.

4. CSF Manometry suggesting progressive increase in intracranial pressure.
5. Obstructive pattern of hydrocephalus.


## 12.7 Pitfalls of Medical Therapy

Continuous monitoring of patient in hospital is required for a prolonged period of time, which increases costs and rapid deterioration may occur with poor outcome, especially if shunt is delayed.


## 12.8 Surgical Management

### 12.8.1 Shunt Surgery

Bhagwati et al. were among the first few to propagate the use of ventriculoatrial (VA) shunt for TBMH [46]. However, VA shunts had a higher risk of dissemination of the disease and possibility of venous thrombosis. Hence, ventriculoperitoneal (VP) shunts became popular since the early 1980s. The Indian Chhabra shunt (Surgiwear, India) is a low price device extensively used in Asia and Africa [48]. The shunt chamber is manually compressible and hence in suspected blockade, it can be pressed to increase the drainage and flush the proteinaceous debris. A shunt malfunction rate of 16% has been reported by Agrawal et al. which is lower than contemporary studies. Singh et al. studied 58 patients and strongly encouraged active intervention to lower raised ICP in patients who failed medical therapy [48, 56].

The indications for shunt surgery are symptomatic hydrocephalus with persistent raised intracranial pressure, radiology showing ventriculomegaly with periventricular ooze and clinical improvement following ventricular tapping.

Ventriculoperitoneal (VP) shunting for postmeningitic hydrocephalus has been a boon as well a nightmare for the neurosurgeons for its potential complications, which can be troublesome. Shunt blockade and shunt infection are two major causes of shunt malfunction. Shunt blockade can be due to increased proteins or cells in the CSF, peritoneal pseudocyst formation, and catheter perforation of the abdominal viscera. Shunt infection is usually due to breach in the aseptic barrier during surgery. A poor general condition and malnutrition due to the TBM are predisposing factors in these patients for infection. The risk of tuberculous dissemination is no longer feared. The incidence of shunt obstruction and shunt infection varies from 16% to 43% and 14% to 15.6%, respectively, in various reported case series. 18.7–22.8% patients require more than one shunt revisions [48, 56]. Antibiotic impregnated shunts are advocated by some groups but not supported by available literature so far. Shunt malfunction should also be suspected in tuberculous spinal arachnoiditis leading to acquired Chiari I malformation and syrinx [49].

Schoeman et al. based their management on ICP monitoring and air encephalogram [65]. Patients found to have noncommunicating hydrocephalus were directly subjected to normalization of ICP in 86% of children who were managed with shunt surgery as against 63% who were managed medically. However, shunt-related complications marred this success. Interestingly, Schoeman et al. found that the ventricular size reduction was significant in shunted patients after first month of treatment but identical to those treated with medical line of treatment at 6 months. There is also the question of how well the ventricular size reduction corresponds to resolution of raised ICP and ultimately improvement in clinical outcome [66]. In HIV-positive patients, a significant relationship is noted between the CD4 counts and outcomes. In a study of a group of 30 patients of TBM with hydrocephalus by Nadvi et al., 15 were HIV positive. They compared outcome between the two groups and reported poorer outcome and higher mortality in HIV-infected group after 1 month of shunt surgery and ATT [67]. They suggested that HIV-positive patients with TBM should undergo a trial of ventricular or lumbar CSF drainage. And only those who show an improvement following EVD should undergo shunt surgery. Asymmetric dilatation of the ventricular system due to meningeal inflammation, high CSF protein content, or ventriculitis is sometimes seen in case of tuberculous meningitis leading to entrapment of one or more ventricular compartment. Trapped temporal horn and isolated fourth ventricle are reported in literature, which require shunt surgery or an endoscopic intervention (Fig. 12.5).

## 12.9  Management of Tuberculoma and Associated Hydrocephalus

Most of the tuberculomas disappear or show substantial resolution on antituberculous treatment (Fig. 12.6). Surgery is rare because of effective antituberculous chemotherapy along with antiedema measures and dexamethasone. The current indications for surgery are large mass especially in the temporal lobe or posterior fossa, uncertain diagnosis in spite of latest advances in neuroimaging, and progressive raised intracranial pressure in spite of adequate medical treatment (Fig. 12.7). Bhagwati et al. reported on 31 children, of whom 5 needed surgical intervention, in 4 of them because they were thought to harbor brain tumors and in the fifth one because of significant mass effect in spite of treatment [25]. Subtotal removal may be done with the aim to establish the diagnosis and reduction of ICP, rather than attempting any radical removal.

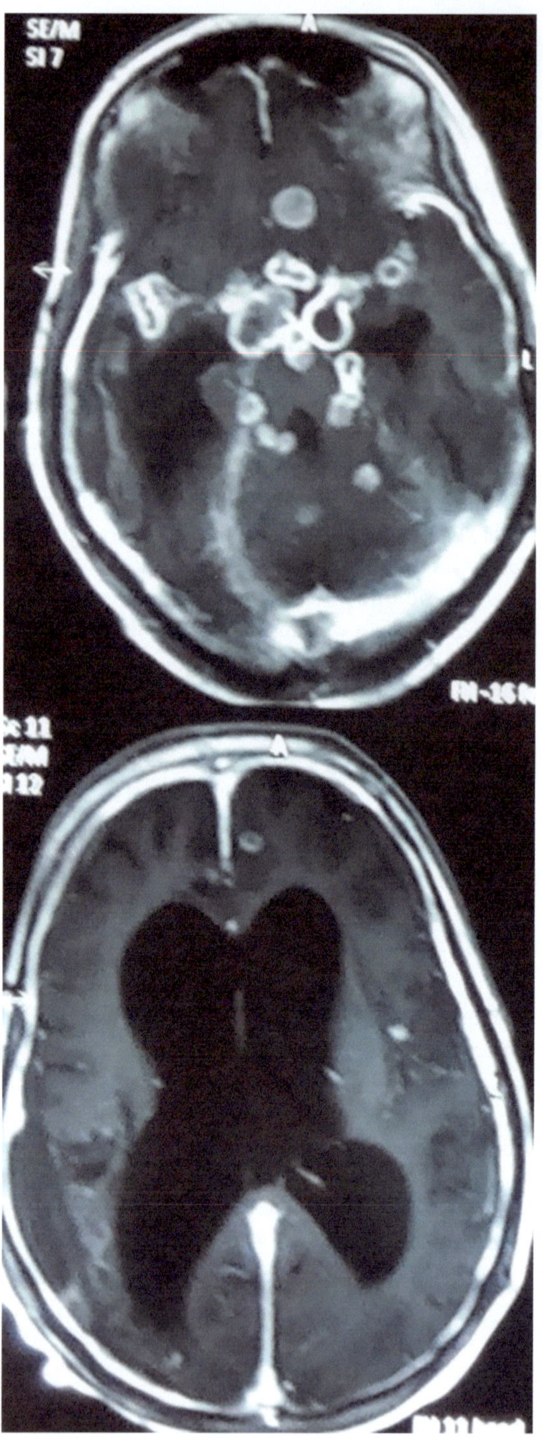

**Fig. 12.6** Axial T1-weighted post contrast MR image showing multiple tuberculomas with significant hydrocephalus

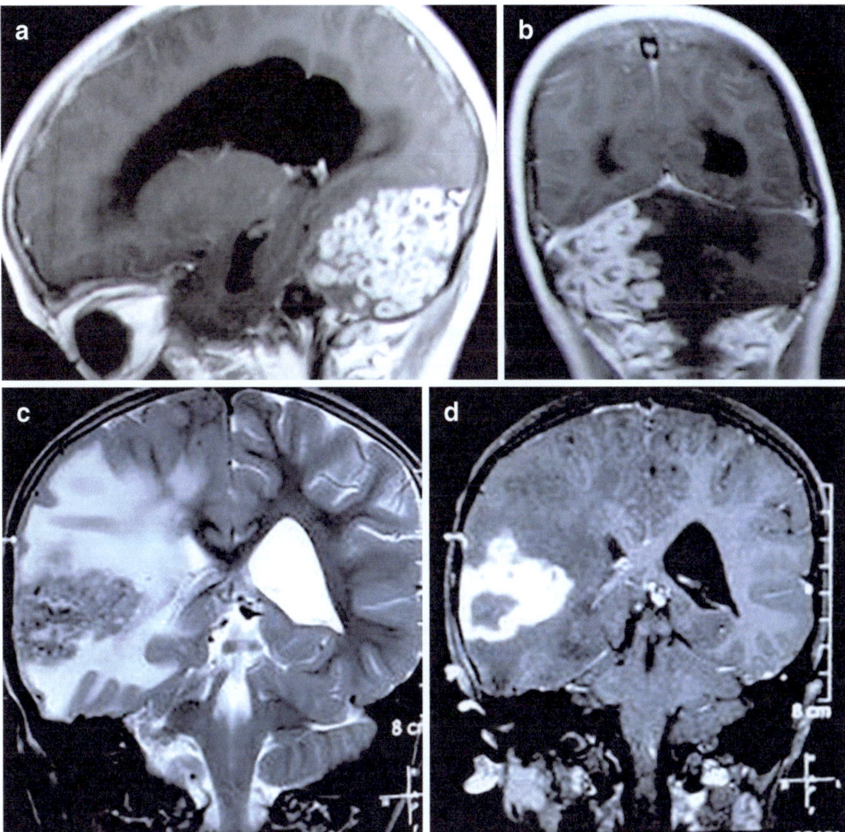

**Fig. 12.7** Large sized tuberculoma in the posterior and middle fossa. (**a**) Axial T1-weighted post contrast MR image showing conglomerate of multiple ring enhancing lesions in the right cerebellum. (**b**) Coronal T1-weighted post contrast MR image showing conglomerate of multiple ring enhancing lesions in the left cerebellum as well. (**c**) Axial T2-weighted MR image showing large hypointense lesion with surrounding extensive edema in the right temporal lobe. (**d**) Axial T1-weighted post contrast MR image showing thick irregular enhancement of the lesion

## 12.10 Endoscopic Interventions

Endoscopic third ventriculostomy (ETV) is now a well-established treatment modality for obstructive hydrocephalus with a success rate of 60–85% in most series [51, 68]. The first use of ETV in TBMH has been reported by Figaji et al., Jonathan et al., and Husain et al. [50, 68, 69]. ETV diverts the CSF to areas which were previously inaccessible and clears exudates from the areas which had impaired absorption [50, 68]. It also decreases the transventricular pressure gradient and the demyelination of periventricular brain parenchyma, which could contribute to some symptoms of hydrocephalus [70–72]. The improved CSF dynamics allow better penetration of antituberculous drugs. Alteration in CSF hemodynamics may also allow better drug delivery [50, 71] Figaji et al. described a simple methodology of success of ETV where entry of air in the ventricular system by lumbar puncture route has been considered a negative predictor due to communicating nature of hydrocephalus [73]. Chugh et al. concluded that endoscopic third ventriculostomy should be considered as the first surgical option for CSF diversion in patients with TBMH. They strongly advocated use of Cine MRI as noninvasive tool of assessment and for comparison postoperatively. They found that patients with chronic disease and longer duration of ATT administration responded well [53].

On the contrary, patients with higher stage of illness and cisternal exudates as observed intraoperatively had a poorer outcome. Singh et al. reported a 77% success rate of ETV—60% early and 17% delayed. They concluded presence of thin and transparent third ventricular floor to be a favorable prognostic indicator [54].

Thus, it seems that success of ETV mainly depends on thickness of third ventricular floor and favorable cisternal anatomy around the third ventricle in this disease [53]. However, TBMH is notorious for thick and almost fibrous exudates in the interpeduncular and the perimesencephalic cisterns. The floor of the third ventricle is frequently thick and the underlying subarachnoid space is often obliterated by exudates (Fig. 12.8). This also adds to the difficulty in identifying the anatomical landmarks and increases the risk of complications. ETV certainly eliminates the need for a shunt but is technically demanding. It should be done by an experienced neurosurgeon who has good training and expertise in ETV [55]. The most commonly reported complications of ETV are failure to perform the ETV due to anatomical distortions and CSF leaks [68].

In summary, ETV has a better success rate in chronic hydrocephalus with obstructive ventricular pattern in our experience in spite of technical difficulties. The role of aqueductoplasty is still unclear.

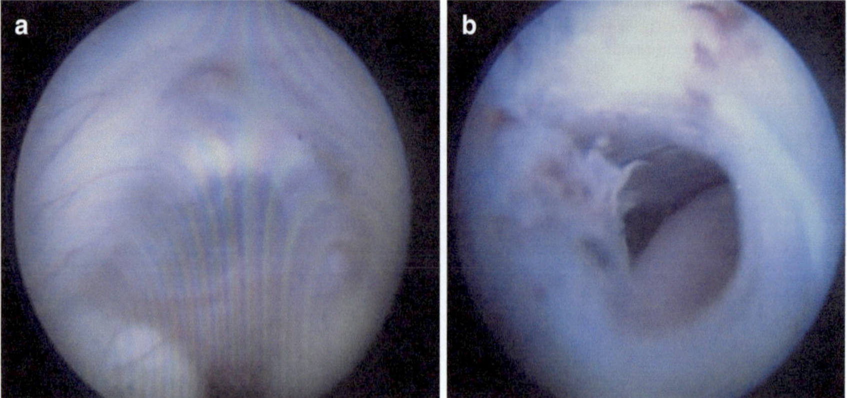

**Fig. 12.8** Endoscopic view of third ventricle floor. (**a**) Opaque third ventricular floor. (**b**) Endoscopic third ventriculostomy done piercing the third ventricular floor showing basilar artery prepontine cistern

Schoeman et al. adopted medical management as the first tier of treatment in patients with communicating hydrocephalus [66]. They were treated with ATT combined with acetazolamide and furosemide. At 1 month of follow-up, should the patient be diagnosed as "medical failure" he or she was subjected to shunt surgery. The lumbar CSF pressure does not correlate with ICP in patients with obstructive hydrocephalus and they are also at the risk of tonsillar herniation. These patients were directly taken up for shunt surgery.

ICP was assumed to have normalized if the following criteria were met:

1.  Normal lumbar CSF pressure, occasional B-waves permitted, and
2.  Ventricular size remaining the same or less and periventricular edema absent or markedly reduced (just visible) after first month.

## 12.11  Outcome Following Shunt Surgery and Endoscopic Third Ventriculostomy

Tubercular hydrocephalus has a high mortality and morbidity. Until 1991, the reported mortality rates for patients with altered sensorium ranged from 10.5% to 57.1% and for those with normal sensorium from 0% to 12.5% [74]. Bhagwati et al. reported mortality in three out of seven patients treated with shunt surgery [21]. Sil and Chatterjee reported that all patients who had a poor outcome following shunt surgery in their series of 37 children had evidence of infarcts on their CT scans [49].

Agrawal et al. reported good outcome in 16 (43%) out of 37 patients included in their study. They had an average follow-up period of 9 months (range 6–24 months). Thirteen (35%) had moderate disability and 6 (16%) had severe disability at 3 months follow-up. Children in grade II had the best results (62%) when compared with grade III patients (good outcome in 40%). All six children with grade IV disease had a poor outcome. Two children, both having multiple infarcts, died and the remaining four were left with severe disability [48].

Palur et al. reported 42.1% mortality with 55% of patients with good outcome or moderate disability. They reported that only admission grade was a statistically significant factor that affected the outcome [44]. The same group has shown that patients with basal ganglia and internal capsular infarcts are also known to have poorer outcome [74]. Modified Vellore grading system is a reliable system to predict outcome following shunt surgery in TBM with hydrocephalus [75]. Schoeman et al. reported that the mortality rate and degree of disability did not differ between patients whose ICP was normalized immediately (surgical group) and those with gradual normalization (medical group) [65]. The final neurological outcome depended on the extent of brain damage and neurological status at presentation.

The overall success rate of ETV in TBM hydrocephalus was 73.1% (19 patients) in a series of 26 patients [53]. The correlation with the stage of illness and presence of intracisternal exudates was statistically significant. They had reported better outcomes in patients who had received ATT for 4 weeks prior to ETV than in those operated earlier [53, 71]. Singh et al. reported a success rate of ETV in 77% of 35 patients of TBM with hydrocephalus [76]. The success rates were not related to the communicating or noncommunicating nature of hydrocephalus. However, the presence of a thin and transparent floor of the third ventricle seemed to be associated with higher success rate of 87%. Figaji et al. concluded that although ETV was technically possible in patients with TBM, only experienced surgeon should perform the surgery, as the procedure is more demanding than in other situations [51, 55, 69].

Early diagnosis of tubercular meningitis is vital for prevention of complications and sequelae. Progressive hydrocephalus should be monitored for timing of surgical intervention. Ventriculoperitoneal (VP) shunt remains the mainstay of treatment in TBMH. ETV is indicated in properly selected cases. Surgical intervention for hydrocephalus not only reduces intracranial pressure but also has independently shown to be useful for better penetration of drugs and reduction in vascular sequelae. Multidrug-resistant tuberculosis should be looked for and aggressively treated, though role of CSF diversion in these patients is not clear. Poor clinical grade has uniformly shown to be a negative predictor, but judicious evaluation of patients for surgery may improve outcome in some cases.

## 12.12 Tuberculoma

Tuberculomas are commonly seen in patients residing in endemic countries [10, 21–25, 34]. They can occur at any age. They can be solitary or multiple and can occur anywhere in the brain parenchyma [23, 25, 34]. In children, they predominate in the infratentorial compartment [10, 77]. Tuberculomas arise when tubercles in the parenchyma of brain enlarge without rupturing into the subarachnoid space. They are usually less than 2–5 mm in size. The occurrence of spinal intramedullary tuberculoma is rare [34, 78–80].

Imaging findings of tuberculoma depends on whether it is noncaseating or caseating with solid or liquid center. A solid noncaseating tuberculoma is isodense or slightly hypodense to the surrounding brain parenchyma on CT and hypointense on both T1W and T2W images on MR imaging. It shows homogeneous enhancement on contrast administration (Fig. 12.9). The cellular components of the noncaseating tuberculomas appear brighter on MT T1W imaging differentiating it from metastases, lymphomas, and other infective granulomas [29–32, 81]. The target sign, a central calcification or nidus surrounded by ring enhancement on postcontrast images, is considered pathognomonic of tuberculoma. Tuberculomas can mimic neurocysticercosis, fungal granulomas, and tumors like lymphomas, gliomas, and metastases. En plaque tuberculomas can mimic meningiomas. In a prospective study, the positive predictive value of CT based diagnosis of brain tuberculoma was found to be only 33% [82]. Newer imaging techniques, like diffusion imaging, MR spectroscopy (MRS) and MT imaging may help in differentiating these conditions [30–32, 81]. Tuberculomas shows a large cellular component appearing bright on

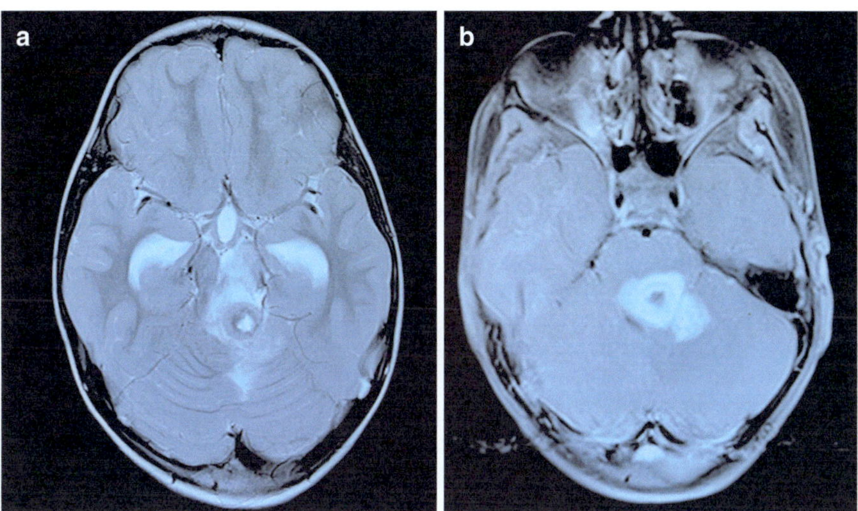

**Fig. 12.9** MR image in a 5-year-old child showing characteristic T2 shortening on T2-weighted images with contrast enhancement on T1 contrast images suggestive of a pontomesencephalic tuberculoma. (**a**) Axial T2-weighted MR image. (**b**) Axial T1-weighted post contrast MR image

MT imaging and with a choline peak on spectroscopy. Fluorodeoxyglucose (FDG) positron emission tomography can be helpful in differentiating an atypical tuberculoma from other neoplastic and non-neoplastic CNS lesions. It can also be used in the follow-up of tuberculomas.

The mainstay of therapy for a brain tuberculoma is antituberculous chemotherapy. Hence, empiric therapy for brain tuberculoma should be considered in selected cases who will comply with periodic clinical and imaging follow-up. The main indication for surgery in children with suspected brain tuberculomas is a doubtful diagnosis of tuberculoma. In patients with a reasonably certain diagnosis, surgical excision of tuberculomas or tuberculous abscess is otherwise generally performed when there is clinical deterioration following optimal medical therapy [23, 77–80, 82–86]. A total excision of the tuberculoma should only be attempted in cases where the tuberculoma is in a non-eloquent region of the brain such as the anterior frontal lobe, anterior temporal lobe or cerebellum. In eloquent and deep seated locations, a partial excision or a biopsy may suffice. A stereotactic biopsy may be a good option in children with deep seated suspected tuberculomas such as those in the thalamus, basal ganglia, and brain stem [87]. Intraventricular tuberculous abscess can cause acute obstructive hydrocephalus or subdural empyema that may necessitate a craniotomy. Biopsy confirmation may be warranted to establish diagnosis in cases of co-infection with HIV contributing to differential diagnosis. Anti-tuberculous drugs should be administered even after total excision of a brain tuberculoma for at least 12 months to sterilize the brain of any tuberculous bacteria. In other patients with a residual tuberculoma, the duration of therapy is dictated by the follow-up imaging findings. Presence of a significant enhancing mass with edema is an indication for continued therapy. Prolonged anti-tuberculous drug therapy (>24 months) is needed in patients who have multiple tuberculomas or tuberculomas larger than 2.5 cm. Surgical debulking of a tuberculoma may be useful to reduce the size to less than 2.5 cm and enable early resolution [7]. Some patients may require anti-tuberculous therapy for up to 4 years [83]. Rarely, a *decompressive surgery* may be needed as a lifesaving procedure in patients with multiple small tuberculomas with severe associated edema and raised intracranial pressure.

## 12.13 Paradoxical Response

There may be an increase in the size of a tuberculous while the patient is on antituberculous therapy which is described as paradoxical response [84]. This phenomenon is probably attributable to an immunological response, which leads to a temporary increase in the size of the lesion that later subsides with further therapy. It is difficult to distinguish paradoxical increase from lack of response to treatment. Paradoxical reaction with increase in the size and number of lesions can occur, usually in the first 3 months of treatment but can happen up to 2 years. In patients undergoing empiric treatment, biopsy confirmation becomes mandatory if the lesion shows growth while on ATT. In patients with a confirmed biopsy report, paradoxical reaction needs to be addressed with steroids, continuation of ATT and possible addition of new second line ATT if the lesion continues to grow [84].

The long-term outcome of patients with intracranial tuberculoma is good in drug sensitive TB with timely and appropriate management. Seizures can persist even after the complete resolution of the lesion in up to 20% of patients. Residual deficits might still be seen in about 20% of patients. Anti-epileptic drugs might be required for several years in these patients. Tuberculoma secondary to MDR or XDR TB bacilli have a poor prognosis and may require concomitant steroids and second line ATT. Home-based treatment of CNS TB is feasible in selected patients under close supervision in areas where there is high incidence of tuberculosis coupled with HIV infection resulting in severe bed shortages in secondary and tertiary hospitals [88].

### 12.13.1 Tuberculous Brain Abscess

Tuberculous brain abscess is rare [89–93]. It can be solitary or multiple. It is an encapsulated collection of pus with abundant viable tubercle bacilli without classic tubercular granuloma formation. The wall is thicker than pyogenic abscess. They can mimic otogenic pyogenic abscesses [90, 91, 93]. The cystic nature of a tuberculoma contains caseous tissue necrosis and liquefaction of the center leading to a straw colored fluid and differs from that of a tuberculous brain abscess which contains true pus [89]. According to the Whitener criteria for tuberculous abscess, it should reveal macroscopic evidence of abscess formation within the brain parenchyma, and, on histologic examination, the abscess wall should be composed of vascular granulation tissue containing acute and chronic inflammatory cells and tubercle bacilli without the typical granulomas associated with tuberculomas [90, 93]. Imaging findings of tuberculous brain abscess are usually nonspecific. They present as large, frequently multiloculated, ring-enhancing lesions with perilesional edema and mass effect (Fig. 12.10). Diffusion-weighted imaging shows restricted diffusion with low apparent diffusion coefficient (ADC) values because of the presence of inflammatory cells in the pus. MRS helps in differentiating tuberculous abscess from those of pyogenic and fungal causes [30–32]. MRS shows lipid, lactate, and phosphoserine without evidence of cytosolic amino acids, in contrast to pyogenic abscess. MT imaging can differentiate tuberculous from pyogenic abscesses. Tuberculous brain abscesses may occur despite anti tuberculous treatment and may rapidly progress to clinical deterioration. Tuberculous brain abscesses are treated with simple aspiration, continuous drainage, fractional drainage, repeated aspiration through burr hole, stereotactic aspiration, subtotal or total excision. Antituberculous medication remains mainstay of therapy [89].

## 12.14  Tuberculosis of the Craniocervical Junction

Craniovertebral junction (CVJ) tuberculosis is a rare form of bone tuberculosis accounting for nearly 0.3–1% of all tubercular spondylitis [94–96] and is caused by secondary infection of the occipito-atlanto-axial complex [97]. The primary source is either lungs or lymph nodes. Rarely, it may start from the bone itself [97, 98]. The osteoligamentous destruction at the craniovertebral junction results in atlanto-axial instability and compression of vital cervico-medullary centers [99]. Often the organisms reach this area via the retropharyngeal lymphatics. Once they gain access,

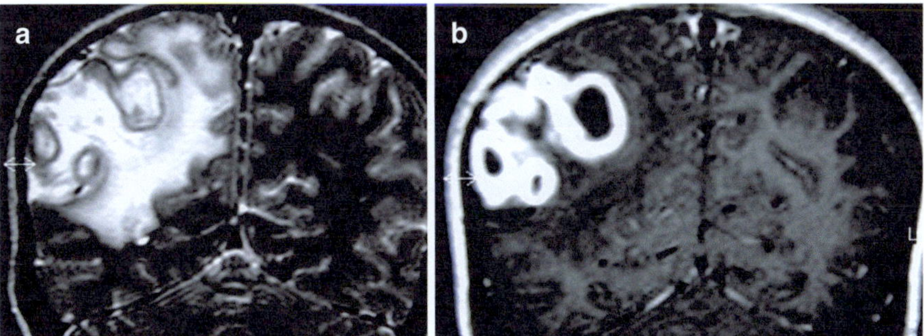

**Fig. 12.10** Tuberculous abscess in the parietal lobe. (**a**) Axial T2-weighted MR image showing multiple hyperintense lesions surrounded by rim of hypointense rim with surrounding extensive edema in the right posterior parietal lobe. (**b**) Axial T1-weighted post contrast MR image showing lesion with hypointense center and thick irregular ring enhancement in the right posterior parietal lobe

they start destroying the bone and ligaments in the local region [97–99]. Being the most mobile segment of the spine, once destruction has started, the instability of CVJ develops quickly [97, 99]. This also leads to a variable amount of soft tissue collection in the epidural, prevertebral, and paravertebral regions [97] (Fig. 12.11). Goel et al. also reported a case of epidural circumferential craniocervical tuberculosis without any vertebral involvement [100]. Patients often present with nonspecific chronic symptoms and a variable amount of neurological deficits and, sometimes, even with sudden death [96, 97, 99]. Neurological deficits develop subsequently, and the cause may be mechanical, vascular, or soft tissue compression [97]. Unfortunately, in spite of well-known clinical and radiological markers for diagnosis, the management is still controversial.

The onset is often insidious [98]. Initial complaints are mild nonspecific neck pain and neck stiffness, which lead to delayed diagnosis and sudden neurological deterioration. Sudden death may also occur due to atlanto-axial instability [101–104]. In a large study from an apex institute in India, Teegala et al. found that all their patients presented with some form of neck pain [97]. In their series, other common symptoms were restriction of neck movements in 77% of patients and constitutional symptoms of tuberculosis in 65% of cases [97]. Same findings were also found in the studies by Sinha et al. and Behari et al. [98, 99].

The clinical features of craniovertebral junction tuberculosis have been described well in the literature [97, 99]. Neck pain is the commonest presenting symptom followed by painful restriction of neck movements. There may be varying degrees of neurological involvement with motor symptoms being more common than sensory symptoms [5, 97]. Myelopathy, manifested in varying grades of weakness and spasticity, is the usual presentation [97, 99]. Sensory manifestations occur due to the involvement of both spinothalamic tract and posterior column. In severe cases, patients sometimes present with respiratory compromise. In Teegala's series, it was found in 10% of cases [97]. Chatterjee et al. found only one patient had respiratory compromise and he fared well after surgical decompression and fixation [105].

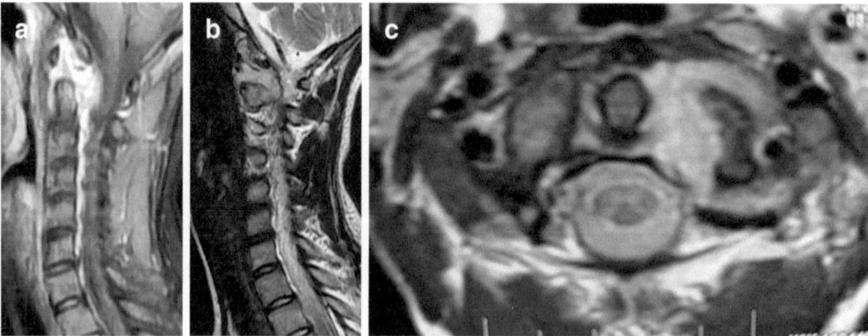

**Fig. 12.11** Craniocervical junction tuberculosis with destruction of left half of anterior arch of C1 and part of left lateral mass, with partial destruction of odontoid process of C2 and epidural collection extending from clivus to T1 in a 16-year-old female. (**a**) Sagittal T1-weighted MR image. (**b**) Sagittal T2-weighted MR image. (**c**) Axial T2-weighted MR image

Sphincter involvement is a rare and late finding. Rarely, one may come with cranial nerve involvement or tuberculous meningitis and encephalopathy [98]. Chatterjee et al. also reported an atypical presentation in a single patient with unilateral hypoglossal nerve palsy [105]. Studies have shown that 20–30% of patients have concomitant tuberculosis at other sites.

The lateral dynamic X-ray of the CVJ and cervical spine is extremely useful for the identification of instability. CT or MRI, the presence of a multilocular, calcified abscess with a thick, enhancing irregular wall in the presence of vertebral body fragmentation is pathognomonic of TB and differentiates it from other lesions at the CVJ, such as rheumatoid arthritis, sarcoidosis, fungal infection, lymphoma, or chordoma.

The management of children with craniovertebral tuberculosis should be individualized. They should be treated according to their clinical presentation and evidence of radiological instability. Patients with gross neurological deficit and instability need early stabilization trans-oral decompression with posterior fixation and four required posterior fixation while those with minimal deficit and no instability. Patients with severe pain or torticollis will need aspiration of the cold abscess with external immobilization. If the patients have no deficit, instability, or severe pain may be managed by external orthoses alone. Antituberculous therapy for tuberculosis is the backbone of the entire treatment plan [105].

## 12.15  Spinal Tuberculosis

### *12.15.1  Tuberculous Meningitis Within Spine*

Tuberculous meningitis within the spine most commonly manifests in decreasing frequency as radiculomyelopathy, intradural extra medullary tuberculomas, syringomyelia, intramedullary tuberculoma, tuberculous myelitis, tuberculous abscess, and infarct. Tuberculous radiculomyelopathy is attributed to tuberculous meningitis of the spinal cord with surrounding arachnoiditis [69, 106]. The severity of the symptoms increases with the degree of exudates seen within the thecal sac. Spinal tuberculomas may present as epidural, intradural extra medullary, or intramedullary lesions [107, 108]. Intradural extramedullary tuberculomas are the most common form of spinal tuberculomas and have features similar to other extra medullary neoplastic lesions. Spinal tuberculomas need surgical intervention when refractory to medical management. Spinal tuberculous abscesses occur following myelitis or tuberculomas and present most commonly as intramedullary lesions [109]. Tuberculous abscess may occur in subarachnoid, subdural, or epidural space. These lesions need surgical biopsy or excision to confirm diagnosis and treat the lesions. Tuberculous myelitis may occur secondary to arachnoiditis and is believed to be due to abnormal immune reaction against mycobacterial antigen. It may present as acute transverse myelitis or longitudinal extensive transverse myelitis. Myelitis commonly affect more than one spinal segment and most commonly involves the thoracic spine with the cervical spine being less frequently involved.

### 12.15.2  Tuberculous Syringomyelia

It is a rare complication of tuberculous arachnoiditis. Patients have a variety of clinical presentations including gait imbalance, sensory disturbances, or sensory loss and motor weakness—flaccid or spastic. Its mechanism has not been fully elucidated. It is believed to be due to disruption of the CSF dynamics by focal arachnoid scarring and thickening at foramen of Magendie and Luschka resulting in increased resistance to CSF flow, as a result of which, additional CSF is pushed into the central canal leading to its dilatation. Other theories such as localised tethering, cord ischemia due to secondary endarteritis are also postulated [110]. It is treated by anti tuberculous therapy with early use of adjunctive corticosteroids and surgical treatment to prevent syrinx formation or reduce the size of existing syrinx. Shunt drainage using syringoperitoneal, syringopleural, and syringosubarachnoidal shunts and central canal decompression by adhesiolysis, detethering, subpial suctioning, and duraplasty have been described. Motor symptoms have been noted to have the best response to treatment with no cases showing complete recovery being reported [111, 112].

### 12.15.3  Multidrug-Resistant CNS Tuberculosis

The emergence of multidrug resistant tuberculosis and extensively drug-resistant tuberculosis has further added to the burden of this disease. Multidrug-resistant tuberculosis is defined as *Mycobacterium tuberculosis* with resistance to at least to isoniazid and rifampicin, and more recently, extensively drug-resistance tuberculosis (XDR-TB), defined as *M. tuberculosis* strains with resistance to both isoniazid and rifampicin plus resistance to a fluoroquinolone and injectable second-line drugs. Drug-resistant tuberculous meningitis is diagnosed when drug-resistant *M. tuberculosis* isolates are found in CSF or in other sites in patients with probable tuberculous meningitis [113]. The resistance is believed to be multifactorial. Acquired resistance was traditionally believed to be due to poor compliance and programmatic failure. There is evidence to suggest that alternative mechanisms such as pharmacokinetic variability, induction of efflux pumps, and poor drug penetration into lesions are likely to be crucial in the pathogenesis of MDR-TB and XDR-TB [113]. In India, 2.1% of new TB cases and 15% of retreatment cases are found to be MDR TB [114].

The diagnosis of drug-resistant tuberculosis is hampered by the unavailability of an affordable, effective, and rapid diagnostic technique. WHO recommends using Line probe assays and Xpert MTB/RIF before conventional tests and use conventional tests if Xpert MTB/RIF is negative. A new Xpert MTB/RIF assay known as

Xpert MTB/RIF Ultra (Cepheid, Sunnyvale, USA) has been recently recommended by the WHO. This assay is more sensitive than the previous generations. Its cartridge can accommodate twice the volume of sample and has two additional molecular targets [115]. Nanotechnology is a new interdisciplinary technology combing basic research and application development. At present, it is a hot issue in medical research, particularly in the field of new diagnosis and treatment tools. The combination of nanomaterials and adaptors has great advantages in regards to detection speed, sensitivity, and accuracy for tuberculosis diagnosis [116].

There are no guidelines for treatment of MDR TB of the CNS. Guidelines have been set for pulmonary MDR TB and are extrapolated to MDR tuberculous meningitis as well. WHO recommends at least use of five effective anti tuberculous drugs during intensive phase which lasts for 8 months followed by a continuation phase of oral drugs lasting 12 months. The drug regime consists of a fluoroquinolone (moxifloxacin or levofloxacin), pyrazinamide, an injectable drug (kanamycin or amikacin), ethionamide/cycloserine, and linezolid [113]. Levofloxacin encapsulated with nanoliposomes has also been designed for MDR-TB with delayed release and longer duration of action, reducing the frequency of drug administration and improving patient compliance. Niosomes, as a carrier of drugs, could be utilized for long-term drug administration to reduce intake of drugs and adverse reactions by improving their bioavailability [116].

## 12.16 Immunotherapy in TB

There is a need to modulate the immune response to tuberculosis. This is true as most of the disease pathogenesis occurs as a result of immune-mediated responses to mycobacterial antigen. The emergence of MDR-TB and XDR-TB has further increased the need for such adjuncts.

Common examples of drugs used for immunosuppression include corticosteroids, thalidomide, and etanercept, which act by reducing the TNF alpha activity. Intravenous immunoglobulin in high doses is believed to reduce the unproductive inflammation by outcompeting the circulating endogenous antibodies [117, 118]. It has been used in pulmonary as well as extra pulmonary tuberculosis. Other agents such as anti-interleukin four neutralizing antibodies, 16a-bromoepiandosterone (HE2000), Heat-killed environmental mycobacterial preparations (*Mycobacterium vaccae, M.w*), RUTI (Mycobacterium tuberculosis liposomal preparation), DNA vaccine (with HSP65, Ag85, MPT-64, and MPT-83), and γ-glutamyl-tryptophan (SCV-07 SciCLone) are some immunomodulators that have been used in humans or in murine models of tuberculosis. Recombinant human cytokines such as IL-2, IL7, IL-15, IL-12, IL-27, and IFN gamma have also been used to enhance the microbicidal effect [119, 120].

# References


1. Be NA, Kim KS, Bishai WR, Jain SK. Pathogenesis of central nervous system tuberculosis. Curr Mol Med. 2009;9(2):94–9.
2. Vadivelu S, Effendi S, Starke JR, Luerssen TG, Jea A. A review of the neurological and neurosurgical implications of tuberculosis in children. Clin Pediatr (Phila). 2013;52(12):1135–43.
3. Sharma SK, Mohan A. Extrapulmonary tuberculosis. Indian J Med Res. 2004;120(4):316–53.
4. Hu J, Li D, Kang Y, Pang X, Wu T, Duan C, et al. Active thoracic and lumbar spinal tuberculosis in children with kyphotic deformity treated by one-stage posterior instrumentation combined anterior debridement: preliminary study. Eur J Orthop Surg Traumatol. 2014;24(Suppl 1):S221–9.
5. Jain AK, Sreenivasan R, Mukunth R, Dhammi IK. Tubercular spondylitis in children. Indian J Orthop. 2014;48(2):136–44.
6. Varatharajah S, Charles YP, Buy X, Walter A, Steib JP. Update on the surgical management of Pott's disease. Orthop Traumatol Surg Res. 2014;100(2):229–35.
7. Navarro-Flores A, Fernandez-Chinguel JE, Pacheco-Barrios N, Soriano-Moreno DR, Pacheco-Barrios K. Global morbidity and mortality of central nervous system tuberculosis: a systematic review and meta-analysis. J Neurol. 2022;269(7):3482–94.
8. Phypers M, Harris T, Power C. CNS tuberculosis: a longitudinal analysis of epidemiological and clinical features. Int J Tuberc Lung Dis. 2006;10(1):99–103.
9. Waecker NJ. Tuberculous meningitis in children. Curr Treat Options Neurol. 2002;4(3):249–57.
10. Parihar V, Yadav YR, Sharma D. Giant extra-axial posterior fossa tuberculoma in a three-year-old child. Neurol India. 2009;57(2):218–20.
11. Diyora B, Kumar R, Modgi R, Sharma A. Calvarial tuberculosis: a report of eleven patients. Neurol India. 2009;57(5):607–12.
12. Ramdurg SR, Gupta DK, Suri A, Sharma BS, Mahapatra AK. Calvarial tuberculosis: uncommon manifestation of common disease—a series of 21 cases. Br J Neurosurg. 2010;24(5):572–7.
13. Gupta PK, Kolluri VR, Chandramouli BA, Venkataramana NK, Das BS. Calvarial tuberculosis: a report of two cases. Neurosurgery. 1989;25(5):830–3.
14. Jadhav RN, Palande DA. Calvarial tuberculosis. Neurosurgery. 1999;45(6):1345–9; discussion 9–50.
15. Dawar P, Gupta DK, Sharma BS, Jyakumar A, Gamanagatti S. Extensive calvarial tuberculosis presenting as exophytic ulcerated growth on scalp in an infant: an interesting case report with review of literature. Childs Nerv Syst. 2013;29(7):1215–8.
16. Garcia-Garcia C, Ibarra V, Azcona-Gutierrez JM, Oteo JA. Calvarial tuberculosis with parenchymal involvement. Travel Med Infect Dis. 2013;11(5):329–31.
17. Singh G, Kumar S, Singh DP, Verma V, Mohammad A. A rare case of primary tuberculous osteomyelitis of skull vault. Indian J Tuberc. 2014;61(1):79–83.
18. Raut AA, Nagar AM, Muzumdar D, Chawla AJ, Narlawar RS, Fattepurkar S, et al. Imaging features of calvarial tuberculosis: a study of 42 cases. AJNR Am J Neuroradiol. 2004;25(3):409–14.
19. Chandir S, Hussain H, Salahuddin N, Amir M, Ali F, Lotia I, et al. Extrapulmonary tuberculosis: a retrospective review of 194 cases at a tertiary care hospital in Karachi, Pakistan. J Pak Med Assoc. 2010;60(2):105–9.
20. Qian X, Nguyen DT, Lyu J, Albers AE, Bi X, Graviss EA. Risk factors for extrapulmonary dissemination of tuberculosis and associated mortality during treatment for extrapulmonary tuberculosis. Emerg Microbes Infect. 2018;7(1):102.
21. Bhagwati SN, Singhal BS. Raised intracranial pressure as a mode of presentation in tuberculous meningitis. Neurol India. 1970;18(2):116–9.
22. Figaji AA, Sandler SI, Fieggen AG, Le Roux PD, Peter JC, Argent AC. Continuous monitoring and intervention for cerebral ischemia in tuberculous meningitis. Pediatr Crit Care Med. 2008;9(4):e25–30.

23. Dastur HM. A tuberculoma review with some personal experiences. I. Brain. Neurol India. 1972;20(3):111–26.
24. Dastur HM. Diagnosis and neurosurgical treatment of tuberculous disease of the CNS. Neurosurg Rev. 1983;6(3):111–7.
25. Bhagwati SN, Parulekar GD. Management of intracranial tuberculoma in children. Childs Nerv Syst. 1986;2(1):32–4.
26. Figaji AA, Fieggen AG. The neurosurgical and acute care management of tuberculous meningitis: evidence and current practice. Tuberculosis (Edinb). 2010;90(6):393–400.
27. Schoeman J, Wait J, Burger M, van Zyl F, Fertig G, van Rensburg AJ, et al. Long-term follow up of childhood tuberculous meningitis. Dev Med Child Neurol. 2002;44(8):522–6.
28. Ramzan A, Nayil K, Asimi R, Wani A, Makhdoomi R, Jain A. Childhood tubercular meningitis: an institutional experience and analysis of predictors of outcome. Pediatr Neurol. 2013;48(1):30–5.
29. Przybojewski S, Andronikou S, Wilmshurst J. Objective CT criteria to determine the presence of abnormal basal enhancement in children with suspected tuberculous meningitis. Pediatr Radiol. 2006;36(7):687–96.
30. Andronikou S, van Toorn R, Boerhout E. MR imaging of the posterior hypophysis in children with tuberculous meningitis. Eur Radiol. 2009;19(9):2249–54.
31. Pienaar M, Andronikou S, van Toorn R. MRI to demonstrate diagnostic features and complications of TBM not seen with CT. Childs Nerv Syst. 2009;25(8):941–7.
32. Chatterjee S, Saini J, Kesavadas C, Arvinda HR, Jolappara M, Gupta AK. Differentiation of tubercular infection and metastasis presenting as ring enhancing lesion by diffusion and perfusion magnetic resonance imaging. J Neuroradiol. 2010;37(3):167–71.
33. Gupta RK, Kathuria MK, Pradhan S. Magnetization transfer MR imaging in CNS tuberculosis. AJNR Am J Neuroradiol. 1999;20(5):867–75.
34. Dastur HM. A tuberculoma review with some personal experiences. II. Spinal cord and its coverings. Neurol India. 1972;20(3):127–31.
35. Tsona A, Metallidis S, Foroglou N, Selviaridis P, Chrysanthidis T, Lazaraki G, et al. Linezolid penetration into cerebrospinal fluid and brain tissue. J Chemother. 2010;22(1):17–9.
36. Sun F, Ruan Q, Wang J, Chen S, Jin J, Shao L, et al. Linezolid manifests a rapid and dramatic therapeutic effect for patients with life-threatening tuberculous meningitis. Antimicrob Agents Chemother. 2014;58(10):6297–301.
37. Akkerman OW, Odish OF, Bolhuis MS, de Lange WC, Kremer HP, Luijckx GJ, et al. Pharmacokinetics of bedaquiline in cerebrospinal fluid and serum in multidrug-resistant tuberculous meningitis. Clin Infect Dis. 2016;62(4):523–4.
38. Stadelman AM, Ellis J, Samuels THA, Mutengesa E, Dobbin J, Ssebambulidde K, et al. Treatment outcomes in adult tuberculous meningitis: a systematic review and meta-analysis. Open Forum Infect Dis. 2020;7(8):ofaa257.
39. Thwaites GE, Lan NT, Dung NH, Quy HT, Oanh DT, Thoa NT, et al. Effect of antituberculosis drug resistance on response to treatment and outcome in adults with tuberculous meningitis. J Infect Dis. 2005;192(1):79–88.
40. Heemskerk AD, Nguyen MTH, Dang HTM, Vinh Nguyen CV, Nguyen LH, Do TDA, et al. Clinical outcomes of patients with drug-resistant tuberculous meningitis treated with an intensified antituberculosis regimen. Clin Infect Dis. 2017;65(1):20–8.
41. Sivakumar V, Rajshekhar V, Chandy MJ. Management of neurosurgical patients with hyponatremia and natriuresis. Neurosurgery. 1994;34(2):269–74; discussion 74.
42. Damaraju SC, Rajshekhar V, Chandy MJ. Validation study of a central venous pressure-based protocol for the management of neurosurgical patients with hyponatremia and natriuresis. Neurosurgery. 1997;40(2):312–6; discussion 6–7.
43. Nagotkar L, Shanbag P, Dasarwar N. Cerebral salt wasting syndrome following neurosurgical intervention in tuberculous meningitis. Indian Pediatr. 2008;45(7):598–601.
44. Palur R, Rajshekhar V, Chandy MJ, Joseph T, Abraham J. Shunt surgery for hydrocephalus in tuberculous meningitis: a long-term follow-up study. J Neurosurg. 1991;74(1):64–9.

45. Lamprecht D, Schoeman J, Donald P, Hartzenberg H. Ventriculoperitoneal shunting in childhood tuberculous meningitis. Br J Neurosurg. 2001;15(2):119–25.
46. Bhagwati SN. Ventriculoatrial shunt in tuberculous meningitis with hydrocephalus. J Neurosurg. 1971;35(3):309–13.
47. Peng J, Deng X, He F, Omran A, Zhang C, Yin F, et al. Role of ventriculoperitoneal shunt surgery in grade IV tubercular meningitis with hydrocephalus. Childs Nerv Syst. 2012;28(2):209–15.
48. Agrawal D, Gupta A, Mehta VS. Role of shunt surgery in pediatric tubercular meningitis with hydrocephalus. Indian Pediatr. 2005;42(3):245–50.
49. Sil K, Chatterjee S. Shunting in tuberculous meningitis: a neurosurgeon's nightmare. Childs Nerv Syst. 2008;24(9):1029–32.
50. Husain M, Jha DK, Rastogi M, Husain N, Gupta RK. Role of neuroendoscopy in the management of patients with tuberculous meningitis hydrocephalus. Neurosurg Rev. 2005;28(4):278–83.
51. Figaji AA, Fieggen AG, Peter JC. Endoscopic third ventriculostomy in tuberculous meningitis. Childs Nerv Syst. 2003;19(4):217–25.
52. Siomin V, Constantini S. Endoscopic third ventriculostomy in tuberculous meningitis. Childs Nerv Syst. 2003;19(5–6):269.
53. Chugh A, Husain M, Gupta RK, Ojha BK, Chandra A, Rastogi M. Surgical outcome of tuberculous meningitis hydrocephalus treated by endoscopic third ventriculostomy: prognostic factors and postoperative neuroimaging for functional assessment of ventriculostomy. J Neurosurg Pediatr. 2009;3(5):371–7.
54. Bhagwati S, Mehta N, Shah S. Use of endoscopic third ventriculostomy in hydrocephalus of tubercular origin. Childs Nerv Syst. 2010;26(12):1675–82.
55. Figaji AA, Fieggen AG. Endoscopic challenges and applications in tuberculous meningitis. World Neurosurg. 2013;79(2 Suppl):S24.e9–14.
56. Singh D, Kumar S. Ventriculoperitoneal shunt in post tubercular hydrocephalus. Indian Pediatr. 1996;33(10):854–5.
57. Bhagwati SN, George K. Use of intrathecal hyaluronidase in the management of tuberculous meningitis with hydrocephalus. Childs Nerv Syst. 1986;2(1):20–5.
58. van Toorn R, Solomons R. Update on the diagnosis and management of tuberculous meningitis in children. Semin Pediatr Neurol. 2014;21(1):12–8.
59. Chee RI, Dinkin MJ. Tuberculous optochiasmatic arachnoiditis and vision loss. Neurology. 2016;87(17):1845.
60. Lee JS, Song GS, Son DW. Surgical management of syringomyelia associated with spinal adhesive arachnoiditis, a late complication of tuberculous meningitis: a case report. Korean J Neurotrauma. 2017;13(1):34–8.
61. Shobha N, Mahadevan A, Taly AB, Sinha S, Srikanth SG, Satish S, et al. Hypertrophic cranial pachymeningitis in countries endemic for tuberculosis: diagnostic and therapeutic dilemmas. J Clin Neurosci. 2008;15(4):418–27.
62. Senapati SB, Mishra SS, Das S, Parida DK, Satapathy MC. Cranio cervical tuberculous hypertrophic pachymeningitis. Surg Neurol Int. 2014;5:52.
63. Kondety SK, Chatterjee S. Acquired Chiari malformation secondary to tuberculous arachnoiditis of the lumbar spine. Neurol India. 2016;64(5):1066–8.
64. Dastur DK, Manghani DK, Udani PM. Pathology and pathogenetic mechanisms in neurotuberculosis. Radiol Clin North Am. 1995;33(4):733–52.
65. Schoeman JF, le Roux D, Bezuidenhout PB, Donald PR. Intracranial pressure monitoring in tuberculous meningitis: clinical and computerized tomographic correlation. Dev Med Child Neurol. 1985;27(5):644–54.
66. Schoeman J, Donald P, van Zyl L, Keet M, Wait J. Tuberculous hydrocephalus: comparison of different treatments with regard to ICP, ventricular size and clinical outcome. Dev Med Child Neurol. 1991;33(5):396–405.

67. Nadvi SS, Nathoo N, Annamalai K, van Dellen JR, Bhigjee AI. Role of cerebrospinal fluid shunting for human immunodeficiency virus-positive patients with tuberculous meningitis and hydrocephalus. Neurosurgery. 2000;47(3):644–9; discussion 9–50.
68. Jonathan A, Rajshekhar V. Endoscopic third ventriculostomy for chronic hydrocephalus after tuberculous meningitis. Surg Neurol. 2005;63(1):32–4; discussion 4–5.
69. Figaji AA, Fieggen AG, Schoeman JF, Peter JC. Endoscopic third ventriculostomy in post-tubercular meningitic hydrocephalus. Minim Invasive Neurosurg. 2006;49(1):60–1.
70. Ghosh S, Chandy MJ. Intrasellar tuberculoma. Clin Neurol Neurosurg. 1992;94(3):251–2.
71. Rajshekhar V, Chandy MJ. Tuberculomas presenting as isolated intrinsic brain stem masses. Br J Neurosurg. 1997;11(2):127–33.
72. Yen HL, Lee RJ, Lin JW, Chen HJ. Multiple tuberculomas in the brain and spinal cord: a case report. Spine (Phila Pa 1976). 2003;28(23):E499–502.
73. Figaji AA, Fieggen AG, Peter JC. Air encephalography for hydrocephalus in the era of neuroendoscopy. Childs Nerv Syst. 2005;21(7):559–65.
74. Rajshekhar V. Management of hydrocephalus in patients with tuberculous meningitis. Neurol India. 2009;57(4):368–74.
75. Mathew JM, Rajshekhar V, Chandy MJ. Shunt surgery in poor grade patients with tuberculous meningitis and hydrocephalus: effects of response to external ventricular drainage and other variables on long term outcome. J Neurol Neurosurg Psychiatry. 1998;65(1):115–8.
76. Singh D, Sachdev V, Singh AK, Sinha S. Endoscopic third ventriculostomy in post-tubercular meningitic hydrocephalus: a preliminary report. Minim Invasive Neurosurg. 2005;48(1):47–52.
77. Jain R, Kumar R. Suprasellar tuberculoma presenting with diabetes insipidus and hypothyroidism—a case report. Neurol India. 2001;49(3):314–6.
78. Dastur HM, Shah MD. Intramedullary tuberculoma of the spinal cord. Indian Pediatr. 1968;5(10):468–71.
79. Kumar R, Kasliwal MK, Srivastava R, Sharma BS. Tuberculoma presenting as an intradural extramedullary lesion. Pediatr Neurosurg. 2007;43(6):541–3.
80. Chitre PS, Tullu MS, Sawant HV, Ghildiyal RG. Co-occurrence of intracerebral tuberculoma with lumbar intramedullary tuberculoma. J Child Neurol. 2009;24(5):606–9.
81. Gupta RKKM, Pradhan S. Magnetization transfer MR imaging in CNS tuberculosis. AJNR Am J Neuroradiol. 1999;20:8.
82. Selvapandian S, Rajshekhar V, Chandy MJ, Idikula J. Predictive value of computed tomography-based diagnosis of intracranial tuberculomas. Neurosurgery. 1994;35(5):845–50; discussion 50.
83. Poonnoose SI, Rajshekhar V. Rate of resolution of histologically verified intracranial tuberculomas. Neurosurgery. 2003;53(4):873–8; discussion 8–9.
84. Kumar R, Prakash M, Jha S. Paradoxical response to chemotherapy in neurotuberculosis. Pediatr Neurosurg. 2006;42(4):214–22.
85. van Toorn R, Schoeman JF, Donald PR. Brainstem tuberculoma presenting as eight-and-a-half syndrome. Eur J Paediatr Neurol. 2006;10(1):41–4.
86. Perez-Alvarez F, Serra C, Mayol L, Liarte A. Unusual central nervous system tuberculosis debut in children: stroke. Childs Nerv Syst. 2008;24(5):539–40.
87. Rajshekhar V, Chandy MJ. CT-guided stereotactic surgery in the management of intracranial tuberculomas. Br J Neurosurg. 1993;7(6):665–71.
88. Schoeman J, Malan G, van Toorn R, Springer P, Parker F, Booysen J. Home-based treatment of childhood neurotuberculosis. J Trop Pediatr. 2009;55(3):149–54.
89. Kumar R, Pandey CK, Bose N, Sahay S. Tuberculous brain abscess: clinical presentation, pathophysiology and treatment (in children). Childs Nerv Syst. 2002;18(3–4):118–23.
90. Abraham R, Kumar S, Scott JX, Agarwal I. Tuberculous brain abscess in a child with tetralogy of Fallot. Neurol India. 2009;57(2):217–8.
91. Andronikou S, Greyling PJ. Devastating yet treatable complication of tuberculous meningitis: the resistant TB abscess. Childs Nerv Syst. 2009;25(9):1105–6; discussion 7, 9–10.

92. Chakraborti S, Mahadevan A, Govindan A, Nagarathna S, Santosh V, Yasha TC, et al. Clinicopathological study of tuberculous brain abscess. Pathol Res Pract. 2009;205(12):815–22.
93. Muzumdar D, Balasubramaniam S, Melkundi S. Tuberculous temporal brain abscess mimicking otogenic pyogenic abscess. Pediatr Neurosurg. 2009;45(3):220–4.
94. Lal AP, Rajshekhar V, Chandy MJ. Management strategies in tuberculous atlanto-axial dislocation. Br J Neurosurg. 1992;6(6):529–35.
95. Desai SS. Early diagnosis of spinal tuberculosis by MRI. J Bone Joint Surg Br. 1994;76(6):863–9.
96. Edwards RJ, David KM, Crockard HA. Management of tuberculomas of the craniovertebral junction. Br J Neurosurg. 2000;14(1):19–22.
97. Teegala R, Kumar P, Kale SS, Sharma BS. Craniovertebral junction tuberculosis: a new comprehensive therapeutic strategy. Neurosurgery. 2008;63(5):946–55; discussion 55.
98. Sinha S, Singh AK, Gupta V, Singh D, Takayasu M, Yoshida J. Surgical management and outcome of tuberculous atlantoaxial dislocation: a 15-year experience. Neurosurgery. 2003;52(2):331–8; discussion 8–9.
99. Behari S, Nayak SR, Bhargava V, Banerji D, Chhabra DK, Jain VK. Craniocervical tuberculosis: protocol of surgical management. Neurosurgery. 2003;52(1):72–80; discussion 1.
100. Shah A, Nadkarni T, Goel N, Goel A. Circumferential craniocervical extradural tuberculous granulations. J Clin Neurosci. 2010;17(6):808–9.
101. Gorse GJ, Pais MJ, Kusske JA, Cesario TC. Tuberculous spondylitis. A report of six cases and a review of the literature. Medicine (Baltimore). 1983;62(3):178–93.
102. Kanaan IU, Ellis M, Safi T, Al Kawi MZ, Coates R. Craniocervical junction tuberculosis: a rare but dangerous disease. Surg Neurol. 1999;51(1):21–5; discussion 6.
103. Dhammi IK, Singh S, Jain AK. Hemiplegic/monoplegic presentation of cervical spine (C1-C2) tuberculosis. Eur Spine J. 2001;10(6):540–4.
104. Raut AA, Narlawar RS, Nagar A, Ahmed N, Hira P. An unusual case of CV junction tuberculosis presenting with quadriplegia. Spine (Phila Pa 1976). 2003;28(15):E309.
105. Chatterjee S, Das A. Craniovertebral tuberculosis in children: experience of 23 cases and proposal for a new classification. Childs Nerv Syst. 2015;31(8):1341–5.
106. Nair BR, Rajshekhar V. Factors predicting the need for prolonged (>24 months) antituberculous treatment in patients with brain tuberculomas. World Neurosurg. 2019;125:e236–47.
107. Tacconi L, Arulampalam T, Johnston FG, Thomas DG. Intramedullary spinal cord abscess: case report. Neurosurgery. 1995;37(4):817–9.
108. Garg RK, Malhotra HS, Gupta R. Spinal cord involvement in tuberculous meningitis. Spinal Cord. 2015;53(9):649–57.
109. Ozates M, Ozkan U, Kemaloglu S, Hosoglu S, Sari I. Spinal subdural tuberculous abscess. Spinal Cord. 2000;38(1):56–8.
110. Kannapadi NV, Alomari SO, Caturegli G, Bydon A, Cho SM. Management of syringomyelia associated with tuberculous meningitis: a case report and systematic review of the literature. J Clin Neurosci. 2021;87:20–5.
111. Kyoshima K, Kuroyanagi T, Toriyama T, Takizawa T, Hirooka Y, Miyama H, et al. Surgical experience of syringomyelia with reference to the findings of magnetic resonance imaging. J Clin Neurosci. 2004;11(3):273–9.
112. Koyanagi I, Iwasaki Y, Hida K, Houkin K. Clinical features and pathomechanisms of syringomyelia associated with spinal arachnoiditis. Surg Neurol. 2005;63(4):350–5; discussion 5–6.
113. WHO treatment guidelines for drug-resistant tuberculosis, 2016 update. WHO guidelines approved by the Guidelines Review Committee. Geneva; 2016.
114. World Health Organization. Global tuberculosis control: WHO report 2011. Geneva: World Health Organization; 2011.
115. Use of Xpert MTB/RIF and Xpert MTB/RIF ultra on GeneXpert 10-colour instruments: WHO policy statement. Geneva: World Health Organization; 2021.

116. Chen W, Huang L, Tang Q, Wang S, Chunmei H, Zhang X. Progress on diagnosis and treatment of central nervous system tuberculosis. Radiol Infect Dis. 2020;7(4):160–9.
117. Ballow M. The IgG molecule as a biological immune response modifier: mechanisms of action of intravenous immune serum globulin in autoimmune and inflammatory disorders. J Allergy Clin Immunol. 2011;127(2):315–23; quiz 24–5.
118. Wen N, Zhao F, Zhu Y, Jia F, Wan C, Wen Y. Acute development of syringomyelia following TBM in a pediatric case. BMC Pediatr. 2021;21(1):36.
119. Churchyard GO, Zumla A. Report of the expert consultation on immunotherapeutic interventions for TB. WHO special programme for research and training in tropical diseases. Geneva: World Health Organization; 2007. p. 143.
120. Churchyard GJ, Kaplan G, Fallows D, Wallis RS, Onyebujoh P, Rook GA. Advances in immunotherapy for tuberculosis treatment. Clin Chest Med. 2009;30(4):769–82, ix.

# Chapter 13
# Novel Surgical Approaches in Childhood Epilepsy: Laser, Brain Stimulation, and Focused Ultrasound

Kalman A. Katlowitz, Daniel J. Curry, and Howard L. Weiner

## Contents




K. A. Katlowitz · D. J. Curry · H. L. Weiner (✉)
Department of Neurosurgery, Baylor College of Medicine, Houston, TX, USA

Department of Neurosurgery, Texas Children's Hospital, Houston, TX, USA
e-mail: hlweiner@texaschildrens.org



© The Author(s), under exclusive license to Springer Nature Switzerland AG 2024
C. Di Rocco (ed.), *Advances and Technical Standards in Neurosurgery*,
Advances and Technical Standards in Neurosurgery 49,
https://doi.org/10.1007/978-3-031-42398-7_13

## 13.1 A Brief History of Epilepsy Surgery

Originally considered to be a disease of the spirit, epilepsy was first proposed to be a biological condition by pioneers such as Hippocrates (480–323 BCE) and Galen (130–200 CE) [1–3]. Yet it took a long time for this idea to become accepted, and epilepsy treatment was firmly in the realm of the spiritual up until the nineteenth century. Once seizures were recognized to represent a biological rather than supernatural process, the hunt began for a way to control them. Antiepileptic drugs, or AEDs, were developed to target seizure networks. These medications are generally designed to suppress neuronal excitability and interrupt pathological activity. Bromide was popularized in the 1850s and phenobarbital was first developed in 1911 [4], but it was not until the latter half of the twentieth century that a true diversity of AEDs was available [4]. Standard of care for epilepsy management currently suggests a trial of at least 2 of these over 40 different drugs. Unfortunately, even with all these options, large-scale studies have suggested that about one out of every three patients with epilepsy will be refractory to medical management, a condition referred to as drug-resistant epilepsy (DRE) [5]. While the ratio is slightly better for pediatric epilepsy [6, 7], there remains a large segment of the epileptic population that requires alternative means of control. These patients often suffer from severe health complications from both the disease itself and the harsh side effects from the escalating doses of the medications that they are taking.

It was clear from the very beginning than an alternative means was needed to treat seizures. At about the same time that these drugs entered the medical literature, pioneers such as Paul Broca, Gustav Fritsch, and Eduard Hitzig were able to correlate neurological functions such as speech and motor activity to select portions of the brain [8]. These scientific advances provided the context for the concept that epilepsy was not only a disease of the brain but also might be localizable to a subset of pathological tissue. Many accredit the beginning of epileptology to John Hughlings Jackson (1835–1911), an English neurologist who attempted to attribute seizures to different areas of the brain, such as the corpus striatum or the cortex [9]. With these ideas in mind, surgeons such as Horseley [10] and Dudley [11] were able to remove lesions and not only treat but in fact cure epilepsy in select patients.

Once these operations were publicized, surgeons hunted for other interventions to cure epilepsy. Not all approaches worked. For example, a surgery to produce a cerebrospinal fluid release "valve" via a galeal flap to release intracranial pressure was demonstrated to have no impact on outcomes [4]. But soon more evidence came out on the definition of a surgical epileptic lesion. Obvious traumatic scars or tumors were easy candidates. Cortical stimulation was used to localize seizure onset zones. With the development of procedures such as the temporal lobectomy [12], epilepsy surgery quickly became an established component of neurosurgical practice. Once the proof of concept was established, surgeons worldwide began to offer surgical treatments for epilepsy.

Yet before they could offer surgery, neurosurgeons first needed to know where to operate. While the field of neurosurgery had been established for decades at this point, it was rarely clear where the epileptic lesion was to be found. Early successful cases had a clear semiology, such as focal motor seizures, but it often was not that simple. New tools for identifying surgical candidates needed to be developed. Localization of epileptogenic lesions significantly improved with the development of electroencephalography in the 1920s [13], followed by electrocorticography (ECoG) in the 1930–1950s [14, 15], and finally stereotactic electroencephalograms (sEEG) in the 1960s [16]. The first video EEG monitoring unit was established in 1976, and the first use of a magnetic resonance imaging (MRI) scanner for epilepsy was reported in the early 1980s [17]. Advanced imaging modalities such as fluoro-deoxyglucose (FDG)-positron emission tomography (PET), single-photon emission computerized tomography (SPECT), magnetoencephalography (MEG), functional MRI (fMRI), and tractography have been developed to aid in the search for the optimal surgical plan [18]. Of course, once the seizure onset zone (SOZ) was established, it was then necessary to act on this knowledge. More importantly, as our ability to monitor the brain expanded, the answer was not always so straightforward. Often there was more than one SOZ, the SOZ was within eloquent cortex and therefore non-resectable, or even no specific SOZ was found at all. More than a way to find seizures, neurosurgeons needed new tools to control them.

Thankfully, innovations did not only happen on the diagnostic front. The rising success rates of open epilepsy surgery combined with the perceived morbidity [19] begged the question of less invasive options. Additionally, fewer than half of those with DRE are candidates for classical focal resection [20], requiring alternative options for control. New approaches were developed to interrupt epilepsy networks that did not depend on classical resection techniques. These developments would not only decrease morbidity but also expand the definition of a surgical candidate.

## 13.2 Laser Ablation

### 13.2.1 History

MRI-guided Laser Interstitial Thermal Therapy (MRgLITT) for pediatric epilepsy was not reported until 2012 [21], but the technological underpinnings have a long history. First came the idea that a lesion could be made through a small incision. The goal of epilepsy surgery is not to remove the offending lesion, but rather interrupt its ability to impact network function. Radiofrequency ablation (RFA) was the first technological advance to make use of this idea, developing as a natural extension of sEEGs. Stereotactic targeting of lesions using RFA was shown to be feasible in 1978 [22] and refined in the early 2000s [23, 24] . The idea was simple—if seizures were noted to be originating with tissue surrounding a specific lesion, then ablation of this tissue would likely lead to the cessation of these seizures.

Unfortunately, there is no real time feedback on the lesioning process with this technique aside from impedance at the electrode tip. This makes it difficult to assess the extent of the lesions with respect to not only the pathological tissue but also to the crucial structures nearby. MRgLITT therefore came in as the natural extension. It offers the same surgical approach, but instead of relying on radiofrequency energy it uses lasers. By using MRI compatible energy delivery (dependent on optical fibers instead of metal electrodes), MRgLITT can ablate pathologic tissue and avoid nearby crucial structures by monitoring three-dimensional temperature in real time. Approved by the FDA in 2007 and first reported in brain tumors [25], it was adapted to pediatric epilepsy in 2012 [21], and then quickly adopted into the adult population.

## 13.2.2  Mechanism

MRgLITT optically delivers thermal energy to cause protein denaturation and cell death via a flexible laser probe inserted into the relevant tissue. The absorbed light energy is converted into heat by surrounding tissues. This heat energy can cause cell death by many modalities. Changes to cell membrane integrity and mitochondrial dysfunction are considered to be the main routes of hyperthermia-induced cell death. At temperatures above 60 °C, rapid protein denaturation occurs, leading to cytotoxicity and coagulative necrosis. At lower temperatures, prolonged exposures still lead to irreversible cell damage [26].

Use of the device is independent of the actual method used to place the probe, reports have used Leksell and CRW frames, BrainLab VarioGuide, ROSA robots, ClearPoint navigation, and more. There are currently two commercially available systems. The Visualase Thermal Therapy System (Medtronic; Minneapolis, Minnesota) was FDA approved in 2007. It uses a 980 nm diode continuous 15 W laser within a 1.6 mm cooling catheter [27] cooled by a saline irrigation system in concert with image processing workstation. To increase the ablation volume, the catheter can be manually advanced or retracted along the insertion tract. The NeuroBlate system (Monteris Medical; Winnipeg, Canada) is a similar system and was approved shortly afterwards. It provides a 1064 nm pulsed 12 W laser using 2.2- or 3.3-mm catheters cooled by carbon dioxide. To improve selectivity, it gives the option of a diffusing tip or a directional probe ("side-fire"). Rather than requiring manual adjustment, it uses a robotic driver to change the catheter depth.

Online software analyzes real time data from the MRI to estimate tissue damage based on the Arrhenius rate process model [28] or cumulative equivalents at 43C (CEM43) [26]. The actual power used depends on the thermography, but reports describe about 10 W over approximately one or two minues [29]. The temperature falloff is precipitous, and the interface between ablated and non-ablated tissue approaches 1 mm. Notably, large vessels and cerebral spinal fluid (CSF) spaces can often act as a heat sink, giving rise to an even sharper cutoff.

### 13.2.3 Indications

Like other lesional approaches to epilepsy, MRgLITT is of limited utility in widespread pathology. Instead, it offers a minimally invasive approach to well localized, small anatomical lesions. It has found particular success among hypothalamic hamartomas (HH) [30], which represent more than half of the published literature [31]. Given its low morbidity and ability to avoid a craniotomy, many are trying to adapt it to both temporal and extratemporal epilepsy [32]. It has been reported for limited multifocal lesions such as focal cortical dysplasia, periventricular heterotopias [33], or tuberous sclerosis complex [34]. That is not to say it cannot be used for widespread networks. For example, recent case reports have used for disconnection surgery such as corpus callosotomies [35] and one systematic review showed that 9/13 patients were able to achieve Engel 1 or 2 outcomes using this approach [36]. Other groups are using it as an initial approach in a possibly two staged procedure [37] to temporal lobe epilepsy in the event of treatment failure due to its low morbidity.

The most intuitive limitation for MRgLITT is the high startup costs requiring an intraoperative MRI, limiting its use to large academic centers and patients with no contraindications to an MRI. Additionally, due to the nature of the current systems available, lesion size is limited to 2–3 cm. Larger lesions would require an alternative approach or multiple fibers, which also significantly increase costs.

### 13.2.4 Outcomes

In well-selected patients, seizure outcomes rates can be similar to or even better than other approaches. Studies have reported about 50–80% Engel 1–2 outcomes after more than a year [29, 31, 32, 38]. For the properly selected patients, however, rates can often exceed traditional surgery. For example, in HH 90% were seizure free at 6 months, versus about 50% with open versus endoscopic options [30].

Of course, the real strength of MRgLITT is the minimization of complications. Large-scale studies have shown that side effects are mostly limited to minor symptoms such as headaches (5%), though they do report a chance of significant deficits such as hemiparesis or visual deficits [38, 39] and even just the placement of the probe can cause subarachnoid or intraventricular hemorrhage [32]. As with all procedures, the complication rate does decrease with experience [40]. One systematic review of over 3000 adult patients found that although outcomes were slightly worse in MRgLITT relative to anterior temporal lobectomies (57% Engel 1 versus 69%), cognitive outcomes were more favorable and the complication rate was less than half (4% versus 11%) [41].

## 13.3  Brain Stimulation

### *13.3.1  History*

As described above, the origins of epilepsy surgery focused on resection of the epileptic tissue. However, oftentimes there either is no lesion found or the area slated for destruction is in eloquent cortex requiring alternative option. While often not as efficacious as directly removing epileptic tissue, direct or indirect neurostimulation can significantly improve quality of life in patients with no other options. This idea is as old as the history of modern epilepsy, with Dr. Corning first popularizing carotid compression in the 1880s [42]. His discovery directly led to the development of vagus nerve stimulation (VNS), an implanted device that reproduces the downstream effects of carotid compression via electrical stimulation of the tenth cranial nerve as it travels within the carotid sheath. First used in 1990 [43], it was approved for adults in 1997 and then expanded to children older than 4 in 2017. It has now been implanted in more than 100,000 patients worldwide [44].

Since that time many different devices, techniques, and targets have been developed for neurostimulation, each with different but often overlapping indications. Responsive neurostimulation (RNS) is a newer technology that offers closed loop stimulation. Similar to a defibrillator, rather than preventing seizures it is designed to abort them [45]. It was approved for adults in 2013, but so far use in the pediatric patient population has been off label.

Next into the lineup came deep brain stimulation (DBS), the archetype of central nervous system stimulation, it was approved for Parkinson's disease in 1997. While DBS was actually first studied in the context of epilepsy in the 1970s [46, 47] and 1980s [48], it was not until 2018 that FDA approval was granted for stimulation of the anterior nucleus of the thalamus (ANT) after the SANTE trial [49]. These targets were then expanded to include the subthalamic nucleus, globus pallidus, cerebellum, caudate nucleus, hippocampus, centromedian nucleus of the thalamus (CMT), and the seizure onset zone itself [50, 51]. Like RNS, DBS is also off label for patients under 18 years old.

### *13.3.2  Mechanism*

In VNS, helical electrodes are wrapped around the left cervical vagus nerve, the right is avoided due to potential cardiac complications. A stimulator implanted in the chest then delivers periodic 20–30 Hz stimulation. Prevailing theories suggest that stimulation of the C fibers within the nerve leads to activation of the nucleus of the solitary tract [52], which in turn has widespread connections such as the locus coeruleus and the raphe nuclei [52–54]. This in turn increases the global levels of norepinephrine and serotonin, which have antiepileptic effects. Given the accrual of efficacy over time [55], it is thought that VNS not only interrupts seizures but also modulates the epileptogenic networks. This device can be used as both a prophylactic treatment with ongoing stimulation and an abortive one by manually increasing stimulation during a clinical seizure. The vagus nerve stimulation (VNS) therapy system (LivaNova, London, UK) has undergone many iterations since its first patient in 1988, with reductions in weight, lead durability, and integrated cardiac assessment. The latest model even includes prone position and bradycardia detection.

RNS ostensibly has a much simpler mechanism. Based on findings that direct cortical stimulation can interrupt intraoperative seizures [56, 57], it was simply an engineering problem to do this on an ambulatory basis. The NeuroPace Responsive Neurostimulator (NeuroPace; Mountainview, California) is the only FDA-approved commercial device available for clinical use. The neurostimulator can currently be hooked up to two sets of four electrode leads, with future devices planned to be able to utilize four leads. Oftentimes sEEG monitoring is performed in advance of implantation to define electrode placement [58]. After the device is implanted, an algorithm is preprogrammed to continuously monitor for seizures. These parameters can be optimized post-implantation to improve the sensitivity and specificity of seizure detection. When a seizure is detected, an electrical pulse is delivered in an attempt to terminate the event. While the system has a wide range of parameters available, typical stimulation is a 100–200 Hz signal at 1.5–3 mA for about 100–200 ms [59]. Interestingly, the impact of RNS is not limited to seizure abortion: recent studies have suggested that responsive neurostimulation can also influence plasticity, enforcing long-term changes in seizure networks [59–61].

The DBS system is set up much like VNS, but instead simulates the central nervous system. Though closed loop stimulation is a key focus of current and future research [62], current clinical models are limited to open loop stimulation. It is thought that constant stimulation of key seizure network nodes at approximately 100 Hz prevents the propagation of seizures. For example, the ANT is a key node within the Papez, or medial limbic, circuit [63]. It has input from the hippocampus via the fornix/mammillothalamic tract with connections to the frontal and cingulate cortices. High frequency stimulation in this area has been suggested to have an inhibitory effect on the network [64], preventing the spread to cortical areas. Stimulation amplitude, frequency, pulse width, and electrode selection can all be optimized in the post-operative clinic visits. While there are a few companies with DBS systems, the Medtronic DBS System for Epilepsy (Medtronic, Minneapolis, MN) is currently the only commercial option designed for epilepsy. Similar to the VNS and RNS devices, these devices also have made significant progress, with a rechargeable model and new abilities to record data for offline analysis.

### 13.3.3  Indications

Neurostimulation was originally designed for patients who do not have a surgical lesion. Due to this distinction, it is considered for palliative rather than curative intent. Yet this is not to say it is an inferior choice. Even minor decreases in seizure frequency can have a significant impact on quality of life, long-term outcomes, and mortality rates. Seizure reduction can also allow for the taper of AEDs, reducing the side effect burden. The choice to pursue neurostimulation and the selection between the different modalities are complex decisions and often depend on many factors including patient baseline function, epileptic circuit localization, and even patient or family preference.

VNS and DBS are particularly well suited toward patients with no clear SOZ. VNS is designed for reducing the frequency of seizures in patients 4 years of age and older with partial-onset seizures that are refractory to antiepileptic medications. It is contraindicated in patients with bilateral or left cervical vagotomies. Current Medtronic guidelines suggest consideration of bilateral ANT DBS stimulation in DRE patients with partial-onset seizures (with or without secondary generalization) who average six or more seizures per month. While the vagal nerve stimulators are classically placed solely on the left vagus nerve, DBS target selection is an active field of research and depends on the indication. For example, ANT or hippocampal stimulation may do best for deep temporal or limbic seizures and CMT for generalized seizure disorders such as Lennox-Gastout [50].

Conversely, RNS is designed for focal epilepsy not amenable to resection. In these cases, the epileptic tissue is either necessary for cognitive function, or surgically inseparable from functional tissue. Notably, given the long-term recording capabilities of RNS, it can also be used for long-term monitoring to guide future surgical planning [65]. This may be especially important in the pediatric population who may not tolerate EMU monitoring [66]. Of course, RNS is not limited to such cases and can be used for targets classically considered for DBS, such as CMT.

### 13.3.4  Outcomes

Early studies in VNS found that about 1/3 of patients receive a greater than 50% reduction in seizure frequency [67, 68] and this number increased to 50% of patients in follow-up studies [55]. Further trials in children found effects in children are similar to adults [58, 69, 70]. While symptomatic bradycardia or even asystole is a feared complication at device initiation, its more common side effect profile is quite favorable, mostly associated with occasional coughing or voice hoarseness.

In RNS, median seizure reduction was about 50–60% for adults [71] and recent pediatric studies have replicated these findings on a smaller scale [72]. These outcomes improved with time [73], lending support to the theory that RNS was not only interrupting seizure networks but was also changing thcm. Given that it is an intracranial procedure, it does come with approximately 10% change of implant site complications such as pain, infection, headache, or dysesthesias [74] and about a 5% chance of intracranial complications such as hemorrhage [71, 75].

Randomized controlled trials in pediatrics are still pending for DBS. Based on adult literature, approximately half of patients who received ANT and HC stimulation had a reduction of 50–90% in seizure frequency [50]. Clinical reports in pediatrics show very similar outcomes [76, 77], though given the wide variety of indications and targets it is difficult to provide a true understanding of its efficacy. Its safety profile is similar to that of DBS for movement disorders. Surgical complications such as hemorrhage, infection, or lead misplacement are usually less than 5%, while rates of stimulation side effects such as psychiatric symptoms or paresthesia are very site dependent and are often temporary [50].

## 13.4  Focused Ultrasound

### 13.4.1  *History*

It was known since the 1940s that ultrasonic waves could be focused to create stereotactic lesions inside the skull [78]. From that initial publication, however, it then took another 70 years for the technology to mature into a practical tool. Most crucial to its development was the addition of MRI monitoring to create safe, focal lesions using MRI-guided Focus Ultrasound (MRgFUS). Like MRgLITT, MRgFUS is dependent on MRI for close monitoring and guidance of the planned lesion. However, this was not the only technical hurdle to be overcome. In addition to accurate monitoring, it was actually quite difficult to produce the energy required at the desired site without causing off target effects. This is due to the significant density difference as ultrasonic waves travel through skull, leading to reflection of the ultrasonic waves. Early versions in fact required the creation of a craniectomy window [79], a stage that is no longer needed.

The current version of the technology was first used for medial thalamotomies for the treatment of chronic neuropathic pain in 2009 [80]. The team was able to create 4 mm lesions with no evidence of treatment-related complications or side effects. The ExAblate Neuro (InSightec, Israel) system was FDA approved for essential tremor in 2016 [81]. Indications have now expanded to include brain tumors [79] and Parkinson's disease [82] and forays are now being made into epilepsy.

## *13.4.2 Mechanism*

Focused ultrasound consists of phased array transducers that allow for the delivery of ultrasound energy. The ExAblate Neuro consists of a 30 cm diameter helmet containing 1,024 650kHz transducers [83] capable of creating a 2–6 mm diameter spherical lesion with 1 mm precision. Treatment planning is highly dependent on the skull anatomy, and special care is taken to avoid heating the skull base. Similar to MRgLITT, MRgFUS is performed within a 3T MRI with the patients' head affixed to a stereotactic frame using MRI thermography to monitor the treatment impact.

In contrast to MRgLITT, the impact of MRgFUS is not limited to the delivery of thermal energy. In addition to heating caused by tissue absorption of ultrasonic waves, mechanical destruction through acoustic cavitation, also known as histotripsy, has been shown to improve the efficiency of the therapy [84, 85]. Lastly, the potential of subtherapeutic energy is an active area of research. Lower energy focused ultrasound can modulate network activity [86–88] and even improve drug delivery by opening the blood–brain barrier (BBB) [89, 90], all without causing permanent damage to the underlying tissue [91].

## *13.4.3 Indications*

The use of MRgFUS in epilepsy is currently in the early research stages, with no clinical trials published to date. Due to technological limitations, it is limited to small lesions of deep brain structures and unable to target larger or more superficial lesions. Even deeper but non-midline structures such as the hippocampus are difficult, as the laterality limits the transducer elements capable of energy delivery. Additionally, patients need to have amenable bony anatomy. One key feature is the skull density ratio (SDR), a metric of the attenuation of ultrasound waves as they travel across the calvarium, as patients with an SDR below a certain threshold are not surgical candidates [92]. As a special consideration possibly more relevant to the pediatric literature, a full head shave is required to minimize interference. This can have significant psychosocial stressors and can lead to patient refusal, though progress is being made into waiving this requirement [93]. Active investigations are underway to investigate its potential for amenable targets such as the medial temporal lobe [94], hypothalamic hamartomas [95], cortical dysplasia, and anterior nucleus of the thalamus.

### 13.4.4   Outcomes

Unfortunately, outcomes for seizure control are limited to the few published case series. One patient with mesial temporal lobe epilepsy was seizure free for 1 year [94]. A similar result was reported in a patient with a hypothalamic hamartoma [95]. Many clinical trials are underway, but reports are still pending. Immediate operative complications rates are significantly lower simply by avoiding the need for a skin incision [83], but a true understanding of the potential risks associated with ultrasonic lesioning of brain tissue will depend on future studies of larger case series. The true strength of the procedure, the ability to non-invasively create immediate and permanent lesions in the brain, will of course be a highlight of these studies. It does this in a manner that is radiation free, a key factor in pediatrics given the long-term complications of pediatric cranial radiation [96].

### 13.4.5   Conclusion

Surgical management of epilepsy is an ever-changing field. The neurosurgical armament continues to grow not only in the evaluation of epileptogenic networks but also in its treatment. Despite a changing disease landscape, our ability to identify, localize, and treat epilepsy has continued to improve. This need is all the more urgent in the pediatric population, as controlling seizure frequency in the developing brain can have long-term implications for quality of life, development, and life expectancy.

Unfortunately, the difficulties of conducting randomized control trials in the pediatric population make high level evidence difficult to find. While pediatric and adult epilepsy are different diseases, they do share enough similarities that extrapolations from adult literature have been shown to hold true in many cases. The unique challenges of pediatric epilepsy can be considered an advantage though, and in fact drive innovation. For example, in contrast to most medications and surgical techniques across the spectrum of medicine, the use of laser ablation in epilepsy was actually transferred from the pediatric to the adult population.

Further work will focus on refining indications for our current tools and developing novel ones. Hand in hand with basic scientists and engineers, the development of these new clinical tools will not only improve outcomes but also can provide new insights into the underpinnings of epilepsy. By perpetuating the cycle of treatment and discovery, we can change epilepsy from an enormous burden on patients, families, and the healthcare system into not only a controllable but also a potentially curable disease.

# References


1. Patel P, Moshé SL. The evolution of the concepts of seizures and epilepsy: what's in a name? Epilepsia Open. 2020;5(1):22–35. https://doi.org/10.1002/epi4.12375.
2. Baloyannis SJ. Epilepsy: a way from Herodotus to Hippocrates. Epilepsy Behav. 2013;28(2):303. https://doi.org/10.1016/j.yebeh.2012.04.003.
3. Temkin O. The doctrine of epilepsy in the Hippocratic writings. Bull Inst Hist Med. 1933;1(8):277–322.
4. Rho JM, Steve HW. Brief history of anti-seizure drug development. Epilepsia Open. 2018;3:114–9. https://doi.org/10.1002/epi4.12268.
5. Kwan P, Brodie MJ. Early identification of refractory epilepsy. N Engl J Med. 2000;342(5):314–9. https://doi.org/10.1056/NEJM200002033420503.
6. Ramos-Lizana J, Rodriguez-Lucenilla MI, Aguilera-López P, Aguirre-Rodríguez J, Cassinello-García E. A study of drug-resistant childhood epilepsy testing the new ILAE criteria. Seizure. 2012;21(4):266–72. https://doi.org/10.1016/j.seizure.2012.01.009.
7. Sillanp M, Schmidt D. Early seizure frequency and aetiology predict long-term medical outcome in childhood-onset epilepsy. Brain. 2009;132(4):989–98. https://doi.org/10.1093/brain/awn357.
8. Feindel W, Leblanc R, de Almeida AN. Epilepsy surgery: historical highlights 1909–2009. Epilepsia. 2009;50(Suppl 3):131–51. https://doi.org/10.1111/J.1528-1167.2009.02043.X.
9. Schijns OEMG, Hoogland G, Kubben PL, Koehler PJ. The start and development of epilepsy surgery in Europe: a historical review. Neurosurg Rev. 2015;38(3):447–61. https://doi.org/10.1007/s10143-015-0641-3.
10. Taylor DC. Occasional historical review one hundred years of epilepsy surgery: Sir Victor Horsley's contribution. J Neurol Neurosurg Psychiatry. 1985;1986(49):485–8.
11. Meador KJ, Loring DW, Flanigin H. History of epilepsy surgery. J Epilepsy. 1989;2(I):19–21.
12. Asadi-Pooya AA, Rostami C. History of surgery for temporal lobe epilepsy. Epilepsy Behav. 2017;70:57–60. https://doi.org/10.1016/j.yebeh.2017.02.020.
13. Stone JL, Hughes JR. Early history of electroencephalography and establishment of the American Clinical Neurophysiology Society. J Clin Neurophysiol. 2013;30(1):28–44. https://doi.org/10.1097/WNP.0b013e31827edb2d.
14. Foerster O, Altenburger H. Elektrobiologische Vorg??nge an der menschlichen Hirnrinde. Deutsche Zeitschrift f??r Nervenheilkunde. 1935;135(5–6):277–88. https://doi.org/10.1007/BF01732786.
15. Palmini A, Kim HI, Mugnol F. Electrocorticography in the definition of the irritative zone: its role in the era of multi-channel EEG and modern neuroimaging. In: Handbook of clinical neurophysiology. Amsterdam: Elsevier; 2003. p. 61–71. https://doi.org/10.1016/S1567-4231(03)03005-3.
16. Bancaud J, Talairach J, Schaub C. Stereotaxic functional exploration of the epilepsies of the supplementary areas of the mesial surface of the hemisphere. Electroencephalogr Clin Neurophysiol. 1962;14:788.
17. Shorvon SD. A history of neuroimaging in epilepsy 1909-2009. Epilepsia. 2009;50:39–49. https://doi.org/10.1111/j.1528-1167.2009.02038.x.
18. Duncan JS. Imaging in the surgical treatment of epilepsy. Nat Rev Neurol. 2010;6(10):537–50. https://doi.org/10.1038/nrneurol.2010.131.
19. Engel J. Why is there still doubt to cut it out? Epilepsy Curr. 2013;13(5):198–204. https://doi.org/10.5698/1535-7597-13.5.198.
20. De Tisi J, Bell GS, Peacock JL, et al. The long-term outcome of adult epilepsy surgery, patterns of seizure remission, and relapse: a cohort study. Lancet. 2011;378(9800):1388–95. https://doi.org/10.1016/S0140-6736(11)60890-8.
21. Curry DJ, Gowda A, McNichols RJ, Wilfong AA. MR-guided stereotactic laser ablation of epileptogenic foci in children. Epilepsy Behav. 2012;24(4):408–14. https://doi.org/10.1016/j.yebeh.2012.04.135.

22. Vladyka V. Surgical treatment of epilepsy and its application in temporal epilepsy. Cesk Neurol Neurochir. 1978;41(2):95–106.
23. Parrent AG, Blume WT. Stereotactic amygdalohippocampotomy for the treatment of medial temporal lobe epilepsy. Epilepsia. 1999;40(10):1408–16. https://doi.org/10.1111/j.1528-1157.1999.tb02013.x.
24. Liscak R, Malikova H, Kalina M, et al. Stereotactic radiofrequency amygdalohippocampectomy in the treatment of mesial temporal lobe epilepsy. Acta Neurochir. 2010;152(8):1291–8. https://doi.org/10.1007/s00701-010-0637-2.
25. Carpentier A, McNichols RJ, Stafford RJ, et al. Real-time magnetic resonance-guided laser thermal therapy for focal metastatic brain Tumors. Oper Neurosurgery. 2008;63(Suppl 1):ONS21–9. https://doi.org/10.1227/01.NEU.0000311254.63848.72.
26. de Almeida Bastos DC, Fuentes DT, Traylor J, et al. The use of laser interstitial thermal therapy in the treatment of brain metastases: a literature review. Int J Hyperthermia. 2020;37(2):53–60. https://doi.org/10.1080/02656736.2020.1748238.
27. McNichols RJ, Gowda A, Kangasniemi M, Bankson JA, Price RE, Hazle JD. MR thermometry-based feedback control of laser interstitial thermal therapy at 980 nm. Lasers Surg Med. 2004;34(1):48–55. https://doi.org/10.1002/lsm.10243.
28. Svaasand LO, Fiskerstrand EJ, Kopstad G, et al. Therapeutic response during pulsed laser treatment of port-wine stains: dependence on vessel diameter and depth in dermis. Lasers Med Sci. 1995;10(4):235–43. https://doi.org/10.1007/BF02133615.
29. Fayed I, Sacino MF, Gaillard WD, Keating RF, Oluigbo CO. MR-guided laser interstitial thermal therapy for medically refractory lesional epilepsy in pediatric patients: experience and outcomes. Pediatr Neurosurg. 2018;53(5):322–9. https://doi.org/10.1159/000491823.
30. Wilfong AA, Curry DJ. Hypothalamic hamartomas: optimal approach to clinical evaluation and diagnosis. Epilepsia. 2013;54(Suppl 9):109–14. https://doi.org/10.1111/epi.12454.
31. Hoppe C, Helmstaedter C. Laser interstitial thermotherapy (LiTT) in pediatric epilepsy surgery. Seizure. 2020;77:69–75. https://doi.org/10.1016/J.SEIZURE.2018.12.010.
32. Lewis EC, Weil AG, Duchowny M, Bhatia S, Ragheb J, Miller I. MR-guided laser interstitial thermal therapy for pediatric drug-resistant lesional epilepsy. Epilepsia. 2015;56(10):1590–8. https://doi.org/10.1111/epi.13106.
33. Ravindra VM, Lee S, Gonda D, et al. Magnetic resonance-guided laser interstitial thermal therapy for pediatric periventricular nodular heterotopia-related epilepsy. J Neurosurg Pediatr. 2021;28(6):657–62. https://doi.org/10.3171/2021.5.PEDS21171.
34. Hooten KG, Werner K, Mikati MA, Muh CR. MRI-guided laser interstitial thermal therapy in an infant with tuberous sclerosis: technical case report. J Neurosurg Pediatr. 2018;23(1):92–7. https://doi.org/10.3171/2018.6.PEDS1828.
35. Roland JL, Akbari SHA, Salehi A, Smyth MD. Corpus callosotomy performed with laser interstitial thermal therapy. J Neurosurg. 2019;134(1):314–22. https://doi.org/10.3171/2019.9.JNS191769.
36. Badger CA, Lopez AJ, Heuer G, Kennedy BC. Systematic review of corpus callosotomy utilizing MRI guided laser interstitial thermal therapy. J Clin Neurosci. 2020;76:67–73. https://doi.org/10.1016/J.JOCN.2020.04.046.
37. Petito GT, Wharen RE, Feyissa AM, Grewal SS, Lucas JA, Tatum WO. The impact of stereotactic laser ablation at a typical epilepsy center. Epilepsy Behav. 2018;78:37–44. https://doi.org/10.1016/j.yebeh.2017.10.041.
38. Perry MS, Donahue DJ, Malik SI, et al. Magnetic resonance imaging guided laser interstitial thermal therapy as treatment for intractable insular epilepsy in children. J Neurosurg Pediatr. 2017;20(6):575–82. https://doi.org/10.3171/2017.6.PEDS17158.
39. Ellis JA, Mejia Munne JC, Wang SH, et al. Staged laser interstitial thermal therapy and topectomy for complete obliteration of complex focal cortical dysplasias. J Clin Neurosci. 2016;31:224–8. https://doi.org/10.1016/j.jocn.2016.02.016.
40. Shao J, Radakovich NR, Grabowski M, et al. Lessons learned in using laser interstitial thermal therapy for treatment of brain tumors: a case series of 238 patients from a single institution. World Neurosurg. 2020;139:e345–54. https://doi.org/10.1016/J.WNEU.2020.03.213.

41. Kohlhase K, Zöllner JP, Tandon N, Strzelczyk A, Rosenow F. Comparison of minimally invasive and traditional surgical approaches for refractory mesial temporal lobe epilepsy: a systematic review and meta-analysis of outcomes. Epilepsia. 2021;62(4):831–45. https://doi.org/10.1111/EPI.16846.

42. Lanska DJ. J.L. Corning and vagal nerve stimulation for seizures in the 1880s. Neurology. 2002;58(3):452–9. https://doi.org/10.1212/WNL.58.3.452.

43. Penry JK, Dean JC. Prevention of intractable partial seizures by intermittent vagal stimulation in humans: preliminary results. Epilepsia. 1990;31(s2):S40–3. https://doi.org/10.1111/j.1528-1157.1990.tb05848.x.

44. Johnson RL, Wilson CG. A review of vagus nerve stimulation as a therapeutic intervention. J Inflamm Res. 2018;11:203–13. https://doi.org/10.2147/JIR.S163248.

45. Geller EB. Responsive neurostimulation: review of clinical trials and insights into focal epilepsy. Epilepsy Behav. 2018;88:11–20. https://doi.org/10.1016/j.yebeh.2018.06.042.

46. Cooper IS, Amin I, Riklan M, Waltz JM, Poon TP. Chronic cerebellar stimulation in epilepsy. Clinical and anatomical studies. Arch Neurol. 1976;33(8):559–70. https://doi.org/10.1001/ARCHNEUR.1976.00500080037006.

47. van Buren JM, Wood JH, Oakley J, Hambrecht F. Preliminary evaluation of cerebellar stimulation by double-blind stimulation and biological criteria in the treatment of epilepsy. J Neurosurg. 1978;48(3):407–16. https://doi.org/10.3171/JNS.1978.48.3.0407.

48. Upton A, Amin I, Garnett S, Springman M, Nahmias C, Cooper IS. Evoked metabolic responses in the limbic-striate system produced by stimulation of anterior thalamic nucleus in man. Pacing Clin Electrophysiol. 1987;10(1 Pt 2):217–25. https://doi.org/10.1111/J.1540-8159.1987.TB05952.X.

49. Fisher R, Salanova V, Witt T, et al. Electrical stimulation of the anterior nucleus of thalamus for treatment of refractory epilepsy. Epilepsia. 2010;51(5):899–908. https://doi.org/10.1111/J.1528-1167.2010.02536.X.

50. Li MCH, Cook MJ. Deep brain stimulation for drug-resistant epilepsy. Epilepsia. 2018;59(2):273–90. https://doi.org/10.1111/epi.13964.

51. Laxpati NG, Kasoff WS, Gross RE. Deep brain stimulation for the treatment of epilepsy: circuits, targets, and trials. Neurotherapeutics. 2014;11(3):508–26. https://doi.org/10.1007/s13311-014-0279-9.

52. Krahl S. Vagus nerve stimulation for epilepsy: a review of the peripheral mechanisms. Surg Neurol Int. 2012;3(2):47. https://doi.org/10.4103/2152-7806.91610.

53. Fornai F, Ruffoli R, Giorgi FS, Paparelli A. The role of locus coeruleus in the antiepileptic activity induced by vagus nerve stimulation. Eur J Neurosci. 2011;33(12):2169–78. https://doi.org/10.1111/j.1460-9568.2011.07707.x.

54. Krahl SE, Clark KB. Vagus nerve stimulation for epilepsy: a review of central mechanisms. Surg Neurol Int. 2012;3(Suppl 4):S255–9. https://doi.org/10.4103/2152-7806.103015.

55. Englot DJ, Chang EF, Auguste KI. Vagus nerve stimulation for epilepsy: a meta-analysis of efficacy and predictors of response. J Neurosurg. 2011;115(6):1248–55. https://doi.org/10.3171/2011.7.JNS11977.

56. Motamedi GK, Lesser RP, Miglioretti DL, et al. Optimizing parameters for terminating cortical after discharges with pulse stimulation. Epilepsia. 2002;43(8):836–46. https://doi.org/10.1046/j.1528-1157.2002.24901.x.

57. Penfield W, Herbert J. Epilepsy and the functional anatomy of the human brain. Boston: Little, Brown and Company; 1954.

58. Kokoszka MA, Panov F, la Vega-Talbott M, McGoldrick PE, Wolf SM, Ghatan S. Treatment of medically refractory seizures with responsive neurostimulation: 2 pediatric cases. J Neurosurg Pediatr. 2018;21(4):421–7. https://doi.org/10.3171/2017.10.PEDS17353.

59. Thomas GP, Jobst BC. Critical review of the responsive neurostimulator system for epilepsy. Med Devices (Auckl). 2015;8:405. https://doi.org/10.2147/MDER.S62853.

60. Kokkinos V, Sisterson ND, Wozny TA, Richardson RM. Association of closed-loop brain stimulation neurophysiological features with seizure control among patients with focal epilepsy. JAMA Neurol. 2019;76(7):800. https://doi.org/10.1001/jamaneurol.2019.0658.

61. Sohal VS, Sun FT. Responsive neurostimulation suppresses synchronized cortical rhythms in patients with epilepsy. Neurosurg Clin N Am. 2011;22(4):481–8. https://doi.org/10.1016/j.nec.2011.07.007.
62. Rosin B, Slovik M, Mitelman R, et al. Closed-loop deep brain stimulation is superior in ameliorating parkinsonism. Neuron. 2011;72(2):370–84. https://doi.org/10.1016/J.NEURON.2011.08.023.
63. Shah A, Jhawar SS, Goel A. Analysis of the anatomy of the Papez circuit and adjoining limbic system by fiber dissection techniques. J Clin Neurosci. 2012;19(2):289–98. https://doi.org/10.1016/J.JOCN.2011.04.039.
64. Mohan UR, Watrous AJ, Miller JF, et al. The effects of direct brain stimulation in humans depend on frequency, amplitude, and white-matter proximity. Brain Stimul. 2020;13(5):1183–95. https://doi.org/10.1016/J.BRS.2020.05.009.
65. Chan AY, Knowlton RC, Chang EF, Rao VR. Seizure localization by chronic ambulatory electrocorticography. Clin Neurophysiol Pract. 2018;3:174–6. https://doi.org/10.1016/j.cnp.2018.03.007.
66. King-Stephens D, Mirro E, Weber PB, et al. Lateralization of mesial temporal lobe epilepsy with chronic ambulatory electrocorticography. Epilepsia. 2015;56(6):959–67. https://doi.org/10.1111/EPI.13010.
67. Handforth A, DeGiorgio CM, Schachter SC, et al. Vagus nerve stimulation therapy for partial-onset seizures: a randomized active-control trial. Neurology. 1998;51(1):48–55. https://doi.org/10.1212/WNL.51.1.48.
68. A randomized controlled trial of chronic vagus nerve stimulation for treatment of medically intractable seizures: the Vagus Nerve Stimulation Study Group. Neurology. 1995;45(2):224–30. https://doi.org/10.1212/WNL.45.2.224.
69. Orosz I, McCormick D, Zamponi N, et al. Vagus nerve stimulation for drug-resistant epilepsy: a European long-term study up to 24 months in 347 children. Epilepsia. 2014;55(10):1576–84. https://doi.org/10.1111/epi.12762.
70. Singhal NS, Numis AL, Lee MB, et al. Responsive neurostimulation for treatment of pediatric drug-resistant epilepsy. Epilepsy Behav Case Rep. 2018;10:21–4. https://doi.org/10.1016/j.ebcr.2018.02.002.
71. Bergey GK, Morrell MJ, Mizrahi EM, Goldman A, King-Stephens D, et al. Long-term treatment with responsive brain stimulation in adults with refractory partial seizures. Neurology. 2015;84(8):810–7. http://hsrc.himmelfarb.gwu.edu/smhs_neurosurg_facpubs.
72. Mortazavi A, Elliott RJS, Phan TN, Schreiber J, Gaillard WD, Oluigbo CO. Responsive neurostimulation for the treatment of medically refractory epilepsy in pediatric patients: strategies, outcomes, and technical considerations. J Neurosurg Pediatr. 2021;28(1):54–61. https://doi.org/10.3171/2020.11.PEDS20660.
73. Heck CN, King-Stephens D, Massey AD, et al. Two-year seizure reduction in adults with medically intractable partial onset epilepsy treated with responsive neurostimulation: final results of the RNS System Pivotal trial. Epilepsia. 2014;55(3):432. https://doi.org/10.1111/EPI.12534.
74. Morrell MJ. Responsive cortical stimulation for the treatment of medically intractable partial epilepsy. Neurology. 2011;77(13):1295–304. https://doi.org/10.1212/WNL.0B013E3182302056.
75. Nair DR, Laxer KD, Weber PB, et al. Nine-year prospective efficacy and safety of brain-responsive neurostimulation for focal epilepsy. Neurology. 2020;95(9):e1244–56. https://doi.org/10.1212/WNL.0000000000010154.
76. Velasco AL, Velasco F, Jiménez F, et al. Neuromodulation of the centromedian thalamic nuclei in the treatment of generalized seizures and the improvement of the quality of life in patients with Lennox–Gastaut syndrome. Epilepsia. 2006;47(7):1203–12. https://doi.org/10.1111/J.1528-1167.2006.00593.X.
77. Yan H, Toyota E, Anderson M, et al. A systematic review of deep brain stimulation for the treatment of drug-resistant epilepsy in childhood. J Neurosurg Pediatr. 2018;23(3):274–84. https://doi.org/10.3171/2018.9.PEDS18417.

78. Lynn JG, Putnam TJ. Histology of cerebral lesions produced by focused ultrasound. Am J Pathol. 1944;20(3):637–49. https://doi.org/10.2176/nmc.ra.2017-0024.

79. Ram Z, Cohen ZR, Harnof S, et al. Magnetic resonance imaging-guided, high-intensity focused ultrasound for brain tumor therapy. Neurosurgery. 2006;59(5):949–55. https://doi.org/10.1227/01.NEU.0000254439.02736.D8; discussion 955–6.

80. Martin E, Jeanmonod D, Morel A, Zadicario E, Werner B. High-intensity focused ultrasound for noninvasive functional neurosurgery. Ann Neurol. 2009;66(6):858–61. https://doi.org/10.1002/ana.21801.

81. Elias WJ, Lipsman N, Ondo WG, et al. A randomized trial of focused ultrasound thalamotomy for essential tremor. N Engl J Med. 2016;375(8):730–9. https://doi.org/10.1056/NEJMoa1600159.

82. Magara A, Bühler R, Moser D, Kowalski M, Pourtehrani P, Jeanmonod D. First experience with MR-guided focused ultrasound in the treatment of Parkinson's disease. J Ther Ultrasound. 2014;2(1):1–8. https://doi.org/10.1186/2050-5736-2-11.

83. Abe K, Taira T. Focused ultrasound treatment, present and future. Neurol Med Chir. 2017;57(8):386–91. https://doi.org/10.2176/nmc.ra.2017-0024.

84. Clement GT. Perspectives in clinical uses of high-intensity focused ultrasound. Ultrasonics. 2004;42(10):1087–93. https://doi.org/10.1016/J.ULTRAS.2004.04.003.

85. Kim YS, Rhim H, Min JC, Hyo KL, Choi D. High-intensity focused ultrasound therapy: an overview for radiologists. Korean J Radiol. 2008;9(4):291. https://doi.org/10.3348/KJR.2008.9.4.291.

86. Zhang M, Li B, Liu Y, et al. Different modes of low-frequency focused ultrasound-mediated attenuation of epilepsy based on the topological theory. Micromachines (Basel). 2021;12(8):1001. https://doi.org/10.3390/MI12081001.

87. Ranjan M, Boutet A, Bhatia S, et al. Neuromodulation beyond neurostimulation for epilepsy: scope for focused ultrasound. Expert Rev Neurother. 2019;19(10):937–43. https://doi.org/10.1080/14737175.2019.1635013.

88. Lee CC, Chou CC, Hsiao FJ, et al. Pilot study of focused ultrasound for drug-resistant epilepsy. Epilepsia. 2022;63(1):162–75. https://doi.org/10.1111/EPI.17105.

89. Lev-Tov L, Barbosa DAN, Ghanouni P, Halpern CH, Buch VP. Focused ultrasound for functional neurosurgery. J Neuro Oncol. 2022;156(1):17–22. https://doi.org/10.1007/S11060-021-03818-3.

90. Zhang Y, Tan H, Bertram EH, et al. Non-invasive, focal disconnection of brain circuitry using magnetic resonance-guided low-intensity focused ultrasound to deliver a neurotoxin. Ultrasound Med Biol. 2016;42(9):2261–9. https://doi.org/10.1016/J.ULTRASMEDBIO.2016.04.019.

91. Stern JM, Spivak NM, Becerra SA, et al. Safety of focused ultrasound neuromodulation in humans with temporal lobe epilepsy. Brain Stimul. 2021;14(4):1022–31. https://doi.org/10.1016/J.BRS.2021.06.003.

92. D'Souza M, Chen KS, Rosenberg J, et al. Impact of skull density ratio on efficacy and safety of magnetic resonance–guided focused ultrasound treatment of essential tremor. J Neurosurg. 2019;132(5):1392–7. https://doi.org/10.3171/2019.2.JNS183517.

93. Eames MDC, Hananel A, Snell JW, Kassell NF, Aubry JF. Trans-cranial focused ultrasound without hair shaving: feasibility study in an ex vivo cadaver model. J Ther Ultrasound. 2013;1(1):24. https://doi.org/10.1186/2050-5736-1-24.

94. Abe K, Yamaguchi T, Hori H, et al. Magnetic resonance-guided focused ultrasound for mesial temporal lobe epilepsy: a case report. BMC Neurol. 2020;20(1):1–7. https://doi.org/10.1186/S12883-020-01744-X/FIGURES/6.

95. Yamaguchi T, Hori T, Hori H, et al. Magnetic resonance-guided focused ultrasound ablation of hypothalamic hamartoma as a disconnection surgery: a case report. Acta Neurochir. 2020;162(10):2513–7. https://doi.org/10.1007/S00701-020-04468-6.

96. Duffner PK, Cohen ME, Thomas PR, Lansky SB. The long-term effects of cranial irradiation on the central nervous system. Cancer. 1985;56(Suppl 7):1841–6. https://doi.org/10.1002/1097-0142.

# Chapter 14
# Cranial Repair in Children: Techniques, Materials, and Peculiar Issues

Paolo Frassanito ⓘ and Thomas Beez

## Contents




P. Frassanito (✉)
Pediatric Neurosurgery, Fondazione Policlinico Universitario Agostino Gemelli IRCCS, Rome, Italy

T. Beez
Department of Neurosurgery, Medical Faculty, Heinrich-Heine-Universität, Düsseldorf, Germany
e-mail: thomas.beez@med.uni-duesseldorf.de



© The Author(s), under exclusive license to Springer Nature Switzerland AG 2024
C. Di Rocco (ed.), *Advances and Technical Standards in Neurosurgery*, Advances and Technical Standards in Neurosurgery 49, https://doi.org/10.1007/978-3-031-42398-7_14

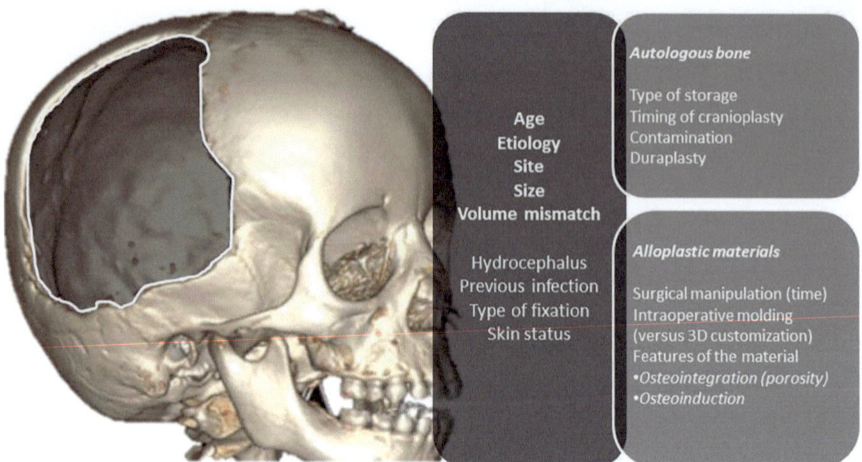



**Fig. 14.1** Factors associated to the outcome of cranioplasty

## 14.1  Introduction

The interest in cranial repair has raised constantly in the last years, as confirmed by the large number of scientific papers and events focused on this topic. Despite several risk factors have been recognized (Fig. 14.1), doubts and controversial issues are still many in particular in the pediatric population.

This pushed to the attempt of reaching a consensus with an expert panel dedicated to pediatric cranioplasty within the Consensus Conference on Cranioplasty (C3) during the International Conference on Recent Advances on Neurotraumatology (ICRAN), held in Naples (Italy) from 20th to 22nd June 2018 [1].

The higher risk of bone resorption in pediatric population is fairly established, with a clear involvement of age-related factors that is maximal in infants and decreases with age along with the incidence of this complication [2–6]. On these grounds, it is essential to define what is pediatric in cranial repair [7] and to stratify the outcome of cranioplasty by age within the pediatric population [8, 9].

However, cranioplasty based on the use of autologous bone is still preferred in pediatric population due to the complications of other cranioplasty solutions and the absence of an ideal material for cranial repair [10]. A large volume of literature deals with new materials, usually claiming good results in the short term, whereas the long-term results are less enthusiastic or even lacking. In daily clinical practice, it is not unusual to encounter extrusion of cranial implants even 20–30 years after initial implantation [11], leading us to conclude that the risk of complication lasts through the whole life of the patient. Moreover, this kind of cases are more easily and frequently reported on unofficial channels, such as online groups of physicians, rather on scientific journals, thus altering the perception of complications of these devices.

A different approach relies on biomimetic materials, namely bioceramics, which try to overcome the limits of synthetic materials, by aiming to osteointegration, through osteoinduction and osteoconduction. This has obvious implications in particular in children, with special regard to the growth of the skull and to the longer life expectancy.

However, the rate of osteointegration is difficult to predict so far, and effective strategies to accelerate and enhance this process are still lacking. Tissue engineering will eventually overcome these limitations.

Although the choice of the material and the timing of the cranioplasty are largely discussed, other factors are increasingly claiming attention and deserve further consideration.

This paper aims to review and discuss the most recent evidences on cranial repair in children.

## 14.2  Choice of the Technique

The techniques for cranial repair mainly focus on the way to close the bone defect and eventually harvest bone autograft. However, soft tissue preservation deserves particular attention. On these grounds, modified trauma flap and other technical nuances [12] are used to reduce the injury to temporal muscle and soft tissues in particular in the pretragal region. Similarly, T-shaped skin incision should be avoided, albeit this option is almost mandatory if urgent decompression is required after elective fronto-temporal surgery.

Whenever autologous bone flap is available, its replacement is still favored in children, as confirmed by consensus statement of C3 [1]. However, this statement can be argued under the age of 7 years, since in the still growing skull, the risk of resorption is higher than 80% [13].

When autologous bone flap is unavailable, harvesting an autologous bone graft could represent an effective option in children. The skull still represents the favored site for harvesting autograft, since the use of ribs and other bone districts is limited by the risk of additional morbidity and in particular of deformity during the future growth of the child [4].

### 14.2.1  Bone Splitting

In case of bone defect with a maximum diameter <5 cm, splitting the cranial bone by its thickness is a valid surgical technique. The parietal region is usually preferred as donor site because of its generally higher thickness and lower esthetical impact compared to the rest of the skull.

The main limitation is represented by the skull thickness at the donor site, as development of diploic layer has been generally considered a factor necessary to allow splitting. This event usually starts at 3 years, the age of the patient thus representing a factor.

Modern technology, such as piezoelectric bone scalpel, allows to split bone graft as thin as 3 mm, thus enhancing the possibility to perform this technique [14].

Healing of the graft, either at the receiving and at the donor sites, relies on the osteogenic potential of dura mater and periosteal layer. Thus, this cranioplasty solution warrants good outcome in case of etiology of bone defect with preserved dura mater and periosteal layer. On the opposite side, when duraplasty allograft coexists with the bone defect (e.g., trauma), the risk of bone graft resorption and failure is higher (Fig. 14.2).

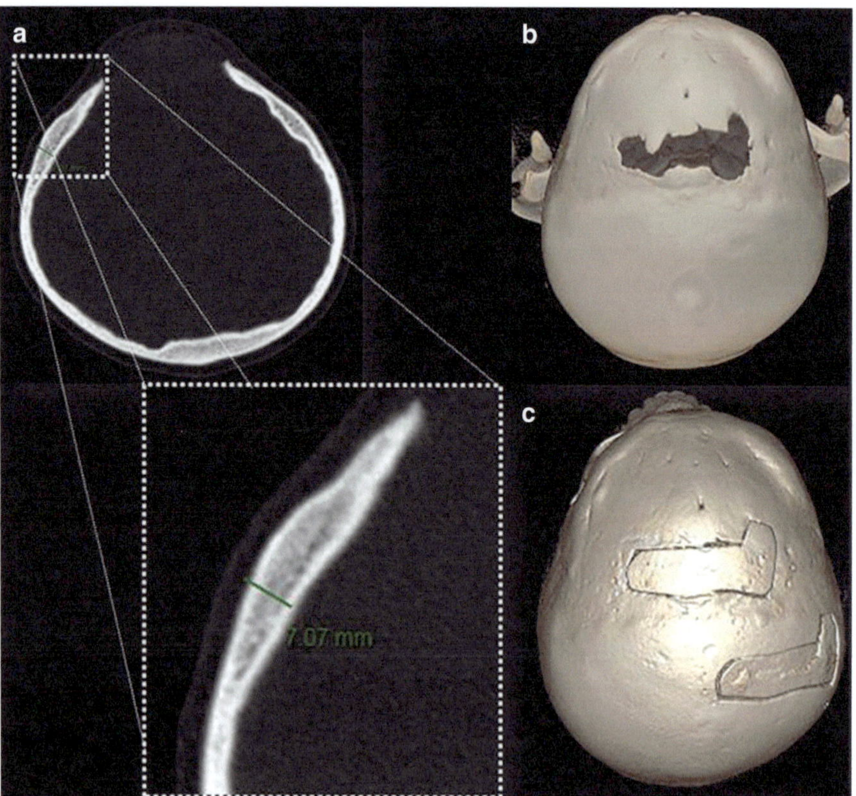


**Fig. 14.2** Three-year-old boy with bregmatic bone defect following surgical correction of trigonocephaly (**a**). 3D-CT scan before and after cranial repair with bone splitting after harvesting bone graft in the right parietal region (**b, c,** respectively)

### *14.2.2  Exchange Cranioplasty*

Exchange cranioplasty (EC) represents an alternative option to harvest autologous bone graft. EC is a technique for cranial repair in children that consists of three steps: (a) harvesting a full-thickness bone graft in an unaffected region of the skull, (b) using the full-thickness bone graft to repair the cranial defect, and (c) repairing the cranial defect at the donor site relying on the preservation of the autologous dura mater and periosteal layer. The osteogenic role of these structures has been already highlighted by Rodgers et al., since in their series the only patients who had residual defects large enough for repeated grafting to be considered were those that had undergone extensive prior surgical manipulation of the entire cranium, leaving no areas of virgin dura or pericranium [15]. The main advantage of this procedure is considered the possibility to exploit a full-thickness calvarial graft, whereas particulate autologous bone may enhance and drive ossification at the donor site.

Though the efficacy of this option has been showed in defects of different etiology, the use of this procedure in post-traumatic defects remains anecdotal and limited to defects of small to medium size (4 cases, ranging from 10 to 72 cm$^2$) [15–17].

The main limitation of these two techniques is the risk of potentially additional morbidity on an unaffected region of the skull and eventually additional surgical wound, if the donor site is not exposed by the initial surgical wound [4].

## 14.3  Choice of the Material

The choice of the material for cranial repair should be carefully balanced on the age of the patient, the features of the bone defect, the availability of autologous bone, either previously stored or eventually harvested, and indication to other heterologous material for cranial repair.

After decompressive craniectomy, autologous bone is preferred for all ages of children, according to C3 consensus statements.

If autologous bone is not available, an osteoconductive material should be preferred for reconstruction.

Below 3 years of age, the best option for osteoconductive material remains unclear.

If a child is more than 3 years of age and an osteoconductive material is not available, a synthetic material can be used but the best option for synthetic material remains unclear [1].

## *14.3.1  Autologous Bone*

Autologous bone as a "biomaterial" is available in the form of autologous bone flaps or autografts from cranial or extracranial donor sites, as described in technical detail above. It is in many aspects the ideal material for cranial reconstruction: By definition, it is the most physiological biomaterial for this purpose and offers the highest (theoretical) potential for osteointegration, i.e., bone healing without interposed scar tissue, to obtain optimal biomechanical properties of the implanted bone flap [18]. In contrast to artificial materials, autologous bone is also compatible with the skull growth in young children [19]. To achieve direct bone healing, viable bone cells, viable dura mater, and periosteum, a minimum gap between bone edge and implant as well as stability of the autologous implant are required [18]. While the latter two aspects can often be achieved by meticulous surgical technique, the viability of autologous bone flaps is uncertain especially after prolonged storage. The main reason for large iatrogenic skull defects is decompressive craniectomy for treatment of raised intracranial pressure. With this procedure, temporary storage of the bone flap is required until reimplantation can be safely performed once the acute phase of brain injury and raised intracranial pressure has passed [20]. While the optimal time window between craniectomy and cranioplasty as well as its influence on complication rates is a matter of scientific debate and data remains inconclusive, this interval generally reflects many weeks of bone flap storage. The common storage techniques are cryoconservation and temporary implantation into an abdominal subcutaneous pocket. However, both means of storage have significant drawbacks: Cryoconservation preserves the structure of the mineralized parts, but causes devitalization of cellular components [21, 22]. The subcutaneous pocket leads to additional surgical morbidity, bone resorption can occur and in small children the subcutaneous space may simply be too small [23]. There are no standardized best practice guidelines for skull flap storage from craniectomy to cranioplasty. Furthermore, clinical studies, either based upon culture versus swab, failed so far to define the role of germ colonization in the resorption of the autologous bone flap. Therefore, tissue banks must implement protocols to provide products with the highest possible clinical effectiveness, without compromising safety [24].

In addition to the aspects related to storage, the dura mater is often opened and widened with an artificial dural substitute during decompressive craniectomy, further impairing the environment for bone healing. Additional factors appear to be the extent of structural brain damage and the presence of hydrocephalus or hygroma [23, 25, 26]. While such patient-specific factors might not be avoidable, the drawbacks related to viability after bone flap storage do not apply to autologous bone harvested as an autograft. However, the surgical autograft techniques described above, i.e., bone splitting, exchange cranioplasty or extracranial grafts, all have additional donor site morbidity, are sometimes hampered by suboptimal spatial fit and coverage, for example, in case of rib grafts, and rely on intact dura mater and periosteum.

In addition to the considerations regarding individual sources and techniques of autologous bone reconstruction, a major problem is inherent to the biomaterial itself and cannot be completely eliminated at present: Bone resorption or aseptic bone necrosis can lead to partial or complete destruction of autologous bone implants and thus loss of biomechanical properties and esthetic outcomes [27, 28]. This phenomenon is most evident in cryoconserved autologous bone flaps after decompressive craniectomy and occurs after a mean period of 19 months following reimplantation [29]. The risk is age dependent, with resorption rates of up to 100% in children under 1 year of age, gradually decreasing to 80% in children under 8 years of age and 50% in older children and adults [30]. A recent study enrolling mainly adult patients provides interesting insights through histopathological examination of residual bone flaps explanted due to significant resorption: A coexistence of osteoblastic and osteoclastic activity was observed and the thinning of the bone flaps was most evident at the edges and the outer surface [22]. Osteoclastic activity was pronounced in areas of bone marrow cavity fibrosis. These observations might stimulate research into focused graft modifications, such as lavage techniques to remove bone marrow as already used in osteochondral allografts or pro-osteoblastic signalling through bone morphogenetic proteins [31–33]. In addition to biological factors, the iatrogenic aspects remain unclear as well. The roles of cranioplasty timing, dural substitutes, conservation protocols, and surgical techniques are incompletely understood and currently investigated in collaborative projects [34–36].

In summary, autologous bone is a very promising biomaterial for cranial reconstruction in children, with the main advantages being osteointegration and compatibility with skull growth. A main problem is bone resorption, which is incompletely understood but probably influenced by storage, surgical technique, and patient age. Future research is required to optimize outcomes in this field.

### *14.3.2 Alloplastic Materials*

Cranial implants made of alloplastic materials are created with CAD–CAM technology (computer aided design–computer aided manufacturing). Such patient-specific implants are designed based on a computed tomography scan and produced by either subtraction methods or additive manufacturing [37, 38]. There is a broad spectrum of alloplastic materials currently available on the market, comprising metal, polymers, mineral-based materials, and composite materials [11].

Titanium is the most common metal currently in use for cranial implants, either as a solid CAD-CAM implant or as a mesh [11, 39, 40]. It is biocompatible and appears to have a lower infection rate. A solid titanium implant leads to significant artifacts in cranial imaging, is very rigid, and cannot be easily modified during surgery, and it has thermoconductive properties that are sometimes felt uncomfortable by patients. A titanium mesh can be modified by the surgeon, but offers little mechanical strength.

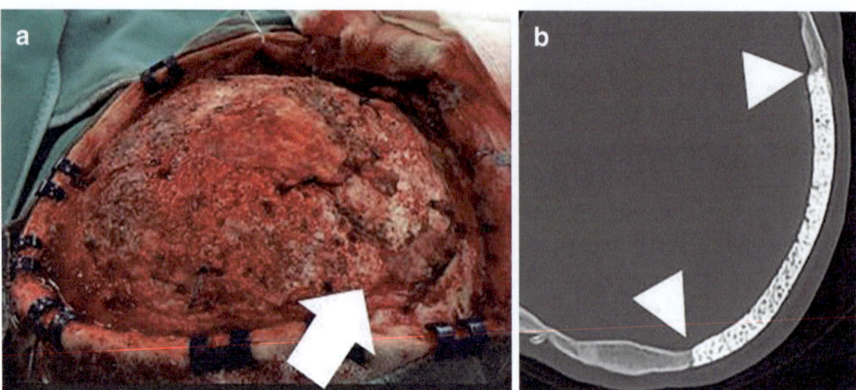

**Fig. 14.3** Hydroxyapatite implant surgically revised because of multiple fractures of the device after a minor trauma occurred in the first months after cranioplasty (**a**, *arrow*). Hydroxyapatite implant with fair signs of osteointegration at 5 years follow-up, in particular at the edges of the bone defect (*arrowheads*) thus warranting characteristics similar to autologous bone (**b**)

The most common polymers are polyetheretherketone (PEEK), polyetherketoneketone (PEKK), and polymethyl methacrylate (PMMA) [11, 41]. PEEK has high elasticity and strength, positive thermoconductive properties, and allows a certain degree of intraoperative modification using high-speed drills. However, its inert surface does not allow for tissue integration or osteointegration. PEKK and PMMA are more porous and might break more easily, but are slightly less inert compared to PEEK. PMMA-based bone cement in combination with CAD-CAM moulds can also be used to produce patient-specific implants in the operation room [42].

Hydroxyapatite is mineral-based material that has a porous structure encouraging tissue ingrowth and osteointegration (Fig. 14.3), but is burdened by a reduced implant strength until osteintegration occurs [8, 11].

Composite materials include for example fiberglass or calcium phosphate within a titanium matrix [43–45]. The aim is to provide properties more similar to bone and encourage tissue integration and osteointegration, although the level of scientific evidence is generally low. The material can be manufactured into very thin implants, and the surface structure is less inert (Fig. 14.4). In contrast to solid titanium implants, most other materials allow for postoperative neuroimaging without significant artifacts.

Clinical data on alloplastic cranioplasty for iatrogenic skull defects in children, especially with regard to comparison of different materials, is mainly limited to (typically retrospective) series and post-marketing surveillance with often small cohorts. A similar degree of evidence is found for autologous cranioplasty [30]. An evidence-based recommendation is therefore not possible. In a large systematic review of almost 900 pediatric cranioplasty procedures, the revision rate for autologous bone flaps was 13% and for alloplastic implants, mainly hydroxyapatite, it was 3% [30]. Caution is warranted when interpreting these results and when drawing conclusions: The risk of bias is high and missing data as well as

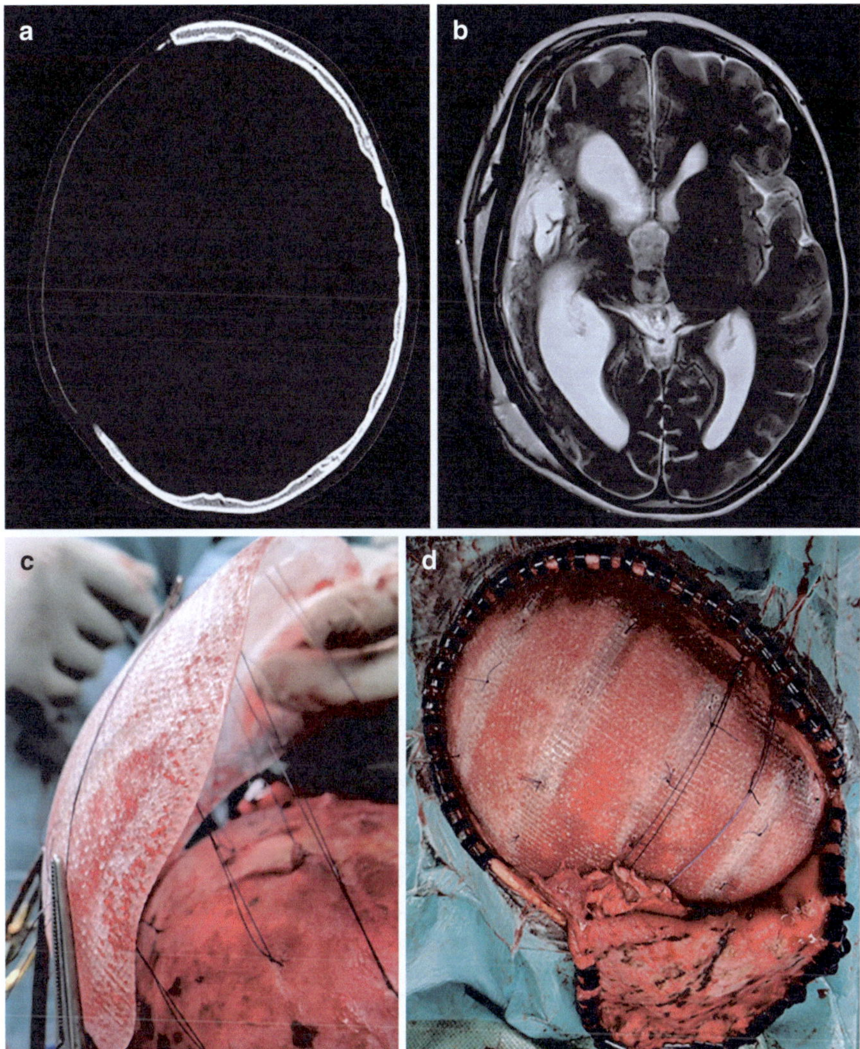

**Fig. 14.4** Eleven-year-old girl with hemicraniectomy defect after severe traumatic brain injury (**a**). Postoperative MRI demonstrates perfect fit of the fiberglass composite implant, with some compensatory ventricular dilatation due to posttraumatic brain volume loss of the right hemisphere (**b**). Note the very thin diameter of the clear implant (**c**) and the sandwich structure allowing instant absorption of blood once put in situ, which is said to encourage osteointegration (**d**)

different outcome parameters hamper pooling of data. However, a recent study comparing complication rates obtained from surgeons on-site with a post-marketing clinical database collected by a manufacturing company of hydroxyapatite found similar results in both groups, indicating reliable data [46]. The revision rate was comparable with the previously mentioned systematic review. For

**Table 14.1** Stratification by age of cranial growth, complications of cranial repair, and strategies to improve the outcome of cranial repair

| Age group [years] | Skull growth | Bone flap resorption rate (%) | Alloplastic implant complication rate | Recommendations |
|---|---|---|---|---|
| <3 | Rapid (~15–17 cm increase in head circumference) | 100 | NA | – Avoid large skull defects, i.e., consider alternatives to decompressive craniectomy<br>– Prefer autografts, e.g., exchange cranioplasty |
| 3–5/7 | Slow (~2–4 cm increase in head circumference) | 80 | 20% | – Assume equipoise between autografts and allografts |
| >5/7 | Very slow (<4 cm increase in head circumference) | 30–50 | 6–8% | – Same considerations as in adults, alloplastic implants appear to be valid and probably superior alternative to cryoconserved bone flaps |

autologous bone flaps, the higher revision rate is largely explained by bone resorption. In our series, the bone flap resorption rate was 70% after a mean follow-up of 19 months, compared with rates obtained from the literature ranging from 20% to more than 80% [29]. Even when taking into account differences in research methodology and reporting, the bone flap resorption rate is high and a main reason for revision surgery.

Across studies, age appears to be a very important and consistent factor significantly influencing complication rates: For autologous cranioplasty with cryoconserved bone flaps, the resorption rate is certainly age dependent, as detailed above [19, 47]. For alloplastic cranioplasty, most data is available for hydroxyapatite implants, and the complication rate in children under 7 years of age is significantly higher (20%) compared to children aged 7–13 years (6.6%) or to adults (8%) [8, 46]. This is explained by conflicts between skull growth dynamics and alloplastic implants. Skull growth is most dynamic and rapid within the first 2 years of life, becomes slower and less extensive afterwards, until the skull volume almost reaches the adult level between 5 and 7 years of life [19].

Table 14.1 attempts to unify the above-mentioned considerations and study results into a cranioplasty strategy and subsequent recommendation (Table 14.1).

Furthermore, the choice of the material obviously influences the choice of the method for cranioplasty fixation. This aspect deserves particular attention in children. Indeed, metal and plastic devices may be potentially fixed with titanium microplates and screws. Once again, titanium may interfere with the still growing skull leading to the lost of stability of the devices and eventual migration or extrusion through the skin. Thus, titanium means are avoided under the age of 7 years. Regardless the age of the patient, these could be not used to secure bioceramics. Sutures are commonly used as an alternative to titanium means, regardless the material used for cranioplasty. Nonresorbable sutures should be used since resorbable sutures may lose their strength and affects the stability of the device. However, silk sutures may extrude through the skin in children due to their allergenic effect, while nylon sutures may be burdened by the same complication for their mechanical rigidity. Biodegradable plates and screws represent also a valid option for bioceramics [4].

## 14.4  Cranioplasty Strategy and Peculiar Issues

The choice of the material received great attention through the literature, but the main risk is to neglect other aspects that may affect the outcome of cranial repair in children or evenly to attribute to the material complications that could recognize other causes. For example, bioceramic warrants lower resistance compared to other synthetic materials, such as plastics and metals. However, some mechanical complications of bioceramic cranioplasty may be attributed to a wrong surgical strategy neglecting some peculiar pediatric aspects, thus configuring a "false-positive" complication of the material [48].

On the other side, the absence of a critical appraisal of the complications related to the use of a particular material may lead to imaginative explanations involving factors unrelated to the failure of cranial repair. As an example, skin dehiscence with exposure of titanium mesh cranioplasty has been related to small new osteogenesis of the dura mater, thus configuring a "false-negative" complication of the material [49].

Finally, planning cranial repair without restoring the physiology of the intracranial system may lead to lethal complication [50].

In conclusion, it is not all about choice of the material and technique, but it is about strategy.

Strategy for cranial repair should carefully consider the etiology of the bone defect. Head injury and decompressive craniectomy represent the most frequent etiology and the most complex picture for reconstruction due to peculiar factors related to the initial disease and surgical aspects.

On the other side, bone tumor is a less frequent etiology and offers the possibility to repair the skull at the same time of surgical demolition, thus avoiding the problems of delayed cranioplasty [51]. In this case, the main issue is a correct planning of the customized implant on the preoperative imaging and a surgical resection that would respect the preoperative planning. In this context, neuronavigation may be used in the demolition phase. Alternatively, the manufacturer of the customized implant may provide osteotomy guide that could help the surgeon to obtain a bone defect perfectly fitting the implant.

In this context, there is still space for intraoperative molding of alloplastic material when there is no time for manufacturing a customized implant (i.e., tumor with clinically significant mass effect and/or malignancy). If the curvature of the outer or

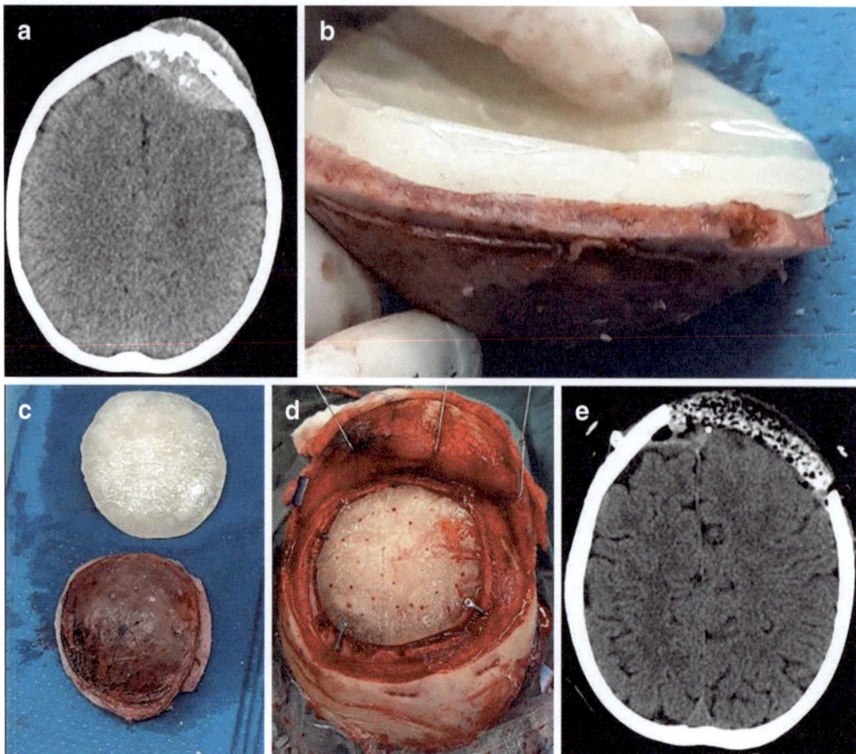

**Fig. 14.5** Sarcomatous lesion of the frontal bone (**a**). PMMA cranioplasty was intraoperatively molded on the inner table of the resected bone flap (**b**, **c**), thus reducing the time of surgical manipulation of the material and obtaining a prosthesis that fits perfectly the defect and the curvature of the skull (**d**), as confirmed by the post-operative CT (**e**)

inner table of the resected bone is not altered by the tumor, the bone flap could be used as a guide for molding the synthetic cranioplasty (Fig. 14.5).

Another frequent cause of cranial defect in children is represented by cranial malformations, in particular bone defects resulting from surgical correction of craniosynostosis [52]. In this context, the features of the defects may largely vary from small defects with preserved dura mater in simple craniosynostosis to large defects in syndromic craniosynostosis with restricted skull volume and herniating dura and intracranial content, requiring an extensive cranial expansion along with skull repair.

Additionally, etiology of the defect may affect the status of soft tissues that should cover the cranioplasty. Once again, trauma etiology may encompass the less favorable condition for cranial repair with additional surgical wound and scarification of soft tissues or loss of substance in the worst case, thus requiring a multidisciplinary approach to cranial repair.

On the other side, in case of syndromic craniosynostosis with multiple previous surgeries and need for cranial expansion, the skin retraction may represent a limit. Acellular dermal matrix has been used to thicken the soft tissue covering cranioplasty with promising results [53, 54]. However, in selected cases, skin expansion is indicated before proceeding to calvarial repair.

Finally, etiology of the defect obviously influences the timing of subsequent cranioplasty. In bone tumors, one-step demolition and reconstruction could be performed and is advocated. In craniosynostosis, it could be recommended to wait for spontaneous bone healing (usually until 3 years of age), before defining the need for cranial repair. In trauma, timing of cranioplasty deserves specific considerations.

A careful knowledge of the etiology of the defect should lead to a careful planning of the cranioplasty strategy.

On these grounds, the presence of a bundle is essential to reduce complications [55].

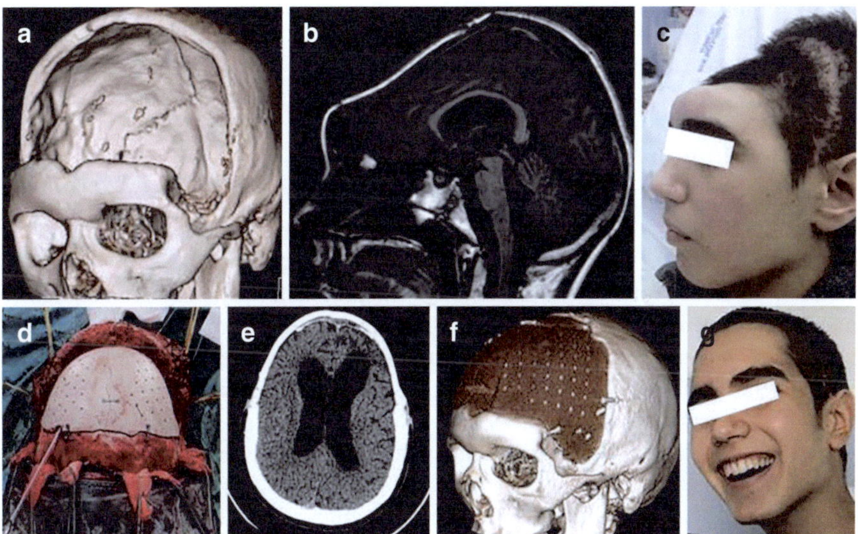

**Fig. 14.6** 3D-CT after bifrontal decompressive craniectomy (**a**) and failure of autologous bone-assisted cranioplasty because of infection. MR and patient picture showing sinking flap associated to syndrome of the trephined (**b**, **c**). Cranioplasty was performed after 2 months, despite the previous history of infection, for the severe neurological disturbances and the risk of skin dehiscence at the edges of bone defect (**d**). CT scan showing expansion of brain parenchyma (**e**) after PEEK cranioplasty (**f**) with good clinical and neurological recovery (**g**)

### *14.4.1  Timing*

Timing of cranioplasty has been largely discussed through the literature. However, discussion focusing the point on early versus late cranial repair does not get to the point.

Restoring the physiological integrity of the skull and its functions is the aim of cranial repair and should be pursued as soon as possible in particular in children and more specifically when the skull is still growing. In other words, as soon as the brain swelling regresses and the general conditions of the patients are suitable to undergo surgery, the skull could and should be repaired.

In our experience, the only real indication to postpone cranioplasty is an infection of the soft tissues of the surgical flap. In that case, we prefer to postpone surgery at least 3 months after curing the infection in order to prevent any further infectious complication of the cranioplasty [56]. On the other side, clinical and neurological conditions of the patients may require to anticipate cranial repair. This is the case of the sinking flap syndrome. Thus, physicians should seek a compromise on timing of cranioplasty (Fig. 14.6).

In children, timing of cranioplasty deserves additional attention under the age of 7 years, namely when the skull is still growing. In this age group, repairing the skull as soon as possible is a priority in order to restore the correct vectors of growth of the skull and avoid any mismatch between the intracranial content and the skull volume related to a deficient growth of the open skull.

### *14.4.2  Management of Hydrocephalus*

Criteria for diagnosis of post-traumatic hydrocephalus are still debated, in particular when the skull is still open, and this issue goes beyond the purpose of the present chapter. On these grounds, extrathecal CSF shunting before cranial repair should be avoided. When progressive dilation of ventricles associated to tense skin flap prevents the placement of cranioplasty, the best management option would be to place a perioperative external ventricular drainage at the time of cranial repair. If hydrocephalus persists after cranioplasty, then CSF shunting is performed. This strategy allows to avoid the concomitant placement of CSF shunting and cranioplasty, which has been associated to a higher risk of complications and to avoid the placement of permanent CSF shunting device in ventriculomegaly related to decompressive craniectomy without overt hydrocephalus [4]. Similarly, subdural collection may be drained at the time of cranial repair and internal subdural shunting device are reserved to cases with recurrent collections after cranioplasty.

The only circumstance, that cannot be avoided, requiring CSF shunting with still open skull is when overt hydrocephalus is treated and cranioplasty is removed because of infection. In this case, patient should be carefully monitored in order to avoid a condition of sinking flap with skin dehiscence at the edges of the bone defect.

### 14.4.3  Age-Related Factors (with Particular Regards to Infant Cranioplasty)

Age is the best established and explained risk factor for cranial reconstruction (Table 14.1). The most problematic age group is children younger than 3 years of age, where an (a) excessively high resorption rate of conserved bone flaps, (b) virtual impossibility of successful repair with alloplastic implant due to the rapid skull growth as well as (c) limitations to bone harvesting procedures (e.g., very thin split bone grafts) are encountered [4, 19]. While exchange cranioplasty as described above might be the most acceptable treatment option, avoiding large iatrogenic defects in this age group is important in our opinion. While the infant skull can accommodate slow intracranial volume increase (e.g., hydrocephalus) by accelerated head growth leading to macrocephaly, this mechanism of compensation does not apply to acute intracranial masses, such as hemorrhage. Therefore in rare circumstances, a decompressive procedure becomes necessary even in infants. However, instead of performing a classic decompressive craniectomy with extracorporeal removal of the bone flap, alternative surgical techniques can be applied to achieve decompression but avoid or at least limit the size of an open skull defect. Such procedures described in the literature are decompressive craniotomies with either a hinge or a free floating bone flap as well as procedures incorporating barrel stave osteotomies (similar to craniofacial surgery) [57, 58].

Once children have reached an age of 3 to 5–7 years, the skull growth will be much slower and less extensive [19]. Alloplastic implants thus become a possible option, whereas conserved bone flaps still have a very high resorption rate, albeit lesser compared to infants. Autografts such as split bone grafts are technically less demanding in this age group compared to infants, as the skull bone is thicker and the diploic space develops by 3 years of age [59]. The degree of evidence is low, and there are advocates of both reconstruction strategies (i.e., alloplastic implants versus autografts). Based on the limited data and the ongoing debate among surgeons, equipoise should be assumed when weighing the risks of alloplastic implants and the risks and donor site morbidity of allografts against each other in this age group.

Thus, it is difficult to define the best option in this age group. Cryoconserved bone flaps are still used as first choice by the first author (PF), while is not the first choice of the second author (TB). However, when reimplanting autologous bone flap, parents must be informed that a revision procedure is highly likely during childhood due to bone flap resorption.

The least problematic pediatric age group with regard to cranial reconstruction are children aged 5–7 years and above, where the skull has almost reached adult dimensions and skull growth is therefore not a factor any more [19]. Here the same considerations apply as in adults, with cryoconserved bone flaps having a resorption rate of 30–50% and alloplastic implants (based on precise data for hydroxyapatite) have a complication rate of 6–8% [46]. The surgical revision rate calculated from the previously mentioned systematic review suggests an advantage of alloplastic over autologous implants, with rates of 3% versus 13% [30]. However, it has to be stressed that the currently available level of evidence is weak and we encourage enrolment of patients in multicentric registries to compare institutional protocols in large cohorts with systematic and prospective data collection [34].

### 14.4.4 The "Volume" Issue (Craniocerebral Disproportion and How to Manage It)

Any mismatch between the skull volume and the intracranial content may favor the occurrence of complications. On this basis, a classification of conditions with volume mismatch was proposed in a previous paper [48].

A negative volume mismatch consists of intracranial content volume minor to skull volume. This condition is easily identified, as the skin flap is sinking, and has been identified as negative prognostic factor eventually related to sudden death after cranioplasty [60]. On these grounds, surgical planning should entail all the measures, aiming to seal the epidural spaces and favor the brain expansion, strictly avoiding closed vacuum suction that could, on the other hand, precipitate the loss of autoregulation of the "sinking" brain [61–63].

A positive volume mismatch consists of intracranial content volume higher than skull volume. This condition could be more subtle and insidious in children when it is not sustained by residual brain edema, or CSF-related disturbances. In fact, in children, a positive volume mismatch may depend on a condition of acquired craniocerebral disproportion.

In craniocerebral disproportion (CCD), the volume of the brain exceeds the intracranial space, leading to inadequate accommodation of the growing brain, failure of physiological regulation mechanism such as cerebral blood volume, and also subsequent anatomical anomalies [64]. This syndrome is best characterized as a complication of chronic overdrainage in children shunted for infant hydrocephalus: The overdraining shunt diminishes the intracranial volume and cerebrospinal fluid (CSF) pulse pressure, thereby negatively modulating calvarial expansive growth, which is basically triggered by brain growth [65]. If this phenomenon is not addressed by increasing the shunt pressure level or adding an anti-siphoning device, the skull remains small and finally microcephaly becomes fixed. Anatomical changes such as copper-beaten inner table, secondary craniosynostosis, or hindbrain herniation become evident. At some point, compensatory mechanisms are exhausted and a clinical picture similar to slit-ventricle syndrome will develop, with episodes of incapacitating headaches being the major symptom. At that point, treatment is often very difficult, as modifications of the shunt can be insufficient and expansion cranioplasty might be indicated.

In the context of iatrogenic skull defects and cranial repair, many aspects of CCD are similar, although aspects of pathogenesis and the problems encountered are somewhat different [48].

The constellation carrying the highest risk for CCD is a child in the first 3 years of life with a large skull defect left open for a prolonged period of time along with fully preserved brain parenchyma (e.g., acute subdural hematoma) [5]. The intracranial pressure and CSF pulsatility are reduced and asymmetrical or even globally reduced skull growth becomes evident. When late cranial repair is finally performed, intraoperative as well as postoperative complications can be encountered. Intraoperative CSF drainage or medical reduction of brain volume (e.g., mannitol administration) might be required to achieve adequate placement of the implant without excessive pressure on the brain. In the postoperative course and during long-term follow up the classical symptoms of CCD can occur. In addition, implant dislocation is a typical sign of CCD in this context. Therapeutic solutions have to be tailored to the individual patient, with surgical interventions ranging from CSF drainage to expansion cranioplasty involving the entire cranium [48, 64, 66].

## 14.5  Conclusions

Cranial repair in children requires a deep understanding of the physiologic mechanism of skull growth. On this basis, careful planning based upon the age of the patient, the etiology of the defect, and the evaluation of brain parenchyma and its residual growth should be performed on a case-by-case basis. A thorough knowledge of the surgical techniques and the characteristics and indications for use of cranioplasty materials is mandatory.

**Conflict of Interest**  PF received consultancy fees from Fin-ceramica spa (producing HA cranioplasty) and Integra-Codman (commercializing HA cranioplasties). TB has no conflicts of interest to declare that are relevant to the content of this article.

## References


1. Iaccarino C, Kolias A, Adelson PD, Rubiano AM, Viaroli E, Buki A, et al. Consensus statement from the international consensus meeting on post-traumatic cranioplasty. Acta Neurochir. 2021;163(2):423–40.
2. Frassanito P, Massimi L, Caldarelli M, Tamburrini G, Di Rocco C. Bone flap resorption in infants. J Neurosurg Pediatr. 2014;13(2):243–4.
3. Rocque BG, Agee BS, Thompson EM, Piedra M, Baird LC, Selden NR, et al. Complications following pediatric cranioplasty after decompressive craniectomy: a multicenter retrospective study. J Neurosurg Pediatr. 2018;22(3):225–32.
4. Frassanito P, Tamburrini G, Massimi L, Peraio S, Caldarelli M, Di Rocco C. Problems of reconstructive cranioplasty after traumatic brain injury in children. Childs Nerv Syst. 2017;33(10):1759–68.
5. Frassanito P, Massimi L, Caldarelli M, Tamburrini G, Di Rocco C. Complications of delayed cranial repair after decompressive craniectomy in children less than 1 year old. Acta Neurochir. 2012;154(5):927–33.
6. Behbahani M, Rosenberg DM, Rosinski CL, Chaudhry NS, Nikas D. Cranioplasty in infants less than 24 months of age: a retrospective case review of pitfalls, outcomes, and complications. World Neurosurg. 2019;132:e479–86.

7. Zaed I, Servadei F. Time to define what is pediatric in cranial reconstruction. Childs Nerv Syst. 2021;37(1):7–8.
8. Frassanito P, Massimi L, Tamburrini G, Bianchi F, Nataloni A, Canella V, et al. Custom-made hydroxyapatite for cranial repair in a specific pediatric age group (7–13 years old): a multicenter post-marketing surveillance study. Childs Nerv Syst. 2018;34(11):2283–9.
9. Frassanito P, Tamburrini G, Massimi L, Di Rocco C, Nataloni A, Fabbri G, et al. Post-marketing surveillance of CustomBone service implanted in children under 7 years old. Acta Neurochir. 2015;157(1):115–21.
10. Klieverik VM, Miller KJ, Singhal A, Han KS, Woerdeman PA. Cranioplasty after craniectomy in pediatric patients—a systematic review. Childs Nerv Syst. 2019;35(9):1481–90.
11. Goodrich JT, Sandler AL, Tepper O. A review of reconstructive materials for use in craniofacial surgery bone fixation materials, bone substitutes, and distractors. Childs Nerv Syst. 2012;28(9):1577–88.
12. Honeybul S. Management of the temporal muscle during cranioplasty: technical note. J Neurosurg Pediatr. 2016;17(6):701–4.
13. Martin KD, Franz B, Kirsch M, Polanski W, von der Hagen M, Schackert G, et al. Autologous bone flap cranioplasty following decompressive craniectomy is combined with a high complication rate in pediatric traumatic brain injury patients. Acta Neurochir. 2014;156(4):813–24.
14. Massimi L, Rapisarda A, Bianchi F, Frassanito P, Tamburrini G, Pelo S, et al. Piezosurgery in pediatric neurosurgery. World Neurosurg. 2019;126:e625–33.
15. Rogers GF, Greene AK, Mulliken JB, Proctor MR, Ridgway EB. Exchange cranioplasty using autologous calvarial particulate bone graft effectively repairs large cranial defects. Plast Reconstr Surg. 2011;127(4):1631–42.
16. Ropper AE, Rogers GF, Ridgway EB, Proctor MR. Repair of a large congenital frontal bone defect with autologous exchange cranioplasty. J Neurosurg Pediatr. 2010;6(5):464–7.
17. Gupta D. Novel solutions to cranioplasty: from exchange cranioplasty to synthetic patient-specific implants. Neurol India. 2021;69(3):618–9.
18. Perren SM. Physical and biological aspects of fracture healing with special reference to internal fixation. Clin Orthop Relat Res. 1979;138:175–96.
19. Frassanito P, Bianchi F, Pennisi G, Massimi L, Tamburrini G, Caldarelli M. The growth of the neurocranium: literature review and implications in cranial repair. Childs Nerv Syst. 2019;35(9):1459–65.
20. Beez T, Munoz-Bendix C, Steiger HJ, Beseoglu K. Decompressive craniectomy for acute ischemic stroke. Crit Care. 2019;23(1):209.
21. Beez T, Sabel M, Ahmadi SA, Beseoglu K, Steiger HJ, Sabel M. Scanning electron microscopic surface analysis of cryoconserved skull bone after decompressive craniectomy. Cell Tissue Bank. 2014;15(1):85–8.
22. Göttsche J, Mende KC, Schram A, Westphal M, Amling M, Regelsberger J, et al. Cranial bone flap resorption-pathological features and their implications for clinical treatment. Neurosurg Rev. 2021;44(4):2253–60.
23. Ernst G, Qeadan F, Carlson AP. Subcutaneous bone flap storage after emergency craniectomy: cost-effectiveness and rate of resorption. J Neurosurg. 2018;129(6):1604–10.
24. Mirabet V, García D, Yagüe N, Larrea LR, Arbona C, Botella C. The storage of skull bone flaps for autologous cranioplasty: literature review. Cell Tissue Bank. 2021;22(3):355–67.
25. Hersh DS, Anderson HJ, Woodworth GF, Martin JE, Khan YM. Bone flap resorption in pediatric patients following autologous cranioplasty. Oper Neurosurg. 2021;20(5):436–43.
26. Schwarz F, Dünisch P, Walter J, Sakr Y, Kalff R, Ewald C. Cranioplasty after decompressive craniectomy: is there a rationale for an initial artificial bone-substitute implant? A single-center experience after 631 procedures. J Neurosurg. 2016;124(3):710–5.
27. Korhonen TK, Salokorpi N, Ohtonen P, Lehenkari P, Serlo W, Niinimäki J, et al. Classification of bone flap resorption after cranioplasty: a proposal for a computed tomography-based scoring system. Acta Neurochir. 2019;161(3):473–81.

28. Korhonen TK, Posti JP, Niinimäki J, Serlo W, Salokorpi N, Tetri S. Two-center validation of the Oulu resorption score for bone flap resorption after autologous cranioplasty. Clin Neurol Neurosurg. 2022;212:107083.
29. Beez T, Munoz-Bendix C, Ahmadi SA, Steiger HJ, Beseoglu K. From decompressive craniectomy to cranioplasty and beyond—a pediatric neurosurgery perspective. Childs Nerv Syst. 2019;35(9):1517–24.
30. Klieverik VM, Miller KJ, Singhal A, Sen HK, Woerdeman PA. Cranioplasty after craniectomy in pediatric patients—a systematic review. Childs Nerv Syst. 2019;35(9):1481–90.
31. Meyer MA, McCarthy MA, Gitelis ME, Poland SG, Urita A, Chubinskaya S, et al. Effectiveness of lavage techniques in removing immunogenic elements from osteochondral allografts. Cartilage. 2017;8(4):369–73.
32. Smith DM, Afifi AM, Cooper GM, Mooney MP, Marra KG, Losee JE. BMP-2-based repair of large-scale calvarial defects in an experimental model: regenerative surgery in cranioplasty. J Craniofac Surg. 2008;19(5):1315–22.
33. Sun Y, Jiang W, Cory E, Caffrey JP, Hsu FH, Chen AC, et al. Pulsed lavage cleansing of osteochondral grafts depends on lavage duration, flow intensity, and graft storage condition. PLoS One. 2017;12(5):e0176934.
34. Beez T, Schuhmann MU, Frassanito P, Di Rocco F, Thomale UW, Bock HC. Protocol for the multicentre prospective paediatric craniectomy and cranioplasty registry (pedCCR) under the auspices of the European Society for Paediatric Neurosurgery (ESPN). Childs Nerv Syst. 2022;38(8):1461–7.
35. Giese H, Sauvigny T, Sakowitz OW, Bierschneider M, Güresir E, Henker C, et al. German Cranial Reconstruction Registry (GCRR): protocol for a prospective, multicentre, open registry. BMJ Open. 2015;5(9):e009273.
36. Kolias AG, Bulters DO, Cowie CJ, Wilson MH, Afshari FT, Helmy A, et al. Proposal for establishment of the UK Cranial Reconstruction Registry (UKCRR). Br J Neurosurg. 2014;28(3):310–4.
37. Moellmann HL, Mehr VN, Karnatz N, Wilkat M, Riedel E, Rana M. Evaluation of the fitting accuracy of CAD/CAM-manufactured patient-specific implants for the reconstruction of cranial defects—a retrospective study. J Clin Med. 2022;11(7):2045.
38. De Santis R, Russo T, Rau JV, Papallo I, Martorelli M, Gloria A. Design of 3D additively manufactured hybrid structures for cranioplasty. Materials. 2021;14(1):181.
39. Dash C, Dasukil S, Boyina KK, Panda R, Ahmad SR. A novel prefabricated patient-specific titanium cranioplasty: reconsideration from a traditional approach. Oral Maxillofac Surg. 2022;26(2):223–8.
40. Cabraja M, Klein M, Lehmann TN. Long-term results following titanium cranioplasty of large skull defects. Neurosurg Focus. 2009;26(6):E10.
41. Punchak M, Chung LK, Lagman C, Bui TT, Lazareff J, Rezzadeh K, et al. Outcomes following polyetheretherketone (PEEK) cranioplasty: systematic review and meta-analysis. J Clin Neurosci. 2017;41:30–5.
42. Abdel Hay J, Smayra T, Moussa R. Customized polymethylmethacrylate cranioplasty implants using 3-dimensional printed polylactic acid molds: technical note with 2 illustrative cases. World Neurosurg. 2017;105:971–979.e1.
43. Vallittu PK. Bioactive glass-containing cranial implants: an overview. J Mater Sci. 2017;52(15):8772–84.
44. Piitulainen JM, Mattila R, Moritz N, Vallittu PK. Load-bearing capacity and fracture behavior of glass fiber-reinforced composite cranioplasty implants. J Appl Biomater Funct Mater. 2017;15(4):e356–61.
45. Sundblom J, Xheka F, Casar-Borota O, Ryttlefors M. Bone formation in custom-made cranioplasty: evidence of early and sustained bone development in bioceramic calcium phosphate implants. Patient series. J Neurosurg Case Lessons. 2021;1(17):CASE20133.

46. Zaed I, Safa A, Spennato P, Mottolese C, Chibbaro S, Cannizzaro D, et al. A multicentric European clinical study on custom-made porous hydroxyapatite cranioplasty in a pediatric population. Front Surg. 2022;9:1–7.
47. Bowers CA, Riva-Cambrin J, Hertzler DA, Walker ML. Risk factors and rates of bone flap resorption in pediatric patients after decompressive craniectomy for traumatic brain injury. J Neurosurg Pediatr. 2013;11(5):526–32.
48. Frassanito P, Bianchi F, Stifano V, Fraschetti F, Massimi L, Tamburrini G, et al. Craniocerebral disproportion after decompressive craniectomy in infants: the hidden enemy of cranial repair? Childs Nerv Syst. 2019;35(9):1467–71.
49. H song S, Shen F, de Wang M, Lin J, F chun L, Yin B, et al. Titanium mesh implants exposure after cranioplasty in two children: involvement of osteogenesis? Chin Neurosurg J. 2017;3(1):8.
50. Dalle Ore CL, Abraham P, Burns LP, Lance S, Gosman A, Meltzer HS. Intracranial hypotension and hypertension associated with reconstructive cranioplasty after decompressive craniectomy: report of a lethal complication with recommended strategies for future avoidance. J Craniofac Surg. 2018;29(7):1862–4.
51. Zaccaria L, Tharakan SJ, Altermatt S. Hydroxyapatite ceramic implants for cranioplasty in children: a single-center experience. Childs Nerv Syst. 2017;33(2):343–8.
52. Szathmari A, Morgado A, Beuriat PA, Petrescu P, Di Rocco F, Mottolese C. Cranioplasty for bone defects after craniosynostosis surgery. Case series with literature review. Neurochirurgie. 2020;66(2):97–101.
53. Madaree A. Use of acellular dermal matrix in craniosynostosis. J Craniofac Surg. 2018;29(1):126–9.
54. du Plessis MI, Cottler PS, Campbell CA. Acellular dermal matrix favorably modulates the healing response after surgery. Plast Reconstr Surg. 2022;150(2):290e–9e.
55. Frassanito P, Fraschetti F, Bianchi F, Giovannenze F, Caldarelli M, Scoppettuolo G. Management and prevention of cranioplasty infections. Childs Nerv Syst. 2019;35(9):1499–506.
56. Lopez J, Zhong SS, Sankey EW, Swanson EW, Susarla H, Jusue-Torres I, et al. Time interval reduction for delayed implant-based cranioplasty reconstruction in the setting of previous bone flap osteomyelitis. Plast Reconstr Surg. 2016;137(2):394e–404e.
57. Yokota H, Sugimoto T, Nishiguchi M, Hashimoto H. Greenstick fracture-hinge decompressive craniotomy in infants: illustrative case and literature review of techniques for decompressive craniotomy without bone removal. Childs Nerv Syst. 2019;35(9):1491–7.
58. Beez T, Munoz-Bendix C, Hänggi D, Beseoglu K, Cornelius JF. Barrel stave osteotomy decompression for acute brain injury in infants: technical note. J Craniofac Surg. 2020;31(7):e707–10.
59. Goodrich JT, Argamaso R, Hall CD. Split-thickness bone grafts in complex craniofacial reconstructions. Pediatr Neurosurg. 1992;18(4):195–201.
60. Robles LA, Cuevas-Solórzano A. Massive brain swelling and death after cranioplasty: a systematic review. World Neurosurg. 2018;111:99–108.
61. Van Roost D, Thees C, Brenke C, Oppel F, Winkler PA, Schramm J. Pseudohypoxic brain swelling: a newly defined complication after uneventful brain surgery, probably related to suction drainage. Neurosurgery. 2003;53(6):1315–26; discussion 1326–1327.
62. Yu KKH, Ghosh K. Letter to the editor: sudden death following cranioplasty: vacuum suction to blame? J Neurosurg. 2016;125(6):1610–2.
63. Anuzis A, Doherty JA, Millward CP, Sinha AK, McMahon CJ. Sudden death associated with the use of suction drains—a report of 2 cases following uneventful cranioplasty and literature review. Is the use of suction drains safe? Br J Neurosurg. 2021:1–6.
64. Beez T, Munoz-Bendix C, Ahmadi SA, Messing-Jünger M, Steiger HJ, Röhrig A. Conservative and operative management of iatrogenic craniocerebral disproportion—a case-based review. Childs Nerv Syst. 2019;35(1):19–27.
65. Sandler AL, Goodrich JT, Daniels LB, Biswas A, Abbott R. Craniocerebral disproportion: a topical review and proposal toward a new definition, diagnosis, and treatment protocol. Childs Nerv Syst. 2013;29(11):1997–2010.
66. Martínez-Lage JF, Ruiz-Espejo Vilar A, Pérez-Espejo MA, Almagro MJ, De San R, Pedro J, Felipe Murcia M. Shunt-related craniocerebral disproportion: treatment with cranial vault expanding procedures. Neurosurg Rev. 2006;29(3):229–35.